VOLUME I

ACLS

CERTIFICATION PREPARATION

Volume I
ACLS
CERTIFICATION PREPARATION
Third Edition

Ken Grauer, M.D., F.A.A.F.P.

Professor
Department of Community Health and Family Medicine
Assistant Director, Family Practice Residency Program
College of Medicine, University of Florida, Gainesville
ACLS National Affiliate Faculty

Daniel Cavallaro, REMT-P

Research Director
The Center for Cardiopulmonary Research
Children's Research Institute
   at All Children's Hospital, St. Petersburg, Florida
Past ACLS National Affiliate Faculty

with 277 illustrations

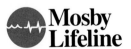

St. Louis Baltimore Boston Chicago London Philadelphia Sydney Toronto

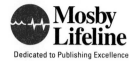
Mosby Lifeline
Dedicated to Publishing Excellence

Publisher: David T. Culverwell
Executive Editor: Richard A. Weimer
Assistant Editor: Julie Scardiglia

Printed in the United States of America

Mosby–Year Book, Inc.
11830 Westline Industrial Drive
St. Louis, Missouri 63146

Library of Congress Cataloging in Publication Data
Grauer, Ken.
    ACLS / Ken Grauer, Daniel L. Cavallaro.—3rd ed.
      p.   cm.
    Includes bibliographical references and index.
    Contents: v. 1. Certification preparation—v. 2. Comprehensive review.
    ISBN 0-8016-7069-1 (v. 1) : $19.95.—ISBN 0-8016-7070-5 (v.2) : $34.95
    1. Cardiovascular emergencies—Problems, exercises, etc.
2. Cardiac arrest—Treatment—Problems, exercises, etc. 3. CPR (First aid)—Problems, exercises, etc. I. Cavallaro, Daniel L.
II. Title.
    [DNLM: 1. Heart Arrest—problems. 2. Life Support Care— problems.
3. Resuscitation—problems.   WG 18 6774a]
RC675.G73 1993
616.1′025′076—dc20
DNLM/DLC
for Library of Congress   92-48248
                                          CIP

93 94 95 96 97 GW/VH 9 8 7 6 5 4 3 2

Authors' Commentary
As This Book Goes to Press
The New Guidelines: *How We Compare*

Revised and updated Guidelines for Cardiopulmonary Resuscitation and Emergency Cardiac Care (put forth by the Emergency Cardiac Care Committee/Subcommittees and American Heart Association) have now been published in the Journal of the American Medical Association (JAMA 268:2171-2295, 1992). The contents of this work reflect proceedings of the 1992 National Conference on Cardiopulmonary Resuscitation (CPR) and Emergency Cardiac Care (ECC)—and forms the basis of the soon-to-be published revised American Heart Association Textbook on ACLS.

As emphasized in its introduction, the new guidelines "do not represent broad changes, nor do they suggest that care provided under past guidelines is either unsafe or ineffective" (ECC/AHA Committee—JAMA, 1992). Note is made in the document of how the term "standards" is conspicuous by its absence from the title of the new recommendations, underscoring a definite lack of "legalistic or prohibitory function" (Paraskos—1992). The authors then go on to openly acknowledge that "deviations from (the new) recommendations and guidelines *may* be warranted when a trained physician (or medical care provider) proficient in CPR and ECC recognizes that such is in the best interest of the patient" (ECC/AHA Committee—JAMA, 1992). Thus the new guidelines are in no way put forth as the sole acceptable approach to cardiopulmonary resuscitation.

For the most part, suggestions and recommendations in our ACLS materials are in close conformance with those presented in the new ECC/AHA guidelines. Nevertheless, *minor differences do exist.* In cases where this occurs, our preferences and opinions are clearly stated as such—based on our approach to clinical integration of existing literature. For purposes of successfully completing the ACLS Provider Course we therefore suggest checking *beforehand* with ACLS faculty of the particular course you are taking *to clarify the range of responses that will be acceptable for the various clinical code simulations of that particular course.*

We summarize below the principle areas where differences arise between our approach and that recommended in the new guidelines:

Use of Magnesium—The new ECC/AHA guidelines primarily favor use of magnesium sulfate for treatment of ventricular arrhythmias (including ventricular fibrillation/tachycardia) in patients with *documented* hypomagnesemia.

In addition to this indication, we favor consideration of magnesium administration for treatment of these arrhythmias in patients with normal (or unknown) serum magnesium levels—especially in lifethreatening situations—when standard antiarrhythmic therapy has been ineffective—and in patients who are *likely to be* intracellularly depleted of this cation.

Use of Epinephrine—The new ECC/AHA guidelines favor administration of **S**tandard-**D**ose **E**pinephrine **(SDE)** in a dose of 1 mg IV as the first agent to be used in cardiac arrest, with repetition of this dose at 3 to 5 minute intervals. Use of **H**igh-**D**ose **E**pinephrine **(HDE)** "is acceptable (after the 1 mg dose has been tried and failed)—but can be neither recommended nor discouraged." Higher doses of epinephrine (of at least 2 to 2.5 times the peripheral IV dose) are likely to be needed when the drug is administered by the *endotracheal route*.

While acknowledging the lack of data demonstrating improved survival from the use of HDE, we nevertheless favor strong consideration for rapidly escalating the dose of epinephrine administered to HDE (i.e., up to a dose of 0.1 to 0.2 mg/kg) for cases of ventricular fibrillation, asystole, and EMD if one (or *at most two*) doses of SDE fail to produce the desired response. We especially favor the use of HDE for treatment of cardiac arrest that occurs outside of the hospital and/or in patients known (or suspected) of having been unresponsive for an extended period of time. Use of HDE should also translate to the use of higher epinephrine doses for *endotracheal route* administration—with increases to 2 mg to 3 mg—or more—if the patient fails to respond to the initial 1 mg ET dose.

Use of Atropine—The new ECC/AHA guidelines allow for an increase in atropine dosing to a total of 0.04 mg/kg (or about 3 mg).

While acknowledging 0.04 mg/kg as the full vagolytic dose, we feel the key concepts are the cautions and reduced indications for the use of this drug—and appreciation of the fact that patients who fail to respond to the previously recommended 2 mg total dose are not very likely to respond to higher atropine doses.

Use of Verapamil/Adenosine—The new ECC/AHA guidelines favor use of adenosine as the antiarrhythmic agent of first choice for pharmacologic treatment of PSVT.

While fully acknowledging the beneficial features of adenosine and the clear need for caution when administering verapamil, we favor consideration of both drugs as *alternative* first-line agents of comparable efficacy for treatment of PSVT. Because each drug has advantages and drawbacks, we base distinction in our selection between these two agents on clinical parameters of the particular case.

Energy Requirements for Defibrillation—Recommendations in the new ECC/AHA guidelines are similar to those put forth in the 1986 Guidelines. Thus, 200 joules are recommended for the *initial* defibrillation attempt—200 to 300 joules are *acceptable* for the second attempt—360 joules are recommended for the third and subsequent attempts—and the recommendation for ventricular fibrillation recurrence is for treatment with countershock at the same energy level that last resulted in successful defibrillation.

We differ slightly from these recommendations by regularly favoring an increase in energy selection for the second defibrillation attempt from 200 to 300 joules (to *ensure* greater current flow)—and in favoring a drop back to 200 joules for the initial countershock delivery if (and when) ventricular fibrillation recurs at a later point in the code.

Approach to Management of a Regular Wide Complex Tachycardia of Uncertain Etiology—Emphasis must always be on "treating the patient and not the monitor." Thus *all* wide complex tachycardias must be assumed ventricular in etiology until proven otherwise. The new ECC/AHA Guidelines downplay the potential role of the 12-lead ECG in the diagnostic process. They recommend treatment initially with lidocaine—to be followed with adenosine if there is no response.

While fully agreeing that the overwhelming majority of wide complex tachycardias of uncertain etiology are ventricular tachycardia (and that they need to be *treated accordingly* until *proven* otherwise), we firmly believe that attention to selected morphologic features on the 12-lead tracing will often be of invaluable assistance for increasing the certainty of one's preliminary diagnosis. As a result, we strongly favor obtaining a 12-lead ECG on all hemodynamically stable patients who present with a wide complex tachycardia *whenever* this is feasible. We also favor stronger consideration of procainamide as a first-line agent for medical treatment of wide complex tachyarrhythmias of uncertain etiology.

Use of the Term Pulseless Electrical Activity (PEA)—The new ECC/AHA guidelines introduce the term **PEA** to encompass EMD (i.e., electromechanical dissociation) *and* a heterogeneous group of rhythms that includes "pseudo-EMD", ventricular escape rhythms, post-defibrillation IVR (idioventricular rhythm), and other bradyasystolic rhythms.

While acknowledging the overlap in definition and management of these entities, we favor continued use of traditional terminology with distinction between EMD, asystole, and other bradyarrhythmias (including slow IVR).

**KEN GRAUER
DAN CAVALLARO**

References

Emergency Cardiac Care Committee and Subcommittees, American Heart Association: Guidelines for Cardiopulmonary Resuscitation and Emergency Cardiac Care, *JAMA* 268:2171-2295, 1992.

Paraskos JA: Emergency Cardiac Care: The Science Behind the Art, *JAMA* 268:2295-2297, 1992.

PREFACE to the Third Edition:
Why This Book Now Consists of Two Volumes
(and How to Find What You're Looking For)

Since publication of the second edition of this book six years ago, numerous advances have been made in the field of cardiopulmonary resuscitation and emergency cardiac care. In response to these advances, to recent revision by the American Heart Association of their guidelines for cardiopulmonary resuscitation, and to feedback received from readers of our second edition, the need was felt to revise this book.

Medical knowledge continues to expand at an exponential rate. Thus, our second edition published in 1987 was double the size of our first edition. This third edition again *doubles* the size of its predecessor. Yet despite the ever increasing size of this book, our dual motivation for writing it remains the same:

i) To provide a practical, easy-to-read *study guide* that facilitates preparation for the ACLS course and *complements* American Heart Association guidelines (and their textbook).

ii) To provide a state-of-the-art, clinically relevant reference source for *comprehensive review* on key topics of interest that relate to cardiopulmonary resuscitation and emergency cardiac care.

Practical space constraints have made these two goals mutually exclusive. There simply was no way to retain the convenient size required of a study guide with the amount of expansion needed to accommodate all of the new material. Fortunately, a solution soon became obvious: *Expand the book into two separate volumes.*

In an attempt to preserve the style and format of our second edition, we have kept the structural organization from that book largely intact. Thus with one exception,* chapter numbers and contents are the same in the third edition as they were in the second edition. **Volume I** of this third edition is therefore now entitled, ***"ACLS: Cer-***

tification Preparation." Its principal aim is to serve as an easy-to-read *study guide* for preparing to take the ACLS course. It also serves as a targeted review of the key components of cardiopulmonary resuscitation. Volume I contains what were the first three parts of our second edition: <u>Part I</u> on the *Essentials of Running a Code* (Chapters 1 through 6), <u>Part II</u> on the *Essentials of Airway and IV Access* (Chapters 7 and 8), and <u>Part III</u> on *Pearls and Pitfalls in Management of Cardiac Arrest* (Chapter 9).

The remaining chapters from our second edition now comprise **Volume II,** which is entitled, ***"ACLS: A Comprehensive Review."*** It includes <u>Part IV</u> on *Topics of General Interest in Emergency Cardiac Care* (Chapters 10 through 13), <u>Part V</u> on *Beyond the Basics* (Chapters 14 through 16), <u>Part VI</u> on *Pediatric Resuscitation* (Chapter 17), and <u>Part VII</u> on *Medicolegal Aspects* (Chapter 18).

How To Use This Book

The entire contents of these two volumes have been rewritten and updated to reflect the *most recent* developments in the field.* *Each volume stands completely on its own.* How each volume may best be used will depend primarily on the needs of the reader:

If the Principal Need is to Review/Prepare for the ACLS Course—*Volume I is the key.* When the time available for review/preparation is exceeding limited (i.e., 3 days or *less*), the primary focus might best be concentrated on Chapter 1. The essence of the ACLS course is now contained in this chapter, which includes an overall perspective for running a code and detailed algorithms with a suggested step-by-step approach for the management of ventricular fibrillation, ventricular tachycardia, bradycardia/asystole/EMD, supraventricular tachyarrhythmias, and use of the AED. Explanatory commentary highlighting key points of interest accompanies each of the treatments recommended. Following each algorithm, concepts are crystallized in a section entitled, *"Questions To Further Understanding."* Thorough review of Chapter 1 may be the most

---

*In the second edition, Chapter 13 was devoted to detailed discussion on the "Use of Lidocaine." To create a place in the third edition for our new chapter on "Special Resuscitation Situations," we have incorporated the information on lidocaine into our greatly expanded chapter on *Acute Myocardial Infarction.*

---

*Numerous references are cited throughout to support our discussion. The sense of currency is conveyed by the fact that many of the sources cited relate to work just recently published (i.e., in 1991 or 1992).

time-effective manner of preparing for the ACLS course (as well as for quickly reviewing the essentials of cardiopulmonary resuscitation).

If after completing Chapter 1 time still remains before the course, preparation (particularly for the MEGA CODE station) might best be facilitated by going through a number of the simulated code scenarios presented in Chapter 4 *(Putting It All Together)*. Additional practice for MEGA CODE is provided in the code vignettes presented in Chapter 5 *(Finding the Error)*. Preparation for the written test is best afforded by working through the *Self-Assessment Section* (Chapter 6), which features 100 multiple choice and true-false questions on various aspects of ACLS. Explained answers provide immediate feedback, and indicate where in the text to refer for additional information.

Readers with the luxury of more time to prepare/review will be rewarded by the wealth of material contained within the remaining chapters of this volume. Essential drugs and treatment modalities are extensively covered in Chapter 2, with suggested recommendations for dosing and a detailed commentary on the use of each agent. Special features included in this chapter are brief overview of the actions of the various alpha- and beta-adrenergic receptors in the autonomic nervous system, full discussion on the pros and cons of using high vs standard dose epinephrine, the "hows and whys" of energy selection for defibrillation, discussion of newer essential drugs expected to have an impact in emergency cardiac care (such as adenosine, magnesium, and amiodarone), explanation of a simplified method for remembering how to calculate IV infusions, and discussion of the role of modalities such as pacing, synchronized cardioversion, the precordial thump, and cough version.

The gamut of cardiac arrhythmias encountered in emergency cardiac care follows in Chapter 3. More than 150 illustrative tracings rapidly advance the reader from basic rhythm interpretation to a fairly high level of sophistication. Clinical relevance and a problem-solving approach aimed to stimulate and actively recruit reader participation is stressed throughout. Numerous practice tracings (with explained answers) have been included to reinforce concepts discussed.

Finishing touches to Volume I are applied in the last three chapters: *Management of the Airway and Ventilation* (Chapter 7), *IV Access* (Chapter 8), and *Pearls and Pitfalls in the Management of Cardiac Arrest* (Chapter 9).

If the Principal Need/Desire is to Explore *Beyond the Basics* in Cardiopulmonary Resuscitation and Emergency Cardiac Care—*Volume II is the key.* This volume begins with Part IV on *Topics of General Interest in Emergency Cardiac Care*, and includes *New Developments in CPR* (Chapter 10), *Sudden Cardiac Death* (Chapter 11), *Acute Myocardial Infarction* (Chapter 12), and *Special Resuscitation Situations* (Chapter 13). This last chapter is completely new and consists of a practical approach to evaluation and management of patients who present with unusual code situations including drowning or near drowning, hypothermia, heat stroke, lightning and electrical injuries, overdose from cocaine or tricyclic antidepressant agents, cardiopulmonary arrest in pregnancy, airplane emergencies, and traumatic cardiac arrest.

Chapters 10 through 12 illustrate the extent to which this third edition has been expanded compared to our previous edition. Thus, our chapter on *Acute Myocardial Infarction* now encompasses six subsections and over 80 pages. Issues that are thoroughly explored include clinical evaluation of the patient with acute ischemic chest pain, standard medical treatments, newer treatments (such as potential use of magnesium for prophylaxis and/or treatment of ventricular arrhythmias), use of thrombolytic therapy, anticoagulation, and antiplatelet agents, when to consider invasive intervention, and an illustra-

tive case study that challenges the reader to clinically apply the material covered. Chapter 11 on *Sudden Cardiac Death* has been similarly expanded, and now includes subsections on out-of-hospital cardiac arrest, the role of electrolytes (potassium and magnesium) in cardiac arrest, in-hospital cardiac arrest, options for management of sudden death survivors, and a special section entitled, *"What To Do If the Patient Dies..."* Features contained in our chapter on *New Developments in CPR* (Chapter 10) include discussion of the mechanisms, efficacy, and potential complications of CPR, clinical application of End-Tidal CO_2 monitoring, a historical review tracing the development of CPR, the rationale for current BLS recommendations, and frank discussion of potential problems that may be encountered in trying to implement CPR. This latter subsection directly confronts controversial issues such as administration of mouth-to-mouth ventilation when you know (or suspect) that the patient may have AIDS.

The additions we have made to Part V of Volume II (on *Beyond the Basics*) should delight the most sophisticated of our readers. Among the new drugs added to Chapter 14 are labetalol, esmolol, IV diltiazem, and discussion on the use of digoxin antibody fragments (for acute treatment of life-threatening digitalis intoxication). Chapters 15 *(Differentiation of PVCs from Aberrancy)* and 16 *(More Advanced Concepts in Arrhythmia Interpretation)* have each nearly doubled in size, and explore their respective topic from every facet imaginable. Numerous clinical examples constantly challenge the reader and illustrate important points that are made.

Chapters 17 *(Pediatric Resuscitation)* and 18 *(Medicolegal Aspects of ACLS)* complete Volume II. Each has been updated and suitably expanded to reflect new developments and advances accomplished since publication of our second edition.

Regardless of one's clinical background and training, there should be more than enough material in these two volumes to satisfy the most demanding of needs. *We emphasize that Volume II is not essential reading for those whose primary concern is successful completion of the ACLS course.* However, the contents of this volume should prove invaluable for those with an interest in delving beyond the core of the ACLS course and/or expanding their horizons in emergency cardiac care.

For the Reader Who Wants More . . . .

IN 1988 we published a series of approximately 350 flash cards in conjunction with the second edition of this book (*ACLS: Mega Code Review/Study Cards*—Mosby–Year Book, St. Louis). The aim of these cards was twofold:

i)   To provide another type of *study aid* that might supplement the second edition of our book.

ii) To provide an additional method of preparing for the challenging MEGA CODE station that would simulate testing conditions, but at the same time allow the student to individualize their preparation, *and proceed at their own pace.*

The first goal was easily accomplished by posing a clinical question or simply listing a drug or arrhythmia on the front of a card, and providing explanatory discussion on the back. The latter goal was attained by incorporating a portion of the cards into simulated code scenarios in which the front of a card presented the patient's rhythm and clinical status, and the back of that card indicated our suggested approach to treatment.

We have completely revised the cards in this study aid (*ACLS: MEGA CODE Review/Study Cards—Second Edition*, Mosby–Year Book, 1993). In addition to updating the cards and greatly expanding the extent of their content, the new set of cards features a much more "user-friendly" format that reinforces *without* duplicating the material we cover in the third edition of our book. Utilization of these *Study Cards* therefore provides an additional, time-effective way of reviewing the essentials of cardiopulmonary resuscitation and preparing for the ACLS course.

We hope you enjoy reading our ACLS material, and find it clinically useful. It was written with YOU—the reader—in mind.

Author's Note

Our recommendations for management in the key algorithms of cardiopulmonary resuscitation are generally very consistent with those put forth by the American Heart Association. However, we do not always adhere strictly to their guidelines. In cases where we differ, we clearly state the rationale for our views, and appropriately reference any points of contention.

We do *not* feel such differences of opinion represent a departure from the objectives of the American Heart Association, since this agency freely acknowledges that their algorithms for treatment are not all inclusive. On the contrary, we firmly believe that acknowledging areas of controversy and presenting potential alternative approaches for selected situations is beneficial and may lead to improved emergency care. Our book is therefore aimed to *complement* the American Heart Association ACLS Textbook. We hope combined use will not only prove insightful, but also add an extra dimension to the learning experience of the reader.

Foreword

The tremendous success of the American Heart Association program on advanced cardiac life support (ACLS) has been evident from the continued demand for this course among the health care professionals. Clearly the course provides the most time-efficient method for improving one's skills in the area of cardiopulmonary resuscitation.

The principal difficulty posed by the ACLS course lies with the large amount of material that the participant is expected to assimilate in a short period of time. Even though the American Heart Association ACLS textbook will ideally be distributed well in advance of the course, this text has not solved the problem of preparing the student for the intensive program to follow. Despite its extensive scope, much of the material in the ACLS textbook is not conveniently organized into a decision-making format for patient care. In addition, practice exercises in arrhythmia interpretation and management of cardiac arrest are entirely lacking.

ACLS: Certification Preparation and a Comprehensive Review by Grauer and Cavallaro was developed in an attempt to meet the educational needs of the reader. Now in its third edition, this book should keenly interest *anyone* who is either taking the ACLS course or involved in emergency cardiac care. Written in a style that transcends medical specialties, the two volumes of this third edition masterfully succeed in accomplishing the authors' goals of producing a practical, easy-to-read study guide that facilitates preparation for the ACLS course, as well as a comprehensive, state-of-the-art review in the field of cardiopulmonary resuscitation.

I find each of the two volumes in this third edition to be stimulating, informative, and invaluable as a *complement* to the American Heart Association ACLS Textbook.

Richard J. Melker, M.D., Ph. D.
Emergency Cardiac Care Committee,
  American Heart Association
Associate Professor
Surgery, Anesthesiology, Pediatrics
University of Florida
College of Medicine
Gainesville, Florida

To my father,

Samuel Grauer

*without whom this book
would not have been possible.*

About the Authors

KEN GRAUER, M.D., F.A.A.F.P., is a professor in the Department of Communicty Health and Family Medicine, College of Medicine, University of Florida, and assistant director of the Family Practice Residency Program in Gainesville. He is board certified in family practice, and is a National ACLS Affiliate Faculty member and former contributor to the American Heart Association ACLS Textbook who served on the Task Force for ACLS Post-Testing. In addition to this book, Dr. Grauer is the principal or sole author of the following books and teaching resources: *ACLS: Mega Code Review/Study Cards* (Second edition—Mosby–Year Book, 1993), *A Practical Guide to ECG Interpretation* (Mosby–Year Book, 1992), *ECG Interpretation Pocket Reference* (Mosby–Year Book, 1992), *Clinical Electrocardiography: A Primary Care Approach* (Second edition—Blackwell Scientific Publications, 1992), and *ACLS Teaching Kit: An Instructor's Resource* (Mosby–Year Book, 1990). He has lectured widely and is primary author of numerous articles on cardiology for family physicians, including several "ECG of the Month" columns that have been published for a period of more than seven years in various primary care journals. He also serves on the Editorial Board of the following journals: ACLS Alert, Family Practice Recertification, Procedural Skills and Office Technology, and Internal Medicine Alert.

Dr. Grauer has become well known throughout Florida and nationally for teaching ACLS courses and ECG/arrhythmia workshops to diverse medical audiences including nurses, paramedics, medical students, physicians in training, and physicians in practice. His trademark has always been the ability to simplify otherwise complicated topics into a concise, practical, and easy-to-remember format.

DAN CAVALLARO, REMT-P, is research director of the Center for Cardiopulmonary Research at All Children's Hospital in St. Petersburg, Florida. He is a former ACLS National Affiliate Faculty member, and a former contributor to the American Heart Association ACLS Textbook who served on the Task Force for ACLS Post-Testing. In addition to co-authoring this book, he has co-authored the following teaching resources: *ACLS: Mega Code Review/Study Cards* (Second edition—Mosby–Year Book, 1993), and *ACLS Teaching Kit: An Instructor's Resource* (Mosby–Year Book, 1990). Clinically, he has worked in the critical care and emergency medical fields for the past 15 years. During that time, he has also been extremely active developing and participating in courses on prehospital care and emergency medicine, and has taught in well over 150 ACLS courses.

Acknowledgments

I am indebted to the following people whose contributions were instrumental to the preparation of this book:

Dan Cavallaro, whose expertise has continued to enrich my knowledge over the years, and whose friendship and enthusiasm helped keep me going during the seemingly "endless" three years it took to complete the writing (and constant rewriting) of this book. His contributions to each of the two volumes in this third edition have truly been *invaluable* to me.

Jorge Giroud, MD, and **Al Saltiel,** MD, for their assistance in helping to write the chapters on intravenous access and pediatrics.

John Gums, Pharm D, for his assistance in helping me write the chapters relating to cardiovascular pharmacology. Nowhere could there possibly be another Pharm D the equal of John, whose encyclopedic, photographic memory and unfathomable clinical insight become the instant envy of all who are lucky enough to work with him.

Fred Langer, RN, for his ingenuity in conceiving our ACLS poetry addendum: *"The Night Before Morning."* The birth of this poem is the result of Fred's labor.

Ellie Green, RN, for her help with the finishing touches of our poem. I'm eternally grateful to Ellie for her assistance in targeting (and retargeting) selected portions of this text to the audience we wanted to reach—as well as for her valued friendship. *Has there ever been a better teacher to bless the nursing profession?*

Arlene Marrin, RN, **Marvin A. Dewar,** MD, JD, and **Ray Moseley,** PhD, for their assistance in helping me write the chapter on medicolegal aspects of ACLS—and for their assistance in the numerous rewritings of this chapter that marked our attempt to keep up with this everchanging field. *What better combination of coauthors could one ask for to write this chapter than a nurse/claims examiner, a doctor/lawyer who happens to be your director, and the best medical ethicist there is?*

Janet Silverstein, MD, Des Schatz, MD, and John Hellrung, MD, for their input in the chapter on pediatrics. To Richard Bucciarelli, MD, Greg Gaar, MD, John Santamaria, MD, and Bonnie Sklaren, for their assistance in helping with the original version of the chapter on pediatrics that appeared in the second edition of our book.

Geno Romano, MD, Brent Leytem, MD, Mike Ware, MD, Karen Hall, MD, Lou Kuritzky, MD, R. Whitney Curry, Jr., MD, René Lee-Pack, MD, Doug Coran, MD, Frank Foster, MD, Boyd Kellet, MD, for their assistance in writing selected portions of the special resuscitation situations chapter.

Larry Kravitz, MD, Harry Sernaker, MD, Jerry Diehr, MD, and Paul Augereau, MD, for their assistance in helping with the original version of the chapter on intravenous access that appeared in the second edition of our book.

Geno Romano, MD, Holly Jensen, RN, Karen Hall, MD, Brent Leytem, MD, Aixa Rey, Pharm D, for reviewing significant portions of the manuscript, and "keeping me honest."

Sherry Wingate, Virginia Hungerford, Steve Roark, MD, Anne Curtis, MD, and Betty Arnette, REMT-P, for their assistance and expertise in reviewing selected portions of this text—and to Jim Nimocks, MD and Garth Vaz, MD for the "fascinoma" tracings they contributed.

J. Daniel Robinson, Pharm D, for contributing the SIMKIN figures which I modified in the chapter on lidocaine.

Robyn Lyemance for her kindness and wonderful patience in the endless photographic sessions needed to prepare the chapters on airway management and IV access.

Kinsey Judkins-Waldron, RN, for her invaluable insight, unfailing support, and tremendously welcome 100%-biased positive feedback during the "middle ages" period of the writing of this book.

Anita Wofford (my career counselor), for dancing into my life during the "final ages" period of this book—and for sustaining me when I needed a friendly attentive "ear" and a caring lifelong friend.

R. Whit Curry, Jr., MD, for allowing me to "pump his brain" on numerous occasions throughout the years on primary care questions about cardiology issues—and for his unwavering support of me in his capacity as Director-Chairman of our Family Practice program.

Rick Weimer of Mosby–Year Book—for his encouragement, enthusiasm, and motivation, out of which this book was born—and out of which came the rebirth of this third edition. **Julie Scardiglia** of Mosby–Year Book, for helping to make the rebirth possible. *Nowhere could there be another pair more deserving of credit (as well as a raise) than Rick and Julie for their positive influence and total involvement in the development and fruition of this project.*

Diana Laulainen of Mosby–Year Book—for jumping in during the "final" stages. *This book would NOT be without Diana!*

Jan and **Jackie Katz** of *Resource Applications,* for making it possible for me to teach (and learn from) nurses across the country.

Mikel Rothenberg, MD—*my favorite pen pal*—for "alerting" me monthly to *What's New in ACLS.*

Pat and **"Tree"** (and the rest of the crew at Sonny's)—and **Phil Heflin** (and the crew at Chaucer's), for their great food and ever EXCELLENT service, and for providing me with a peaceful, pleasant, and inspiring environment for writing (and forever rewriting), and reviewing much of the text. And ditto for Ruby Tuesday.

Maria Alvarez—the BEST dance teacher I know—as well as my other "best" dance teacher, Ray Parris, for their inspiration toward excellence in ballroom dancing, and who together with all my friends at the *Maria Alvarez Imperial Dance Studio,* were instrumental in helping me to maintain my sanity (and still have fun by dancing) for much of the time I was working on this book.

Barney Marriott, MD, and **William P. Nelson,** MD, *for teaching me more about ECGs than I can ever say.*

Brian Kennedy, MD and **Andres Ticzon,** MD, for teaching and inspiring a family physician (= me!) to better appreciate the magic of cardiology.

The Cardiology staff at Alachua General Hospital (Burt Silverstein, MD; Steve Roark, MD; Mike Dillon, MD; Gary Cooper, MD, and Fraser Richards, MD), for their tremendous support of me, and for teaching cardiology to our residents.

ALL of the other excellent cardiologists who have inspired me, and from whom I have learned.

ALL those who have knowingly (and unknowingly) provided me with tracings through the years.

ALL the nurses, medical students, residents, and other paramedical personnel who have allowed me to learn by teaching them.

Ken Grauer, MD

Contents

CONTENTS

PART III Pearls & Pitfalls in the Management of Cardiac Arrest

VOLUME II
Brief Contents

PART VI   Pediatric Resuscitation

CHAPTER 17 PEDIATRIC RESUSCITATION 625

PART VII   Medicolegal Aspects

CHAPTER 18 MEDICOLEGAL ASPECTS OF
ACLS 663

VOLUME I

ACLS

CERTIFICATION PREPARATION

PART I

The Essentials of Running a Code

CHAPTER 1

AN APPROACH TO THE KEY ALGORITHMS FOR CARDIOPULMONARY RESUSCITATION

SECTION A

OVERVIEW OF CARDIAC ARREST

Introduction

The goal of this chapter is to provide a brief overview of the approach to the management of cardiopulmonary arrest and to introduce the **Algorithms for Treatment.** At first glance, the thought of having to learn all the material contained herein may seem to be no less than an overwhelming task. *This need not be the case.* If one breaks down the topic of cardiac arrest into those rhythms that are usually associated with the initial event (i.e., *primary* or precipitating mechanisms of the arrest), and the rhythms that are most likely to follow conversion out of ventricular fibrillation (i.e., *secondary* mechanisms or postconversion rhythms), organization of the problem becomes much simpler *(Figure 1A-1).*

Although it may initially seem like innumerable therapeutic options are available, the essentials of management are contained within the basic algorithms presented in this chapter. Mastery of these algorithms will provide you with the information needed to effectively run most codes (and to do well on the MEGA CODE Station).

Another reason these algorithms are important is that they provide an overall perspective for the management of cardiac arrest. *They are the essential foundation upon which the building blocks of treatment are laid.* Although some may object to the thought of dependence on algorithms (on the grounds that they sometimes restrict thinking and do not always apply to the particular situation at hand)—their use in training emergency care providers to manage cardiac arrest has clearly been shown to *expedite* clinical decision making. Perhaps nowhere in medicine does the ability to rapidly decide on a rational course of therapy have as much impact on survival as it does at the scene of a cardiopulmonary arrest.

With practice and application, recall of the various algorithms becomes automatic. Such "automaticity" is extremely beneficial during an arrest situation, because it helps prevent the emergency care provider from forgetting basic material that was so well known under less stressful circumstances. Algorithms are *not* meant to be a substitute for judgment. On the contrary, reflexive recall of the framework of management *facilitates* organization of one's thinking, the setting of priorities, and institution of appropriate therapeutic measures.

Algorithms do *NOT* account for all possible permutations of management. *They are not meant to*—since doing so would entail specification of an endless number of uncommonly used treatment alternatives that would not only confuse the issue, but would also defeat the original purpose of the algorithm—namely, *organization, simplicity,* and *practicality.*

Primary Mechanisms of Cardiopulmonary Arrest

Most cases of cardiopulmonary arrest occur *outside* the hospital. As suggested by Figure 1A-1, the three principal **primary mechanisms** for out-of-hospital cardiopulmonary arrest are:

1. Ventricular tachycardia
2. Ventricular fibrillation
3. Bradycardia (including electromechanical dissociation [EMD] and asystole).

Of these three primary mechanisms, *ventricular fibrillation* is by far the most common in this setting. It occurs in

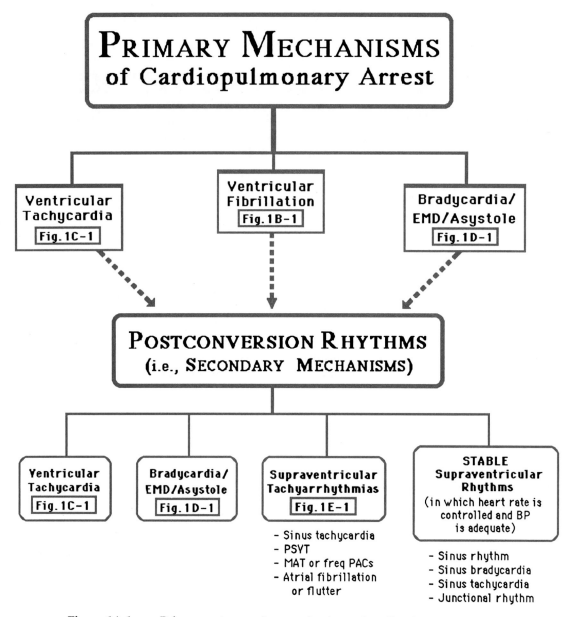

Figure 1A-1.   *Primary* and *secondary* **mechanisms** of cardiopulmonary arrest.

almost two thirds of cases. In contrast, ventricular tachy-cardia is a relatively infrequent mechanism of out-of-hospital cardiac arrest. In only 5% to 10% of cases is ventricular tachycardia documented as the initial rhythm (i.e., as the *presumed* precipitating mechanism of the arrest) by emergency medical service (EMS) personnel at the time of their arrival on the scene. The remaining patients (a little less than one third of the total) are initially found in a bradyarrhythmia (including EMD or asystole).*

The literature suggests that *ventricular tachycardia* is a much more common precipitating mechanism of cardiac arrests that occur *inside* the hospital. Perhaps this is simply a result of the fact that the time from onset of the arrest until discovery by trained personnel is significantly less in a hospital setting. In other words, *it is likely that many cases of out-of-hospital cardiac arrest began as ventricular tachycardia, and have already deteriorated to ventricular fibrillation (and/or to asystole) by the time they are first recognized.*

Primary respiratory arrest is also an important precipitating mechanism of arrests that occur inside the hospital. As is the case for ventricular tachycardia, the finding of *pure* respiratory arrest as a precipitating mechanism is probably a reflection of the earlier discovery that is likely to occur in a hospital

---

*A recent study by Wang et al (1991) suggests that a *supraventricular tachyarrhythmia* may be the precipitating cause of out-of-hospital cardiac arrest in a small but significant percentage of cases. Clinical implications of this finding are discussed in Section A of Chapter 11.

setting (i.e., discovery of the victim at a point *after* breathing has stopped—but *before* there has been progression to full cardiac arrest). In contrast, identification of a victim in *pure* respiratory arrest is much less likely outside of the hospital because deterioration of the rhythm (to ventricular fibrillation or a bradyarrhythmia) has almost always occurred by the time the victim is finally discovered.

Management of the three principal *primary* mechanisms of cardiac arrest is outlined in the treatment algorithms that follow in Figures 1B-1, 1C-1, and 1D-1 (in Sections 1B, 1C, and 1D, respectively).

> The importance of identifying the *precipitating mechanism* of an arrest lies with selection of treatment priorities and assessment of the likely prognostic implications of each rhythm. By far, patients found in *respiratory arrest* or *ventricular tachycardia* have the best chance of being successfully resuscitated. In contrast, those who are initially found in a *bradyarrhythmia* in association with out-of-hospital cardiac arrest have almost no chance of ultimate survival. Patients with *ventricular fibrillation* as the primary mechanism of their arrest have an intermediate chance for long-term survival (estimated to be between 5% to 25%, depending on a host of variables). *Clearly the goal of emergency cardiac care must be to arrive on the scene at a point in the process BEFORE irreversibility has set in* (i.e., ideally *BEFORE* deterioration of the initial rhythm to ventricular fibrillation or asystole).
>
> Treatment priorities may also be a function of the mechanism of the arrest. This is especially true with **epinephrine,** for which the dose of drug required to optimize coronary and cerebral perfusion during resuscitation appears to vary according to *duration* of the arrest and the *initial* (precipitating) rhythm. Thus higher doses of drug (i.e., **HDE** or **H**igh-**D**ose **E**pinephrine) are likely to be needed *sooner* in a patient who has been unresponsive for a longer period of time (as is usually the case for out-of-hospital cardiac arrest). In contrast, a lower dose of epinephrine (i.e., **SDE** or **S**tandard-**D**ose **E**pinephrine) may be adequate (at least some of the time) for treatment of cardiac arrest that is *promptly* attended to in a hospital setting. Patients with no electrical activity at all (i.e., victims who are initially found in asystole) are also likely to require higher doses of drug *sooner* than patients with evidence of partial (albeit inadequate) contractile function (as may be the case for some patients with EMD). *Full discussion on the rationale, indications for use, and dosing of SDE and HDE is found in Sections B and C of Chapter 2.*

Regardless of the precipitating mechanism—*if the decision is made to initially try SDE but the drug fails to produce the desired response, we feel the dose of epinephrine should be rapidly increased (i.e., to HDE).*

Secondary Mechanisms of Cardiopulmonary Arrest

If a patient in ventricular fibrillation is successfully converted out of this rhythm, one of the four *secondary* mech-

anisms of cardiac arrest that are shown in Figure 1A-1 may result:

1. Ventricular tachycardia
2. A *bradyarrhythmia* (including EMD and asystole)
3. A *supraventricular* rhythm with a *rapid* heart rate (i.e., a supraventricular *tachyarrhythmia*)
4. A *supraventricular* rhythm with a *controlled* heart rate (and an adequate blood pressure)

Treatment of either ventricular tachycardia or bradycardia that arises as a *secondary* mechanism (i.e., as a post-conversion rhythm following defibrillation) is similar to the treatment recommended for these rhythms when they arise as the primary mechanism of an arrest.

> In other words, the clinical approach suggested in Figures 1C-1 and 1D-1 (for treatment of ventricular tachycardia and bradyarrhythmias, respectively) retains its applicability *regardless* of when in the code the rhythm occurs.

Alternatively, defibrillation of the patient may convert ventricular fibrillation into a *supraventricular* mechanism *other than bradycardia.* Clinically, the treatment approach will again depend on the specific mechanism of the rhythm and its hemodynamic effect.

> If the heart rate of a post-conversion supraventricular rhythm is controlled and blood pressure is adequate—*no additional treatment may be needed.* On the other hand, if defibrillation produces a supraventricular *tachyarrhythmia* (and/or a supraventricular rhythm associated with hypotension), management according to the treatment algorithm suggested in Figure 1E-1 is indicated.

The ABCs of Cardiopulmonary Resuscitation

The KEY to survival from cardiopulmonary arrest depends on three principal factors: (1) *early recognition* of the clinical state of unresponsiveness (associated with the condition of apnea and/or pulselessness); (2) prompt initiation of **B**asic **L**ife **S**upport **(BLS)** by the lay public; and (3) activation of EMS personnel capable of providing treatment with **A**dvanced **C**ardiac **L**ife **S**upport **(ACLS)** measures.

> Assessment and management of the unconscious victim begins with the **ABC**s (of **A**irway, **B**reathing, and **C**irculation). The following sequence for provision of BLS should be mastered:
>
> 1. Establish unresponsiveness.
> 2. Call for help. Activate the EMS system.
> 3. Position the victim and *open the Airway.*
> 4. Check for the existence and adequacy of *spontaneous Breathing.*
> 5. Perform rescue breathing if needed. Start with two full breaths.

6. Assess *Circulation* (by establishing whether a pulse is present).
7. Begin external chest compression. Combine this with rescue breathing, and continue until EMS personnel arrive.

Once providers capable of ACLS are on the scene, attention can be directed *beyond* BLS measures to the delivery of more definitive care. As soon as the prevailing mechanism of the arrest is identified, treatment may be provided according to the approach suggested by the appropriate algorithm.

We close this section by emphasizing that the **Algorithms for Treatment** that we will present in Sections 1B through 1F need *not* be memorized on this first reading. Instead, the purpose of this chapter is merely to provide an overall perspective of the approach to management of cardiopulmonary arrest.

Rather than tedious memorization at this time, we suggest you simply *familiarize* yourself with the content of this chapter. Then, *feel free to frequently refer back to these algorithms as you work through the rest of the book*. Recall of the material will be greatly facilitated (and will almost become second nature) as the natural result of practice and application.

ALGORITHM FOR VENTRICULAR FIBRILLATION

Identification of Cardiopulmonary Arrest and Initial Patient Assessment

The suggested sequence for management of ventricular fibrillation is shown in *Figure 1B-1*. Although resuscitative efforts begin with *recognition* of the arrest, *calling for help*, and initiating the ABCs, by far the most important treatment modality is *EARLY defibrillation*. Studies have demonstrated that, if EMS personnel are able to do nothing other than defibrillate the patient, the likelihood of survival will be significantly increased. The same urgency for prompt defibrillation carries over to the occurrence of ventricular fibrillation in a hospitalized setting. Endotracheal intubation, establishment of intravenous (IV) access, and administration of medications all play a secondary role.

Time is of the essence. The chances of converting a patient out of ventricular fibrillation are *inversely* proportional to the amount of time from the onset of this arrhythmia, until the time that countershock is applied. Consequently, all efforts must be directed toward rapid establishment of the diagnosis (of ventricular fibrillation) followed by *immediate* defibrillation.

> Quick-look paddles facilitate this process. Quick-look paddles should be applied *before* attempts are made at intubation or securing IV access. This holds true not only for cardiopulmonary arrests that occur in the field, but also for those that take place in the hospital or emergency department when the patient is not being monitored. *Immediate application of quick-look paddles by hospital personnel may save the precious seconds that determine whether resuscitation will be successful.*

Consideration may be given to delivery of a precordial thump *on discovery* of a pulseless victim of cardiac arrest. If quick-look paddles are readily available, delivery of the thump is sometimes *momentarily* delayed to verify the diagnosis (of ventricular fibrillation). Alternatively, if a defibrillator is on the scene, one may perfer to withhold the thump entirely in favor of electrical defibrillation.

> The protocol for treatment of the victim in cardiac arrest is different if an **automatic external defibrillator (AED)** is available. For the purpose of simplicity, we defer discussion of the algorithm for "Use of the AED" to the end of this chapter *(see Figure 1F-1)*.

Initiate Management Sequence for Treatment of Ventricular Fibrillation: *Initial Defibrillation Series*

1) COUNTERSHOCK

The preferred energy level for the 1st countershock attempt in adults is 200 joules.

> The recommendation to use 200 joules for the initial countershock attempt is based on studies that demonstrate fewer post-conversion complications (i.e., AV block, asystole), but comparable survival rates for patients defibrillated with low (175 joules) versus high (320 joules) energy shocks (Weaver et al, 1982).

If pulselessness (and ventricular fibrillation) persist after the first shock, *the defibrillator should be immediately recharged in preparation for repeat defibrillation.* Minimizing the time between countershock attempts in this manner reduces transthoracic resistance (TTR) and allows a greater amount of *current* to pass through the heart with the second shock. The recommended energy level for this 2nd countershock attempt is 300 joules.

> By **BOTH** *increasing the energy level* **AND** *minimizing the time between successive countershocks*, one ensures that a greater amount of current will flow through the heart on the second attempt. This enhances the chance for successful electrical conversion.

If ventricular fibrillation persists, a 3rd countershock attempt (this time with maximal energy, or 360 joules)—should be delivered. *Some patients only respond to defibrillation with maximal energy.*

If Ventricular Fibrillation Persists

2) INTUBATION/IV ACCESS

If ventricular fibrillation is still present after the third countershock attempt, one should *resume CPR*, attempt to intubate the patient, establish IV access, and hook the patient up to a monitor. *A trial of medications is now in order.*

3) EPINEPHRINE

Epinephrine is the drug of choice for treatment of cardiac arrest. The KEY role of the drug during cardiopul-

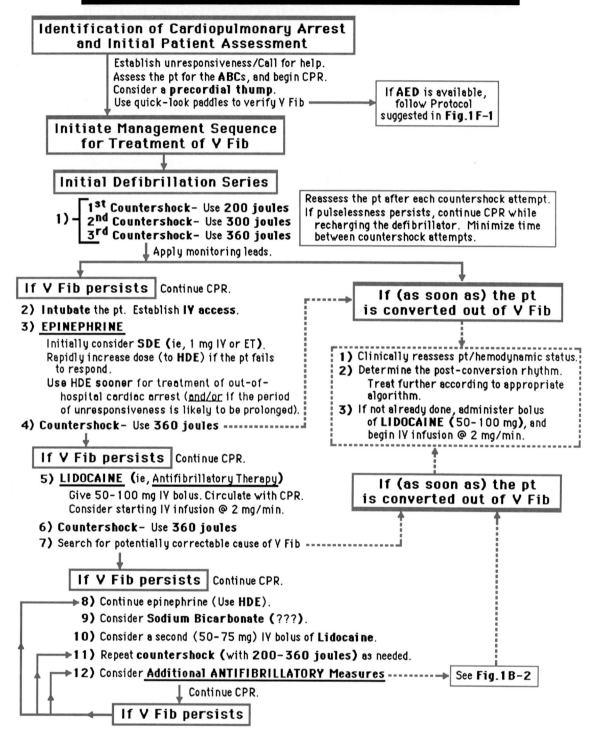

Figure 1B-1.   Algorithm for treatment of **Ventricular Fibrillation.**

monary resuscitation is *not* a result of its potent chronotropic and inotropic effects, but rather from its ability to facilitate blood flow to the coronary and cerebral circulation in the arrested heart.

> Epinephrine may be administered either *intravenously* (IV) or *endotracheally* (ET)—depending on which route of access is established first. **SDE** (i.e., **S**tandard-**D**ose **E**pinephrine = 1 mg of the 1:10,000 solution, by either the IV or ET route) is often tried first. If this is unsuccessful, the dose should be rapidly increased to **HDE** (**H**igh-**D**ose **E**pinephrine—*as described in Section 2B*). As we have already noted, higher doses of epinephrine (i.e., HDE) should probably be used much sooner (if not immediately) for patients with out-of-hospital cardiac arrest (and/or for those in whom the period of unresponsiveness is likely to have been prolonged).

4) COUNTERSHOCK

Following epinephrine administration, another <u>countershock</u> with maximal energy (<u>360 joules</u>) should be delivered in an attempt to convert the patient out of ventricular fibrillation.

If Ventricular Fibrillation Persists

Ventricular fibrillation that fails to respond to the above measures (Steps #1 to #4) is referred to as **REFRACTORY.** Development of this situation should prompt a trial of **antifibrillatory therapy.**

5) LIDOCAINE

<u>Lidocaine</u> is generally accepted as the *initial* antifibrillatory agent of choice for medical treatment of refractory ventricular fibrillation. The recommended dose for the first IV loading bolus of the drug is between <u>50 to 100 mg IV</u> ($\approx$1 mg/kg). Consideration might also be given at this time to beginning a maintenance infusion of the drug (at a rate of <u>2 mg/min</u>).

> In the spontaneously beating heart, a continuous IV infusion of lidocaine (at a rate of 2 mg/min) is typically begun *immediately after* giving the bolus with the aim of maintaining therapeutic serum levels of the drug. Because the effects of a bolus only last a short time, however, additional boluses would have to be repeated *at least* every 10 minutes to maintain the drug's effect in the absence of a continuous infusion.
>
> Lidocaine pharmacokinetics are markedly altered in the arrested heart. Clearance of the drug is significantly *decreased* in this situation, so that as little as one (or at most two) boluses of drug are usually enough to maintain therapeutic lidocaine levels, even *without* a maintenance infusion. As a result, some emergency care providers advocate withholding initiation of the maintenance infusion until *after* the patient is converted out of ventricular fibrillation. The point to emphasize is that *if you choose not to begin the lidocaine maintenance infusion at the time you administer one or more loading boluses of the drug, it is* **imperative** *to remember to do so* **as soon as** *the patient is converted out of ventricular fibrillation.*

6) COUNTERSHOCK

Following administration of lidocaine in Step #5, CPR should be performed for at least 1 to 2 minutes to allow the drug a chance to reach the central circulation. This is followed again by <u>defibrillation</u> with full energy (<u>360 joules</u>).

7) SEARCH FOR A *POTENTIALLY CORRECTABLE* CAUSE OF VENTRICULAR FIBRILLATION

Persistence of ventricular fibrillation at this point should prompt consideration of other factors that could account for the patient's refractory condition. This might include a problem with the **ABC**s (i.e., a nonpatent airway, asymmetric or absent breath sounds, lack of a pulse with CPR), and/or some other predisposing cause.

> *Potentially correctable* predisposing causes of refractory ventricular fibrillation that should be considered include underlying <u>metabolic disturbances</u> (such as diabetic ketoacidosis or hyperkalemia), <u>hypothermia, hypovolemia, drug overdose</u> (especially of cocaine, tricyclic antidepressants, or narcotics), and/or development of a <u>complication of CPR</u> (such as tension pneumothorax or pericardial tamponade).
>
> Clearly, ventricular fibrillation may also be the end result of many other kinds of processes—such as cardiogenic shock (from massive myocardial infarction) or ruptured aortic aneurysm. Practically speaking, however, diagnosis of these conditions is much less important because of the improbability that refractory ventricular fibrillation from such causes would respond to any treatment at this point in the code.

We emphasize that a predisposing, potentially correctable cause of refractory ventricular fibrillation will *NOT* be found in most cases of cardiac arrest. Nevertheless, it is essential to keep this possibility in mind because:

1. Cardiac arrest is potentially reversible if there is a predisposing cause that can be corrected.
2. If there is a predisposing cause, standard treatment measures are unlikely to be successful *unless* (and *until*) that predisposing cause is corrected.

If Ventricular Fibrillation Persists

Clinically, it may be helpful to realize that, if ventricular fibrillation persists *despite* application of these first 7 Steps, remaining therapeutic options are relatively limited. *There is simply not that much more that can be done.* We suggest:

8) CONTINUING EPINEPHRINE (HDE)

Recovery from prolonged cardiopulmonary arrest is unlikely unless coronary perfusion pressure (CPP) is adequate (i.e., ≥15 mm Hg). In the arrested heart, epinephrine in *sufficient amount* appears to be needed to achieve such pressures. The drug should therefore be given liberally (i.e., *at least* every 5 minutes—if not by *continuous* IV infusion), and in high enough doses (i.e., early use of HDE if the patient fails to respond).

9) CONSIDERING SODIUM BICARBONATE

Although sodium bicarbonate has been freely used in the past for the treatment of cardiac arrest, recent data strongly question this practice. In fact, a strong case could be made for *NEVER* administering any sodium bicarbonate during cardiopulmonary resuscitation *regardless* of what the pH value happens to be. Instead, efforts at correcting acidosis might focus on *optimizing ventilation*, especially during the early minutes of a code when the major component of acidosis is likely to be respiratory in nature (from **hypo**ventilation).

Alternatively, one *might* consider empirically administering 1 to 2 ampules of sodium bicarbonate after 10 to 15 minutes in a code on the grounds that sufficient time should have passed for a metabolic component of the acidosis to develop.

If this decision is made (to administer sodium bicarbonate), *it is essential not to overshoot correction of the acidosis*. The body is much less adept at functioning in the presence of alkalosis than it is with a mild acidosis. Thus, a pH reading of between 7.25 and 7.35 would be a perfectly acceptable value in the setting of cardiac arrest. Practically speaking then, sodium bicarbonate administration should probably not even be considered unless the period of arrest is prolonged and/or the drop in pH is significant (i.e., to *below* 7.15 to 7.20)—*if bicarbonate administration is ever considered at all. . . . .*

10) CONSIDERING A SECOND IV BOLUS OF LIDOCAINE

If ventricular fibrillation is still present at this point in the code, it would be reasonable to administer a second (50 to 75 mg) IV bolus of lidocaine *before* turning to other antifibrillatory measures.

As we have already indicated, the altered pharmacokinetics of lidocaine in the arrested heart markedly reduce drug clearance so that no more than one or two boluses of lidocaine are needed in most patients to maintain adequate therapeutic levels for as long as resuscitation is in progress.

11) REPEAT COUNTERSHOCK AS NEEDED

There is *NO LIMIT* to the number of times a patient can be defibrillated. Thus, *as long as ventricular fibrillation persists, a potentially treatable situation is present.* After every intervention, CPR should therefore be performed (for a period of at least 1 to 2 minutes to allow adequate time for drugs to reach the central circulation)—and this should be followed by repeat countershock (at an energy level of between 200 to 360 joules) until there is conclusive evidence of cardiovascular unresponsiveness.

> It is essential to *ALWAYS* check for a pulse after *EVERY* intervention–and/or *WHENEVER* the rhythm changes on the monitor. Forgetting to do so may result in iatrogenic defibrillation of a patient in sinus rhythm whose monitor leads fell off. *(It will probably also result in your failure of the ACLS course!!!)*

12) CONSIDER ADDITIONAL ANTIFIBRILLATORY MEASURES

Failure of Steps #1 to #11 to convert the patient out of ventricular fibrillation should prompt consideration of *additional* Antifibrillatory Measures *(see Figure 1B-2).*

If (As Soon As) the Patient Is Converted OUT of Ventricular Fibrillation

If the patient is converted out of ventricular fibrillation *at any time* during the above treatment process, *prophylactic* lidocaine should be started immediately in the hope that this may prevent a recurrence. If bolus therapy has not yet been given (and/or if more than 5 minutes have elapsed since the time of the last dose), an IV bolus of the drug should also be given.

Because spontaneous circulation has been restored, *lidocaine pharmacokinetics will have changed*. Thus it will be essential to maintain a continuous IV infusion to ensure a lasting drug effect. An infusion rate of 2 mg/min is optimal for most patients.

Clinically, the patient should be fully reassessed after conversion out of ventricular fibrillation. Further management decisions can then be made according to the appropriate treatment algorithm (depending on the mechanism of the post-conversion rhythm and the patient's hemodynamic status).

Additional ANTIFIBRILLATORY Measures

As suggested above, if ventricular fibrillation persists *despite* application of Steps #1 to #11, consideration might be given to a final step *(Step #12)*, which we have labeled: **Consider Additional Antifibrillatory Measures.** For ease of reference, the four alternatives included in this step have been separated into an extension algorithm *(Figure 1B-2)*.

Additional ANTIFIBRILLATORY Measures

If V Fib persists DESPITE application
of Steps #1-11 in Fig.1B-1

Consider **Step #12**

Additional **ANTIFIBRILLATORY** Measures: **✱**

12a) Magnesium Sulfate (consider especially if serum magnesium is likely to be low).
　Give 1-2 g IV over 1-2 minutes.
　May repeat this dose in 5-10 minutes if there is no response.

　and/or

12b) Bretylium Tosylate (consider as antifibrillatory therapy if lidocaine ineffective).
　Give 1 amp (=500 mg) by IV bolus. Circulate with CPR (for 1-2 minutes); then defibrillate.
　May then give 10 mg/kg IV (≈1-2 amps). Resume CPR; then defibrillate again.
　May repeat bretylium thereafter q15-30 minutes (up to a total dose of 30 mg/kg).
　May follow with a maintenance IV infusion (@ 1-2 mg/min) if the drug is effective.

　and/or

12c) IV ß-Blocker (consider especially if increased sympathetic tone/ischemia suspected).
　IV PROPRANOLOL- Give 0.5-1.0 mg by slow IV (over 5 minutes)-
　　　　　　- up to a total dose of 5.0 mg.

　and/or

12d) Amiodarone (might consider empirically if the drug is available).
　IV loading of 150-500 mg (over a 5-10 minute period).
　May repeat this dose in 15-30 minutes.
　If the drug is effective, may consider a maintenance infusion (with 20-50 mg/hr).

If the pt is converted out of V Fib

1) Clinically reassess pt/hemodynamic status.
2) Determine the post-conversion rhythm.
　Treat further according to appropriate algorithm.
3a) If not already done, administer bolus of **LIDOCAINE (50-100 mg)**, and begin IV infusion @ 2 mg/min.

　and/or

3b) Continue maintenance IV infusion of other antifibrillatory agent.

✱ At the time of this writing, there are no definite guidelines for administration of the **Additional ANTIFIBRILLATORY Measures** listed here. The suggested approach that we outline in this algorithm therefore reflects our opinion (based on available literature).

Figure 1B-2.　Algorithm of **Additional Antifibrillatory Measures** to consider if the patient in ventricular fibrillation fails to respond to the management approach suggested in Figure 1B-1.

> At the time of this writing, *no definite guidelines exist for administration of the* **additional Antifibrillatory Measures** *that we list here.* The approach we suggest in this algorithm therefore reflects *our opinion* (based on available literature).

12a) MAGNESIUM SULFATE

The role of magnesium sulfate in the treatment of cardiac arrest has not yet been completely clarified. As a result, use of the drug in this setting is still largely empiric. Although one might expect patients with low serum magnesium levels to benefit most from this form of therapy, *serum levels do not necessarily correlate with body stores of this cation.* Moreover, a beneficial antiarrhythmic effect has clearly been shown to occur in some patients *despite* normal serum magnesium levels at the time of administration.

> Practically speaking, the risk of toxicity from administration of magnesium sulfate to a patient in cardiac arrest is minimal (if not negligible), even if prearrest serum magnesium levels are normal. As a result, we favor *empiric* use of this drug in the setting of cardiac arrest when conventional measures have failed. Clearly, the drug should be given to patients in cardiac arrest who are *known* to be hypomagnesemic. If not used empirically, it should *at least be strongly considered* when suspicion for this electrolyte disturbance is high (as it may be for patients with other electrolyte disturbances, for those who were taking digoxin or diuretics, and/or for patients with a history of alcohol abuse).

For empiric use in the emergency treatment of life-threatening ventricular arrhythmias, a dose of 1 to 2 g of IV magnesium sulfate is often tried initially (given over a period of 1 to 2 minutes), and repeated in 5 to 10 minutes if there is no response.

12b) BRETYLIUM TOSYLATE

Bretylium is an effective antifibrillatory agent. Although administration of the drug rarely results in spontaneous conversion of ventricular fibrillation to sinus rhythm, it may facilitate conversion to sinus rhythm with subsequent countershocks.

> The antifibrillatory effect of bretylium usually begins to act within a few minutes. On occasion, however, this effect may be significantly delayed (for as long as 10 to 15 minutes!). As a result, once a decision is made to try bretylium, resuscitation efforts should probably not be terminated until adequate time has been allowed to give the drug a chance to work.

The recommended initial dose of bretylium for treatment of ventricular fibrillation is an IV bolus of 5 mg/kg. Considering the empiric nature of dosing in the setting of cardiac arrest (and in the interest of facilitating calculations in this situation), we favor administration of one complete ampule (= 500 mg) for the initial IV bolus (rather than strict calculation on a bodyweight basis).

The initial bolus of bretylium should be circulated (with CPR for 1 to 2 minutes), and then followed by repeat defibrillation. If unsuccessful, a second IV bolus (of 10 mg/kg–or *approximately* 1 to 2 ampules) may be tried several minutes later. Additional (10 mg/kg) boluses may be given as needed (up to a total dose of 30 mg/kg).

> While still a matter of controversy, it is possible that the effects of lidocaine and bretylium in refractory ventricular fibrillation may be *additive*. Thus, even if a maximal dose of the first agent (which is usually lidocaine) doesn't work, addition of the second drug (bretylium) could result in a *combination* that is now effective.
>
> Because the duration of action of a bretylium bolus is relatively prolonged (usually lasting for 2 to 6 hours), some protection against immediate recurrence of ventricular fibrillation is automatically provided by this form of administration. Most emergency care providers also tend to initiate a *prophylactic* maintenance infusion (of either bretylium *and/or* lidocaine) as soon as the patient is converted to a normal rhythm in the hope of providing additional protection.

12c) IV β-BLOCKER

The most difficult part about suggesting recommendations for the use of IV β-blockers in the setting of cardiopulmonary arrest is knowing when to administer these drugs. Clearly, there are times when all other treatment measures will fail, and *only* IV β-blockers may save the patient.

> Situations in which the use of an IV β-blocker is most likely to be lifesaving are those in which excessive sympathetic tone is implicated as an important etiologic factor in the arrest (i.e., in a setting of known ischemia or acute *anterior* infarction—especially when cardiac arrest was preceded by a period of tachycardia or hypertension—and/or in the setting of cocaine overdose or severe stress during the prearrest period). Empiric use of an IV β-blocker is encouraged if refractory ventricular fibrillation occurs in association with any of these factors.

Because of ease of administration and familiarity with its use, propranolol is the IV β-blocker most commonly selected for treatment of patients in cardiac arrest. The recommended dose of this drug for IV administration is 0.5 to 1 mg given *slowly* (i.e., over a 5-minute period). This dose may be repeated as needed (up to a total dose of 5 mg).

> Alternatively, *other* IV β-blockers (i.e., metoprolol, esmolol) could be used instead of propranolol.

12d) AMIODARONE

Amiodarone is a class III antiarrhythmic agent. Although the drug is remarkably effective as an oral agent in the long-term management of supraventricular and ventricular arrhythmias, experience with IV use of amiodarone in the setting of cardiac arrest is limited. A small, retrospective study by Williams et al (1989) is extremely encouraging, and suggests that the drug could be much more effective as an antifibrillatory agent than either lidocaine or bretylium.

> At the time of this writing, IV amiodarone remains an investigational agent that is not yet available for general use. Additional studies are clearly needed to determine the true role (if any) of the drug in the treatment of cardiac arrest. Nevertheless, the future may see IV amiodarone assume an increasingly important role in this emergency setting. Empiric administration of the drug (in the dose range suggested in Step 12d of Figure 1B-2) may well prove to be a reasonable option to consider when confronted with a patient in refractory ventricular fibrillation that has not responded to other measures— or for a patient with cardiac arrest from recurrent ventricular tachycardia who is unable to maintain sinus rhythm with conventional antiarrhythmic therapy.

If the Patient Is Converted *OUT* of Ventricular Fibrillation

If any of the above antifibrillatory measures are successful, antiarrhythmic prophylaxis should be immediately started in the hope of preventing a recurrence. Although lidocaine (IV bolus and continuous infusion) is usually used for this purpose, another agent (i.e., bretylium, amiodarone) could be substituted if alternative therapy was needed to convert the patient out of ventricular fibrillation.

Questions to Further Understanding

WHAT ENERGY IS OPTIMAL FOR DEFIBRILLATION?

Although the current recommendation for defibrillation of adults on the initial countershock attempt is 200 joules, this is not necessarily the optimal energy level for all patients. *Defibrillation is NOT benign.* On the contrary, use of excessive energy with countershock attempts can sometimes produce an adverse result (in the form of additional conduction system damage and/or conversion of ventricular fibrillation to asystole).

> When transthoracic resistance (TTR) values are low, as little as 100 joules will successfully defibrillate the overwhelming majority of patients. Use of excessive energy in such individuals (i.e., 300 or more joules) is likely to be *counterproductive* and result in a decreased chance of converting the patient out of ventricular fibrillation (Kerber et al, 1988). In contrast, higher energy levels (of *at least* 300 to 360 joules) are much more likely to be needed for defibrillation to be successful when TTR is high. The problem is that *there is no practical way to determine TTR at the moment of countershock delivery with the types of defibrillators in current use.* Until **current-based defibrillators** (that are able to *instantaneously* measure TTR, and adjust current delivery accordingly) become generally available, empiric use of 200 joules for the initial countershock attempt in adults may represent the most reasonable compromise.

WHAT IF VENTRICULAR FIBRILLATION RECURS DURING THE CODE?

Although official recommendations are to repeat countershock with the same amount of energy that successfully converted the patient the last time they were defibrillated, we generally prefer to drop back to 200 joules. As noted above, *defibrillation is not benign.* Use of an excessive energy level for defibrillation may produce additional conduction system damage and/or precipitate conversion of ventricular fibrillation to asystole.

> Clinically, it is very possible that a patient who didn't initially respond to 200 joules may do so later in the code. This is because of a number of factors, including reduction of TTR (as a *cumulative* effect of all previous countershock attempts), and therapeutic benefits that may accrue from medications given since the last countershock attempt.

There is no drawback to reducing the energy level selected for defibrillation of ventricular fibrillation that recurs later during the code. If this lower energy level (of 200 joules) is unsuccessful, the solution is simple: Immediately recharge the defibrillator to a higher energy level (i.e., 360 joules), and then defibrillate again.

SHOULD A PRECORDIAL *THUMP* BE USED?

Although the precordial thump may occasionally convert a patient out of either ventricular fibrillation or ventricular tachycardia, the maneuver appears to be much more likely to either have no effect, or to exacerbate the rhythm (i.e., precipitate a pulseless rhythm or produce asystole). This is because the emergency care provider has absolutely no control over when in the cardiac cycle the energy will be delivered with the thump. Aggravation of the rhythm is likely if the thump is inadvertently delivered during the vulnerable period.

> We find it easiest to think of the thump as a *"No-Lose" Procedure.* As a result, we generally reserve use of the thump for treatment of rhythms *without* a pulse—since *there is really "nothing to lose" from treatment of such rhythms.* In contrast, we are *against* using the thump to treat a patient in sustained ventricular tachycardia in which a pulse is present—since there is "too much to lose" in this situation (i.e., you may lose the pulse). Programmed delivery of an electrical impulse at a *designated* point in the cardiac cycle (i.e., use of *synchronized cardioversion*) is a far more preferable form of treatment for sustained ventricular tachycardia associated with a palpable pulse.
>
> Other instances in which the use of a precordial thump is reasonable include treatment of *pulseless* ventricular tachycardia and/or ventricular fibrillation. Practically speaking, however, if a defibrillator is readily available (or will *very soon* be available), we feel it is equally reasonable to withhold the thump in favor of delivery of an electrical impulse (i.e., defibrillation).

WILL PROMPT DEFIBRILLATION CAUSE ASYSTOLE?

Admittedly, shocking a patient in ventricular fibrillation *DOES* run the risk of precipitating asystole—*especially* if a patient has already been in ventricular fibrillation for a period of time. However, the chance that a patient in ventricular fibrillation will ultimately survive is significantly greater if they are immediately defibrillated (*BEFORE* attempting intubation and/or drug administration!), than if these other interventions are attempted first (Martin et al, 1986).

> It is important to appreciate that the *realistic* chance for meaningful (i.e., neurologically intact) *long-term survival* is relatively small when a patient is found in out-of-hospital cardiac arrest with ventricular fibrillation as the initial mechanism. Nevertheless, a chance for survival does exist—and *it is maximized by immediately defibrillating the patient as soon as this is possible* (i.e., BEFORE attempting intubation and/or drug administration).

WHAT TO REMEMBER ABOUT CPR?

CPR—in and of itself—will unfortunately *not* prevent ventricular fibrillation from deteriorating to asystole (Enns et al, 1983). However, performance of CPR may *delay* deterioration of the rhythm to asystole—and in so doing preserve the period of *viability* (i.e., *potential* responsiveness to defibrillation) for a short amount of time (perhaps 1 to 2 minutes?).

> Although the precise mechanism of CPR remains uncertain—and *several* mechanisms may be operative at the same time to varying degrees—what *DOES* seem clear is that the efficacy of CPR can be enhanced by attention to *four* factors:
>
> 1. *Compressing with proper form and sufficient force*—*NOT* "rib-breaking" force, but enough force to adequately depress the sternum.
> 2. *Compressing at the higher end of the recommended rate range*—or as close to 100 compressions per minute as possible.
> 3. *Giving epinephrine ASAP during resuscitation*—since this is the KEY drug for favoring blood flow to the coronary and cerebral circulations.
> 4. *Optimizing ventilation*—being sure to deliver slow, full respirations.

WHY HAS SODIUM BICARBONATE BEEN DEEMPHASIZED?

The acidosis that occurs during the initial minutes of cardiac arrest is primarily respiratory in nature (due to *hypoventilation*). Recommended treatment for this respiratory acidosis is to improve ventilation—*NOT to give sodium bicarbonate!* Treatment with sodium bicarbonate has *never* been shown to improve survival. On the contrary, early administration of sodium bicarbonate may *aggravate* the situation by producing a *paradoxical intracellular acidosis* (that may lead to further depression of myocardial func-

tion). As a result, use of sodium bicarbonate in the usual code situation is to be strongly discouraged for *AT LEAST* the first 5 to 10 minutes of the arrest!

> A possible exception to this general rule may be if a severe preexisting metabolic acidosis was known to be present at the time of the arrest (as might be the case for a patient with diabetic ketoacidosis or lactic acidosis)—especially if the metabolic acidosis could be a contributing cause of the arrest. However, *recent data now question whether sodium bicarbonate should even be given under these circumstances (because of its potentially deleterious effects).*

WHICH ROUTE IS <u>BEST</u> FOR GIVING DRUGS?

A **central line** inserted *ABOVE* the diaphragm (i.e., a *subclavian* or *internal jugular line*) is the optimal route for drug delivery during cardiac arrest (assuming a provider is present who can rapidly insert the line with a minimal chance of causing pneumothorax). In contrast, a *femoral line* is an ineffective route for drug delivery in the arrested heart (unless a long enough catheter is used that can be threaded *above* the diaphragm).

> The **ET route** is an excellent alternative option (and the access route of choice) for medication administration in patients who are intubated *before* IV access is achieved. It should be noted that higher than usual doses of epinephrine (2 to 3 times the peripheral dose–*or more!*) may be needed when the drug is administered by the ET route.

In the absence of a central line, use of a **peripheral IV** may be adequate in most cases of cardiac arrest provided: (1) a *large-bore* IV catheter is used; and (2) a *proximal* site (such as the anticubital fossa) is chosen for insertion. Drug delivery from a peripheral IV during cardiopulmonary resuscitation may further be optimized by: (3) *flushing the IV line* (with 50 to 100 ml of fluid); and (4) *raising the arm* after drug administration.

> It should be emphasized that placement of a small "butterfly" in the dorsum of the wrist is *not* an effective route for drug administration in the arrested heart.

> *We suggest initially using whatever access route is established first.* If this happens to be a central line *above* the diaphragm, we'll continue to administer drugs such as epinephrine by this route. If it is a peripheral IV line, we'll tend to follow with the next dose of epinephrine by the ET route (as soon as the patient is intubated). In contrast, if the ET route is established first, we'll tend to follow with the next dose of epinephrine by peripheral IV (as soon as the line is inserted).

WHICH DRUGS CAN BE GIVEN BY THE ET ROUTE?

The drugs that can be given by the ET route are easily remembered with the assistance of one or more mnemonics:

ALE—**A**tropine, **L**idocaine, and **E**pinephrine

ALOE—**A**tropine, **L**idocaine, **O**xygen (which *IS* a drug), and **E**pinephrine

NAVEL—**N**arcan (for cardiac arrest due to narcotic overdose), **A**tropine, **V**alium (if seizures accompany the arrest), **E**pinephrine, and **L**idocaine

HOW TO GIVE EPINEPHRINE?

The optimal way to dose epinephrine during cardiac arrest remains uncertain. What has become clear is that epinephrine is essential for increasing coronary perfusion pressure (CPP) in the arrested heart—and that higher doses of drug (i.e., HDE) may be needed in certain patients to achieve CPPs that are adequate for resuscitation.

> SDE (i.e., 1 mg of the 1:10,000 solution by either the IV or ET route) is often tried first—especially when the rhythm is ventricular fibrillation and the duration of the arrest is likely to be short. If unsuccessful, we feel consideration should be given to increasing the dose of epinephrine rapidly (to HDE). Higher doses of epinephrine are likely to be needed much sooner for patients initially found in asystole and/or when arrest duration prior to arrival of the health care team is prolonged (as is usually the case for arrests that occur out-of-hospital).

The point to emphasize is that if SDE is selected first, the dose of epinephrine should probably be increased (to HDE) if the patient fails to respond.

IS THERE AN <u>EASY</u> WAY TO REMEMBER HOW TO PREPARE IV INFUSIONS?

We devote Section C of Chapter 2 to *"Simplified Calculation of IV Infusions."* As a *preview* to this section, we introduce here the ***Rule of 250 ml.*** This rule greatly facilitates recall of an easy-to-learn method for estimating the appropriate *initial* IV infusion rate for *most* of the essential drugs used in ACLS. Adjustments in dosing can then be made based on the patient's clinical response. The rule is as follows:

Mix **1 unit** of *whatever* drug you are using in **250 ml** of D5W, and set the IV infusion to run at **15 to 30 drops/min.**

The KEY to application of the **"Rule of 250 ml"** lies with determining the amount of drug contained in one "unit." *Our calculations assume the following:*

For the *antiarrhythmic agents*, **1 unit of drug** = 1 g of **lidocaine**
= 1 g of **procainamide**
= 1 g of **bretylium**

For the *catecholamines*, **1 unit of drug** = 1 mg (= 1 vial) of **isoproterenol**
= 1 mg (= 1 ampule) of **epinephrine** (in a 1:10,000 concentration for **SDE**)

For *dopamine*, **1 unit of drug** = 200 mg (= 1 ampule) of **dopamine**

Substitution into the **Rule of 250 ml** of the quantities listed above for "1 unit" of drug (for any of the three *antiarrhythmic agents*, two *catecholamines*, or for *dopamine*) automatically results in an appropriately prepared initial IV infusion rate. Thus one might proceed in the following manner to prepare an IV infusion of these drugs:

> **Lidocaine**—Mix **1 g** (= 1 unit) of *lidocaine* in **250 ml** of D5W (or 2 g in 500 ml), and set the infusion to run at **30 drops/ min** (= 2 mg/min).

> **Procainamide**—Mix **1 g** (= 1 unit) of *procainamide* in **250 ml** of D5W (or 2 g in 500 ml), and set the infusion to run at **30 drops/min** (= 2 mg/min).

> **Bretylium**—Mix **1 g** (= 1 unit) of *bretylium* in **250 ml** of D5W (or 2 g in 500 ml), and set the infusion to run at **15 drops/ min** (= 1 mg/min).

> **Isoproterenol**—Mix **1 mg** (i.e., 1 vial = 1 unit) of *isoproterenol* in **250 ml** of D5W, and set the infusion to run at **30 drops/min** (= 2 μg/min).

> **Standard-Dose Epinephrine (SDE)**—Mix **1 mg** (i.e., 1 ampule = 1 unit) of a *1 : 10,000 solution of epinephrine* in **250 ml** of D5W, and set the infusion to run at between **15 to 30 drops/min** (i.e., 1 to 2 μg/min).

Discussion on preparation of an IV infusion for **High-Dose Epinephrine (HDE)** is deferred until Sections 2B and 2C.

> **Dopamine**—Mix **200 mg** (i.e., 1 ampule = 1 unit) of *dopamine* in **250 ml** of D5W, and set the infusion to run at between **15 to 30 drops/min** ($\approx$2 to 5 μg/kg/min for most patients).

WHAT IF VENTRICULAR FIBRILLATION IS REFRACTORY?

We refer to ventricular fibrillation as being *refractory* if it fails to respond to initial attempts at defibrillation and treatment with epinephrine (Steps #1 to #4 in the algorithm shown in Figure 1B-1).

Treatment options for refractory ventricular fibrillation are included in the remaining steps of this algorithm and in Figure 1B-2.

- A trial of *antifibrillatory* therapy (initially with lidocaine)
- A search for an underlying cause of ventricular fibrillation
- Continued epinephrine administration (using HDE)
- Continued countershock (as needed)
- Consideration of sodium bicarbonate (?)
- Consideration of *other antifibrillatory measures* (such as magnesium sulfate, bretylium, an IV β-blocker, and/or amiodarone)

WHAT IS THE MAXIMUM NUMBER OF TIMES YOU CAN DEFIBRILLATE A PATIENT?

There is *NO* maximum number. *As long as the rhythm is ventricular fibrillation, the mechanism of cardiac arrest is potentially treatable (and may respond to defibrillation).* Search for a *potentially correctable* underlying cause of ventricular fibrillation, and *continued* application of Steps #8, #11, and #12 in Figures 1B-1 and 1B-2 (i.e., HDE, repeat countershock, and additional antifibrillatory measures) are indicated *UNTIL cardiovascular unresponsiveness can be conclusively demonstrated.*

WHEN SHOULD RESUSCITATION EFFORTS BE TERMINATED?

If a patient has remained in ventricular fibrillation for *more than* 30 minutes *despite* application of appropriate treatment measures (i.e., application of Steps #1 through #12 in Figure 1B-1), the chance that resuscitation will be successful, *and* that the patient will survive to *ultimately leave the hospital neurologically intact* is exceedingly small (if not negligible!). As a result, we feel it reasonable to declare "cardiovascular unresponsiveness" (and terminate resuscitation efforts) *after* this period of time.

> Practically speaking, the chance of neurologically intact long-term survival is exceedingly small if the patient fails to respond to appropriate resuscitation efforts after 20 minutes!

Exceptions to this general rule (when you may want to continue resuscitation efforts *beyond* 20 to 30 minutes) include:

1. Resuscitation of *children* (who may sometimes fully recover after far longer periods of time)
2. *Hypothermia* (in which a patient should *NEVER* be pronounced dead "until they are *warm* and dead")
3. Victims of *drowning* (especially *cold water drowning*)
4. Patients with *recurrent* ventricular fibrillation (i.e., when the patient goes "in and out" of ventricular fibrillation *multiple* times)

WHAT SHOULD BE DONE AFTER THE CODE IS "OVER"?

The checklist of "things to do" at the end of a successful resuscitation effort includes the following:

1. Verify the adequacy of the **A**irway and **B**reathing (i.e., the adequacy of ventilation and oxygenation, the presence of bilateral and symmetric breath sounds, lung excursion, patient color, and ABGs).
2. Verify the adequacy of **C**irculation (i.e., the presence of a pulse, adequacy of blood pressure, intravascular volume status).
3. Verify that a lidocaine bolus has been given, and that the patient is on a continuous IV infusion of the drug (and/or of another antifibrillatory agent).
4. Determine what (if any) other medications that the patient is receiving.
5. Be sure "routine" laboratory tests have been ordered including:
   - Chest x-ray (for ET tube, central line placement, assessment of hemodynamic status)
   - 12-lead ECG (for evidence of acute infarction/ischemia)
   - Blood work (e.g., CBC, SMAC-25, serum electrolytes including magnesium)
6. Be sure the patient's family has been spoken to (and that they are satisfied with the explanation of events of the code that was given to them).
7. Acknowledge the efforts of your coworkers.
8. Write a note in the chart.
9. Notify the patient's attending physician (if this is not you).
10. Spend a moment reflecting on how things went during the code—*how things might have gone better*—and what you might do differently (if anything) next time.
11. Update the patient's code status (in case they arrest again).

Items #6 through #10 on this list should be done *regardless* of whether or not the resuscitation effort was successful.

IS LONG-TERM SURVIVAL FROM OUT-OF-HOSPITAL CARDIAC ARREST LIKELY IF EMS/PARAMEDIC EFFORTS FAIL TO RESTORE SPONTANEOUS CIRCULATION ON THE SCENE?

No. Practically speaking, the chances for long-term, neurologically intact survival from out-of-hospital cardiac arrest are exceedingly small if adequately performed BLS and ACLS measures (including defibrillation) fail to restore a spontaneous pulse in the field. This sobering fact provides the rationale for full application of ACLS procedures by trained paramedical personnel *at the scene—* rather than prematurely rushing the pulseless patient to an emergency department.

The opposite situation holds true for the victim of severe trauma—for whom expeditious transfer to a capable facility after field stabilization offers the greatest chance for meaningful survival.

The moral is clear. Early defibrillation is the *KEY* determinant of survival from out-of-hospital cardiac arrest. Although every effort *MUST* always be made to resuscitate a patient (until there is *definitive* evidence of cardiovascular unresponsiveness), realistic chances for long-term survival are small if properly performed BLS/ACLS in the field fails to restore spontaneous circulation.

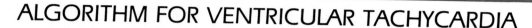

SECTION C

ALGORITHM FOR VENTRICULAR TACHYCARDIA

Identification of Sustained Ventricular Tachycardia: *Assessment of Hemodynamic Status*

The KEY to management of sustained ventricular tachycardia hinges on assessment of the patient's hemodynamic status. This is reflected in the recommendations shown in *Figure 1C-1* for treatment of this condition. Thus, the *FIRST* (and most basic) decision is to determine if there is a pulse.

If There Is NO PULSE

Pulseless ventricular tachycardia should generally be treated in the same manner as ventricular fibrillation— by immediate *unsynchronized* countershock (with 200 joules).

There may be one exception to this general approach. If you are familiar enough with your equipment to be able to activate the synchronizer switch in about the same amount of time it would take to deliver an unsynchronized countershock, it may be reasonable to attempt synchronized cardioversion first. Unsynchronized countershock can always be used if synchronized cardioversion is either ineffective and/or if the machine fails to readily discharge the synchronized impulse.

A word of caution is in order. The reason unsynchronized countershock has been recommended when no pulse is palpable is that, at the more rapid rates of ventricular tachycardia usually associated with these unstable patients, distinction between the QRS complex and the T wave often becomes exceedingly difficult (if not impossible). Under such circumstances, delivery of a "synchronized" discharge becomes equally likely to fall on a T wave (during the vulnerable period) as not. Delivery of unsynchronized countershock for pulseless ventricular tachycardia may obviate the need for you (and the defibrillator) to try to make such a decision.

If There IS a PULSE

If a pulse is present, it becomes essential to determine if the patient is *HEMODYNAMICALLY STABLE* or not. If the patient is unstable, the need for immediate action is urgent. However, if the patient is hemodynamically stable, there is a little more time to reflect on the process.

A patient is said to be **"hemodynamically stable"** when blood pressure is adequate (i.e., ≥90 mm Hg systolic) and no symptoms (such as chest pain, dyspnea, or altered mental status) are present. *NOT all patients with sustained ventricular tachycardia are (or immediately become) hemodynamically unstable!* In fact, some patients with ventricular tachycardia are able to

remain alert and maintain an adequate blood pressure for minutes, hours *(and even days!) without* showing any signs of decompensation. This is especially likely to occur when the rate of the ventricular tachycardia is not excessively rapid (i.e., between 140 to 170 beats/min).

If a pulse is present and the patient is alert, one should strongly consider the use of cough version.

Whether the mechanism for **cough version** is improved coronary perfusion (from the increase in intrathoracic pressure generated by the cough), activation of the autonomic nervous system, or conversion of mechanical energy from the cough (into an electrical depolarization) is unknown. What has been shown is that the cough may effectively convert ventricular tachycardia to normal sinus rhythm in a surprising number of cases.

In practice, cough version appears to be vastly under-utilized. The technique should probably be the *FIRST* intervention for treatment of the conscious patient who presents in sustained ventricular tachycardia.

In contrast to cough version, use of the *precordial thump* has been strongly deemphasized as a treatment modality for ventricular tachycardia. The problem with the thump is that even though the maneuver may occasionally convert ventricular tachycardia to sinus rhythm, it is equally likely (if not more so) to convert this rhythm to ventricular fibrillation, asystole, or pulseless idioventricular rhythm. Thus, if synchronized cardioversion is readily available, it would seem to be far preferable to delivery of 2 to 5 joules at a random (and possibly vulnerable) point in the cardiac cycle, as is provided by the thump.

If There IS a Pulse, BUT the Patient IS (or at ANY Time Becomes) Hemodynamically UNSTABLE

If the patient has a pulse, but is hemodynamically unstable, *immediate* cardioversion must take precedence over antiarrhythmic therapy. Delay for the several minutes needed to draw up and administer medications is *unacceptable* in this urgent situation. An energy level of *at least* 100 joules should probably be chosen for emergency cardioversion.

It should be emphasized that if the patient shows signs of hemodynamic compromise *at any time* during administration of antiarrhythmic therapy, synchronized cardioversion must be *immediately* performed.

VENTRICULAR TACHYCARDIA

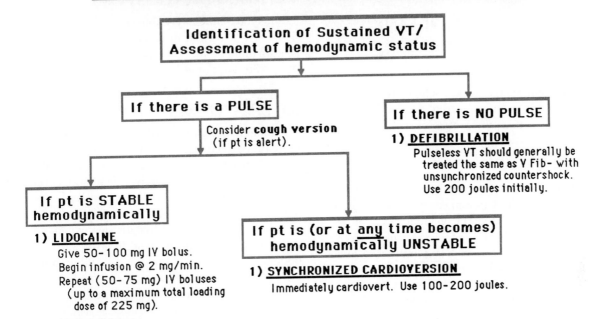

**Identification of Sustained VT/
Assessment of hemodynamic status**

If there is a PULSE

Consider **cough version**
(if pt is alert).

If there is NO PULSE

1) DEFIBRILLATION
Pulseless VT should generally be
treated the same as V Fib– with
unsynchronized countershock.
Use 200 joules initially.

**If pt is STABLE
hemodynamically**

1) LIDOCAINE
Give 50–100 mg IV bolus.
Begin infusion @ 2 mg/min.
Repeat (50–75 mg) IV boluses
(up to a maximum total loading
dose of 225 mg).

2) PROCAINAMIDE
Give 100 mg IV q 5 min (up to
1 g loading dose).
Alternatively, may load pt with
500–1,000 mg (mixed in 100 ml
of D5W), to infuse over 30–60 min.
If IV loading is effective, may start a
maintenance infusion @ 2mg/min.

**If pt is (or at any time becomes)
hemodynamically UNSTABLE**

1) SYNCHRONIZED CARDIOVERSION
Immediately cardiovert. Use 100–200 joules.

If hemodynamically stable VT persists:

3a) BRETYLIUM
IV infusion of 500 mg (mixed in 50 ml of D5W) given over a 10 minute period.
If IV loading is effective, may start a maintenance infusion @ 1–2 mg/min.

3b) SYNCHRONIZED CARDIOVERSION
"Semielective" cardioversion– ie, sedate the pt, call anesthesia to the bedside, consider
use of a lower energy level (of 50–100 joules) for initial cardioversion attempt.

and/or

3c) Alternative Measures:
Search for potentially correctable cause of sustained VT.
Consider use of an IV ß-blocker such as **propranolol (** 0.5–1.0 mg by slow IV
over 5 minutes– up to a total dose of 5.0 mg**)**.
Magnesium sulfate– 1–2 g IV (over 1–2 min). May repeat dose in 5–10 min
if there is no response.

Figure 1C-1.   Algorithm for treatment of **Sustained** Ventricular Tachycardia.

Although ventricular tachycardia frequently responds to cardioversion with energy levels of as low as 20 joules, the use of *at least* 100 joules may be preferable for treatment of a hemodynamically compromised patient. With a more stable patient, time is less critical and a trial at a lower energy level (i.e., with 50 joules) may be reasonable.

If There IS a Pulse AND the Patient IS Hemodynamically STABLE

If a pulse is present *and* the patient is hemodynamically stable, it is reasonable to initiate a trial of antiarrhythmic therapy.

1) LIDOCAINE

Lidocaine is generally accepted as the antiarrhythmic agent of choice for medical treatment of sustained ventricular tachycardia. An initial IV loading dose (of between 50 to 100 mg–or about 1 mg/kg) is usually given, and an IV infusion (at a rate of 2 mg/min) is begun. Additional 50- to 75-mg IV boluses may follow every 5 to 10 minutes thereafter (either as needed—and/or until a total loading dose of 225 mg has been given).

Although many clinicians tend to increase the lidocaine infusion rate with each additional bolus of the drug that is given, this is *not* essential during the period of lidocaine loading. On the contrary, routinely increasing the infusion rate after administration of each lidocaine bolus may *unnecessarily* increase the risk of developing lidocaine toxicity.

On the other hand, if the ventricular arrhythmia rapidly resolves after bolus administration—*only to recur AFTER steady state conditions have been achieved* (i.e., at an infusion rate of 2 mg/min)—administration of an *additional* 50-mg bolus AND an increase in the infusion rate (i.e., to 3 mg/min) may be warranted. *(See Section 12E for a more detailed discussion on the pharmacokinetic rationale for lidocaine dosing).*

2) PROCAINAMIDE

If lidocaine is ineffective, procainamide is generally recommended as the *second-line* agent for medical treatment of sustained ventricular tachycardia. IV procainamide is usually given in 100-mg increments (administered *slowly* over a 5-minute period) until one of the following *end points* is achieved:

1. The patient has received a total loading dose of 500 to 1,000 mg.
2. The arrhythmia is suppressed.
3. Hypotension develops.
4. QRS widening occurs.

Alternatively, 500 to 1,000 mg of procainamide may be diluted in 100 ml of D5W and administered as a loading IV infusion over 30 to 60 minutes.

If either loading regimen of procainamide is successful, a continuous *IV maintenance* infusion of the drug may be started at a rate of 2 mg/min.

If Hemodynamically Stable Ventricular Tachycardia Persists

If hemodynamically stable ventricular tachycardia persists *despite* a trial of medical therapy with lidocaine and procainamide, *three* therapeutic options remain (Steps #3a, #3b, and/or #3c in Figure 1C-1):

3a) BRETYLIUM

Although frequently used in the past, administration of bretylium tosylate for medical treatment of ventricular ectopy/ventricular tachycardia has been deemphasized. In reality, the drug appears to be much more effective as an *antifibrillatory* agent than as an *antiarrhythmic* agent. Moreover, the most common long-term adverse effect associated with bretylium therapy is hypotension, which further limits its use. As a result, we tend to favor other therapeutic options (i.e., Steps #3b and/or #3c) if lidocaine and procainamide are ineffective.

If bretylium is used for treatment of ventricular tachycardia, the drug should be given as an IV loading infusion rather than as bolus therapy. To do this, one ampule of bretylium (=500 mg) is mixed in 50 ml of D5W, and then infused over a 10-minute period. Following IV loading, a maintenance IV infusion (at a rate of between 1 to 2 mg/min) may be continued to sustain the drug's effect.

3b) SYNCHRONIZED CARDIOVERSION

In the event that medical therapy is unsuccessful in converting the patient out of sustained ventricular tachycardia, *synchronized cardioversion* may be tried. If the patient shows no signs of hemodynamic compromise, this may be carried out under **"semi-elective"** circumstances. This entails:

1. Sedation of the patient (with IV diazepam or another agent)
2. Calling anesthesia to the bedside (to assist with intubation if needed)—so as to leave you free to concentrate on managing the arrhythmia
3. A trial at a lower energy level (i.e., 50 joules initially–increasing to 100 to 200 joules as needed)

As already emphasized, should the patient show signs of hemodynamic compromise *at any time* during the treatment process, synchronized cardioversion must be *immediately* performed. Use of a higher initial energy level (of at least 100 to 200 joules) becomes preferable in this situation.

3c) ALTERNATIVE MEASURES

As suggested in Figure 1C-1, _alternative_ measures to consider for treatment of sustained ventricular tachycardia that has not responded to lidocaine and procainamide include:

1. Searching for a _potentially_ correctable cause of the rhythm
2. Use of an IV β-blocker
3. Use of magnesium sulfate

The rationale for use and the dosing recommendations we favor for these alternative measures are similar to those stated in our explanation to Steps #7, #12a, and #12c in Figures 1B-1 and 1B-2.

Questions to Further Understanding

WHAT SHOULD BE DONE FIRST IF THE PATIENT IS IN SUSTAINED VENTRICULAR TACHYCARDIA?

If the patient is in sustained ventricular tachycardia:

1. Don't _PANIC!!!!_
2. Assess the patient in the manner suggested by Figure 1C-1.

The _KEY_ to evaluation and management of sustained ventricular tachycardia lies with determining whether a pulse is present. If it is not, then _immediate_ countershock (i.e., _unsynchronized_ defibrillation) is in order.

If a palpable pulse is present, then the next order of business is to determine whether the patient is hemodynamically stable. If not, _synchronized cardioversion_ takes precedence over all other forms of therapy. On the other hand, if the patient in sustained ventricular tachycardia is hemodynamically stable, a trial of medical therapy (with lidocaine, procainamide, and/or other measures as suggested in Figure 1C-1) is reasonable.

DOES THE PATIENT HAVE TO BE ALERT TO BE HEMODYNAMICALLY STABLE?

No. Clearly, many patients with cardiac arrest will not regain consciousness the moment a hemodynamically stable rhythm develops. A host of factors may account for a persistent unconscious state in the setting of cardiac arrest (including severe hypoxia and/or metabolic insult, residual effects from drug overdose, associated seizure activity, etc.). Thus, despite continued unresponsiveness, a patient

in sustained ventricular tachycardia may remain _"hemodynamically stable"_ as long as the rhythm is associated with evidence of good perfusion (i.e., good peripheral pulses and a systolic blood pressure of at least 90 mm Hg).

WHAT IF YOU ARE UNCERTAIN WHAT THE RHYTHM IS?

If the rhythm is a regular, wide complex tachycardia— _ASSUME VENTRICULAR TACHYCARDIA UNTIL PROVEN OTHERWISE_—and treat the patient accordingly.

Don't be dissuaded from the diagnosis of ventricular tachycardia because of a patient's hemodynamic status. Statistically, ventricular tachycardia is a much more likely diagnosis than supraventricular tachycardia (SVT) with either aberration or bundle branch block. This is especially true in older adults with a history of underlying heart disease (i.e., angina, prior myocardial infarction, and/or heart failure)— _regardless_ of whether the patient is alert or not, and what the blood pressure happens to be.

If you are in doubt about the etiology of the rhythm— and the patient is hemodynamically stable (at least temporarily)—you have the luxury of a little extra time to reflect on the process. In this situation, obtaining a _12-lead ECG_ may provide invaluable clues to the true cause of the arrhythmia.

A pearl to remember is that empiric use of **procainamide** may be effective in converting _both_ SVT _and_ ventricular tachycardia. Even if unsuccessful in converting the latter, procainamide may still slow the ventricular response of ventricular tachycardia, thus allowing the patient to remain hemodynamically stable for a longer period of time.

It should be emphasized that if the patient is (or _at any time_ becomes) hemodynamically unstable, _it no longer matters what the rhythm is._ Synchronized cardioversion now becomes _immediately_ indicated.

SHOULD EPINEPHRINE BE GIVEN IF SUSTAINED VENTRICULAR TACHYCARDIA IS ASSOCIATED WITH HYPOTENSION?

Although epinephrine is termed a _"pressor agent,"_ it is _CONTRAINDICATED_ for treatment of ventricular tachycardia.

By definition, sustained ventricular tachycardia that is associated with hypotension is hemodynamically unstable. As a result, the treatment of choice is _immediate_ cardioversion— _NOT_ administration of a catecholamine (such as epinephrine or dopamine) that may further exacerbate the ventricular arrhythmia.

WHAT IF MEDICAL THERAPY OF A PATIENT WITH HEMODYNAMICALLY STABLE VENTRICULAR TACHYCARDIA IS INEFFECTIVE?

If the patient fails to respond to a full trial of medical therapy (with lidocaine, procainamide, and other measures such as bretylium, an IV β-blocker, and/or magnesium sulfate)—then *synchronized cardioversion* may be in order *(see Fig. 1C-1).*

> As long as a patient in sustained ventricular tachycardia remains hemodynamically stable, synchronized cardioversion may be performed under "semielective" circumstances (i.e., with sedation, assistance from anesthesia, and selection of a lower energy level for the initial cardioversion attempt).

WHAT IF SYNCHRONIZED CARDIOVERSION PRODUCES VENTRICULAR FIBRILLATION?

Although synchronization to the upstroke of the R wave miniumizes the chance that the electrical impulse will be delivered during the "vulnerable period," it still does not eliminate the possibility of cardioversion precipitating development of ventricular fibrillation.

> Comfort can be taken in the fact that, even if ventricular fibrillation is produced by cardioversion, the chance for converting the patient out of this rhythm is excellent. This is because you are right on the scene—*and the time from recognition of this complication until action (i.e., defibrillation) should be minimal.* Anticipate this possibility. Know that even if synchronized cardioversion precipitates development of ventricular fibrillation, you will probably be able to save the patient by deactivating the synchronizer mode and immediately defibrillating the patient (with 200 to 360 joules).

WHAT IF THE CARDIOVERTER WON'T WORK?

There are numerous cardioverter/defibrillators on the market. Each features nuances in operation that distinguish one particular model from the next. In many hospitals, different types of defibrillators are present in different patient care areas. *The time to learn about operation of all of the various types of defibrillators that are used in your hospital is NOT in the middle of a code.*

If you do find yourself confronted with a patient in sustained ventricular tachycardia who is in need of electrical therapy—*and you are unable to get the defibrillator to deliver a synchronized impulse (for whatever reason). . . .*—do *NOT* spend more than a *few* moments trying to get the device to work. Instead, simply turn off the synchronizer switch and defibrillate the patient.

> Delivery of an unsynchronized countershock will successfully convert most cases of ventricular tachycardia (albeit at a slightly increased risk compared to the use of synchronized cardioversion). The reason for not delaying defibrillation for more than a few moments is that delivery of an unsynchronized countershock to a hemodynamically unstable patient in ventricular tachycardia is far preferable to delivery of no electrical energy at all.

WHAT IF THE RHYTHM IS TORSADE?

"Torsade de pointes" is an unusual type of ventricular tachycardia that was first described by the French in 1966. The term literally means *"twisting of the points."* As implied by its name, the rhythm is recognized by a changing polarity of the QRS complex (from positive to negative, and back to positive again). This differs morphologically from the usual type of ventricular tachycardia in which QRS complexes tend to be of similar orientation.

> The importance of prompt recognition of "torsade" lies with the approach to management—*which is quite different from that for the usual type of ventricular tachycardia!*
>
> 1. Torsade is often caused by drugs that lengthen the QT interval (such as quinidine, procainamide, tricyclic antidepressants, and phenothiazines). *As a result, use of the antiarrhythmic agents quinidine and procainamide is contraindicated in these patients.*
> 2. Lidocaine may occasionally be effective in treatment—*but not consistently.*
> 3. The *KEY* to management of torsade is to identify and eliminate the underlying (precipitating) cause of the arrhythmia (i.e., use of quinidine, tricyclic antidepressant overdose). Unfortunately, *it may take hours for the effects of the precipitating agent to wear off!*
> 4. Synchronized cardioversion may be effective in converting torsade. Unfortunately, the arrhythmia has a disturbing tendency to revert back *immediately* after conversion. As a result, *multiple cardioversion attempts are often needed until the underlying cause is corrected.*
> 5. IV administration of magnesium sulfate has become generally accepted as the medical treatment of choice. *(See Sections 2B and 16C for additional information on the evaluation and management of Torsade de pointes.)*

ALGORITHM FOR BRADYARRHYTHMIAS (INCLUDING EMD/ASYSTOLE)

The bradyarrhythmias encompass a wide range of rhythm disturbances ranging from the often innocent *sinus bradycardia*, to the usually lethal *asystole* and *electromechanical dissociation (EMD)*. Prognosis and treatment depend on the rhythm, the clinical setting, and the patient's hemodynamic status. Recommendations for management are summarized in the treatment algorithm shown in *Figure 1D-1*.

If There Is SINUS BRADYCARDIA with a Pulse *and* Blood Pressure Is ADEQUATE

No specific treatment other than routine supportive measures (i.e., observation, oxygen, and establishment of IV access) are needed for sinus bradycardia when a pulse is present and the patient has an adequate blood pressure.

If There Is SINUS BRADYCARDIA with a Pulse, BUT Blood Pressure Is INADEQUATE

If a pulse is present, but the patient's blood pressure is insufficient to maintain adequate perfusion (i.e., <90 mm Hg), *hemodynamic compromise* is said to exist. Treatment is therefore in order.

1) ATROPINE

Atropine should not be used for treatment of the asymptomatic individual with bradycardia. Instead, the drug is reserved for *symptomatic* bradycardia (i.e., bradycardia associated with chest pain or dyspnea), and/or bradycardia accompanied by signs of *hemodynamic compromise* (i.e., hypotension, congestive heart failure, ventricular ectopy, or altered mental status).

> The recommended initial dose of atropine for treatment of sinus bradycardia is 0.5 mg IV. This may be repeated every 5 minutes until either a favorable clinical response occurs, or a total of 2 mg have been administered.

2) DOPAMINE

If the patient's volume status is judged to be adequate and atropine has not been effective in achieving the desired clinical response, infusion of a *pressor agent* should be started. For the patient with sinus bradycardia and a less severe degree of hypotension, dopamine is the agent most commonly preferred.

> A dopamine infusion may be prepared by mixing 1 ampule (=200 mg) of drug in 250 ml of D5W, and beginning the infusion at a rate of between 15 to 30 drops/min. This will provide an initial infusion rate of between 2 to 5 μg/kg/min for most patients. The rate of infusion may then be titrated according to clinical effect.

3) VOLUME INFUSION

The patient with bradycardia and hypotension may be *volume depleted*—either from volume loss (due to hemorrhage or dehydration), or as a result of inappropriate vasodilatation (from acute myocardial infarction, septic, or neurogenic shock).

> Although most individuals with hypotension will be *tachycardic*, this is not always the case. In particular, patients with acute *inferior* infarction frequently manifest excessive parasympathetic tone, which commonly leads to bradycardia and hypotension. Placing such patients in Trendelenburg position, and cautious volume infusion is the treatment of choice.

Because it may often be difficult to adequately assess the patient's volume status clinically, it is important to maintain a high index of suspicion for the possibility of hypovolemia.

Hypotension is a common problem in emergency cardiac care. Patients with hypotension may be tachycardic, bradycardic—or have a normal heart rate. Ideal management entails identification and correction of the underlying cause of the disorder. Although these goals often extend beyond immediate capabilities of the emergency care provider faced with a patient in extremis, the point to emphasize is that *empiric volume infusion* should *ALWAYS* be strongly considered as a potential therapeutic intervention for patients with hypotension of uncertain etiology, and/or not responding to other measures.

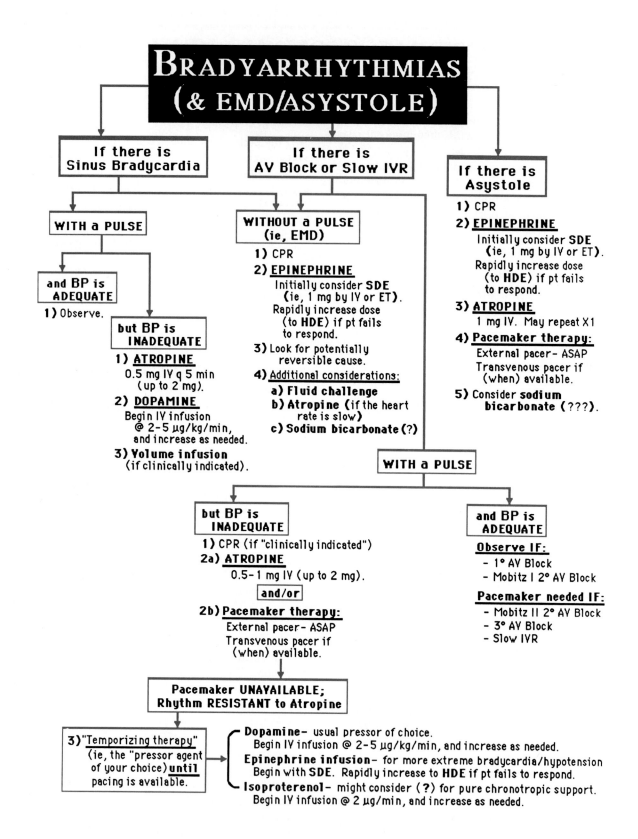

Figure 1D-1.   Algorithm for treatment of **Bradycardia/EMD/Asystole.**

If There Is SINUS BRADYCARDIA *without* a Pulse (i.e., EMD)

If sinus bradycardia is present on the monitor (i.e., presence of organized *electrical* activity), but there is no pulse (i.e., lack of *mechanical* activity), the patient is in *EMD*. The *KEY* points to emphasize about this disorder are:

1. By definition, EMD is a *nonperfusing* rhythm.
2. EMD is almost always *secondary* to (i.e., the result of) some other underlying condition.

Management considerations reflect these KEY points. There are *three* main *PRIORITIES* to keep in mind:

1) RESUME CPR

The *first* priority in management *MUST be* to resume CPR (since by definition EMD is a *nonperfusing* rhythm).

2) EPINEPHRINE

Administration of epinephrine is the next priority. SDE (i.e., 1 mg by IV or ET) may be tried initially, but the dose should be increased rapidly (to HDE) if the patient fails to respond.

> The principal reason for recommending epinephrine as the drug of choice for treatment of EMD is that it favors perfusion to the heart and brain. It is therefore the most effective pharmacologic way to optimize blood flow to these vital organs. However, because EMD is almost always a *secondary* condition, administration of epinephrine *by itself* will usually not resolve the problem *UNLESS the precipitating cause of the disorder can be identified and corrected.*

Occasionally, EMD may be a *primary* disorder. In such cases, instead of an underlying precipitating cause, the principal problem is *inadequate coronary perfusion*. Recent evidence suggests that some degree of *purposeful* cardiac contraction is often present—*albeit inadequate to generate a palpable pulse*— or at least inadequate to provide effective organ perfusion (Callaham and Barton, 1990; Paradis et al, 1992). Epinephrine's preferential shunting effect (which favors blood flow to the coronary and cerebral circulation), together with its potent chronotropic and inotropic effect (which increases contractility) may be lifesaving in such instances.

3) LOOK FOR POTENTIALLY REVERSIBLE CAUSES

As implied above, success in treating EMD will usually depend on identifying and correcting the underlying (precipitating) cause of the disorder. The most common *potentially treatable* causes of EMD to consider are the result of:

- *Inadequate ventilation*—i.e., intubation of the right mainstem bronchus, tension pneumothorax
- *Inadequate perfusion*—i.e., pericardial tamponade and especially *hypovolemia* (from any of a number of causes including dehydration, blood loss, or other forms of shock)
- *Metabolic abnormalities*—i.e., persistent severe acidosis, hyperkalemia

4) ADDITIONAL CONSIDERATIONS:
a) *Consideration* of a Fluid Challenge

Hypovolemia is one of the most common (and most easily treated) causes of EMD. AS a result, an *empiric* trial of *fluid infusion* may be indicated if EMD fails to respond to epinephrine (even if there is no obvious reason for the patient to be hypovolemic).

b) *Consideration* of Atropine

Because bradycardia is *not* the principal problem with EMD, treatment with atropine will usually not restore perfusion. Nevertheless, administration of atropine may help when EMD is associated with an excessively slow heart rate—and *empiric* use of the drug is indicated in such cases.

> Not reflected by the algorithm shown in Figure 1D-1 is the fact that EMD can also occur in association with normal (or even tachycardic) heart rates. Although atropine administration is clearly *not* indicated in such cases, other treatment considerations for EMD are the same as when the heart rate is slow.

> Clinically, the electrical rhythm associated with EMD may provide some insight as to the likelihood of resuscitation. Assuming underlying (precipitating) factors have been identified (and corrected if possible), prognosis tends to be best when there is organized atrial activity (in the form of definite P waves), and when the QRS complex is narrow. Prognosis tends to be poorest when P waves are absent and the QRS complex is markedly widened (Stueven et al, 1989).

c) *Consideration* of Sodium Bicarbonate

Because of questionable benefit (and a potential to be counterproductive), sodium bicarbonate should probably *not* be administered for EMD unless the period of arrest has been extended and/or the patient is strongly suspected of having a severe underlying acidosis that could be the precipitating *cause* of the EMD.

If There Is AV BLOCK or SLOW IVR *without* a Pulse (i.e., EMD)

The presence of AV block or slow IVR *without* a palpable pulse again defines the condition of EMD (i.e., presence of organized electrical activity without a pulse). The treatment approach is therefore *identical* to that outlined above for EMD that occurs in association with sinus bradycardia.

If There Is AV BLOCK or SLOW IVR *with* a Pulse *and* Blood Pressure Is ADEQUATE

Pharmacologic therapy is generally *not* needed if either AV block or slow IVR occur in a patient who is *hemodynamically stable* (i.e., *with* a pulse *and* adequate blood pressure). Instead, the principal question is whether a pacemaker is needed. The answer depends on the specific type of conduction disturbance and continued assessment of its hemodynamic consequences.

Pacemaker therapy is unnecessary for treatment of a hemodynamically stable patient with either 1° AV block, or 2° AV block of the Mobitz I (Wenckebach) type. These conduction disorders typically occur in association with acute *inferior* infarction. As long as heart rate is not excessively slow *and* the patient remains hemodynamically stable, careful <u>observation</u> should be all that is needed.

In contrast, 2° AV block of the Mobitz II type, high-grade or complete 3° AV block, and slow IVR tend to be much more severe conduction system disturbances. As a result, <u>pacemaker insertion</u> will generally be required when these conduction defects occur in the setting of cardiac arrest *regardless* of whether the patient is hemodynamically stable or not. Use (or ready stand-by) of an external pacer may be extremely helpful while preparation for transvenous pacemaker insertion is made.

If There Is AV BLOCK or SLOW IVR *with* a Pulse, BUT Blood Pressure Is INADEQUATE

Treatment is definitely indicated for the patient with either AV block or slow IVR if there is accompanying hypotension. Measures to consider include the following:

1) CPR

As suggested by the algorithm, <u>CPR</u> should be performed ***"if clinically indicated."***

The need to perform CPR in addition to other therapeutic measures will depend on the severity of hypotension and the degree of hemodynamic compromise. Thus, it would *not* be needed for treatment of 2° or 3° AV block if the patient was alert, asymptomatic, and had only borderline hypotension (i.e., a systolic pressure of between 80 to 85 mm Hg). On the other hand, continuation of CPR would be an essential component of therapy for an unresponsive patient in a slow IVR associated with a systolic blood pressure of *less than* 60 mm Hg. *Whether to perform CPR in less clearcut situations is a matter of clinical judgment.*

2a) ATROPINE

As discussed above, the use of atropine is *only* indicated for treatment of bradyarrhythmias that are associated with evidence of hemodynamic compromise.

Clinically, a dosing schedule for administering atropine in which 0.5 mg of the drug is given IV every 5 minutes (up to a maximum dose of 2 mg) may *not* be practical for management of conduction disorders associated with an extremely slow heart rate and/or significant hypotension (i.e., a systolic pressure of *less than* 80 mm Hg). Dosing according to this protocol would require *no less* than 15 minutes to administer the full 2 mg of the drug! As a result, it may be preferable to administer a larger dose of drug to such patients (i.e., 1 mg of atropine at a time), repeating the dose in several minutes if the desired clinical response is not achieved.

2b) PACEMAKER THERAPY

Optimal management of hemodynamically significant AV block or slow IVR that occurs in the setting of cardiac arrest entails the use of <u>pacemaker therapy</u>. Ideally, a *transvenous pacemaker* should probably be inserted as soon as this is possible. The problem is the need for the proper equipment, facilities, and personnel qualified to perform the procedure.

The most exciting advance in the field of pacemaker therapy has been refinement and the increased use of the *external pacemaker*. Obvious advantages of this modality are speed of application and the fact that the device is entirely noninvasive—features that make external pacing the treatment measure of choice when transvenous pacemaker insertion is not immediately possible.

As suggested by Step #2a in the algorithm, *atropine* is often administered prior to pacing—*primarily because of the rapidity with which the drug can be given.* Factors to consider when deciding whether to try atropine before (and/or instead of) pacemaker therapy include:

1. The patient's clinical condition and the urgency of the need for treatment (i.e., the degree of hemodynamic compromise imposed by the conduction defect)
2. The feasibility of immediate transvenous pacemaker insertion (i.e., availability of appropriate equipment, facilities, and personnel)
3. The availability of an external pacemaker
4. The potential for atropine administration to produce an adverse clinical effect (i.e., "unmasking" of underlying and previously opposed sympathetic tone, precipitation of tachycardia, ventricular arrhythmias, and/or paradoxical exacerbation of the degree of AV block)

If a Pacemaker Is UNAVAILABLE *and the* Rhythm Is RESISTANT to Atropine

If pacemaker therapy is not immediately available and there has been no response to full doses of atropine, a trial with a pressor agent is indicated. It should be emphasized that when hypotension accompanies AV block or slow IVR in the setting of cardiac arrest, pressor agents should *ONLY* be used as a *stopgap measure* (i.e., as *"temporizing therapy"*) to tide the patient over until more definitive measures (i.e., pacemaker therapy) can be instituted.

3) TEMPORIZING THERAPY

We refer to temporizing therapy in this setting as use of the ***"pressor agent of your choice"*** because selection between the various agents is really a function of hemo-dynamic parameters, clinical circumstances, *and* personal preference.

Under most clinical circumstances, we favor use of **dopamine** as our pressor agent of choice. A decided advantage of this drug is that adjustment of the rate of infusion allows manipulation of the relative amount of dopaminergic, β-ad-renergic, and α-adrenergic receptor activity. Thus, at low in-fusion rates (i.e., *less than* 2 μg/kg/min), the *dopaminergic* (renal vasodilatory) effect prevails. At moderate infusion rates (i.e., between 2 to 10 μg/kg/min), the β-adrenergic stimulating effect predominates. At higher infusion rates, the α-adrenergic (vasoconstrictor) stimulating effect becomes increasingly more important until ultimately (i.e., at infusion rates of greater than 15 to 20 μg/kg/min) the effects of dopamine are virtually the same as those of epinephrine and norepinephrine.

In contrast to dopamine, indications for the use of **isopro-terenol** have become quite limited. Problems with the drug are that it increases myocardial oxygen consumption, is ex-tremely arrythmogenic, and produces peripheral vasodilata-tion. This latter effect is particularly deleterious in the arrested heart because it serves to divert blood flow from the coronary circulation. Isoproterenol does provide effective *chronotropic sup-port* when administered cautiously (i.e., at low infusion rates) to normotensive patients with significant bradycardia. How-ever, because of the peripheral vasodilatation it produces, it tends to be much less effective if hypotension is present in addition to bradycardia. It would therefore seem that use of other pressor agents should be preferable to isoproterenol in most clinical situations.

Epinephrine may also be used as a "pressor" agent for treatment of the patient with hemodynamically significant bradycardia. Administration of the drug in the form of a *con-tinuous **IV infusion*** is preferable in this situation because it allows fine adjustments in dosing to be made instead of the "all-or-none" effect that is seen with bolus therapy. Lower doses (i.e., SDE) should be tried first. The rate of infusion can then be progressively increased as needed according to the clinical response. In general, we tend to reserve use of epi-nephrine infusion for patients with more severe bradyarrhyth-mias and/or when dopamine has been ineffective.

Appropriate *initial* infusion rates for dopamine, isopro-terenol, and epinephrine can be easily calculated by ap-plying the **Rule of 250 ml.** Thus, preparation of a con-tinuous IV infusion for these pressor agents might proceed as follows:

Isoproterenol—Mix **1 mg** (=1 vial = 1 "unit") of iso-proterenol in **250 ml** of D5W, and set the infusion to run at **30 drops/min** (=2 μg/min).

Standard-**D**ose **E**pinephrine (**SDE**)—Mix **1 mg** (=1 am-pule = 1 "unit") of a *1:10,000 solution of epinephrine* in **250 ml** of D5W, and set the infusion to run at between **15** to **30 drops/min** (=1 to 2 μg/min).

Dopamine—Mix **200 mg** (=1 ampule = 1 "unit") of do-pamine in **250 ml** of D5W, and set the infusion to run at between **15** to **30 drops/min** (≈2 to 5 μg/kg/min for most patients).

Complete discussion of the *Rule of 250 ml* is covered in Section 2C. Recommendations for use of **H**igh-**D**ose **E**pinephrine (**HDE**) is discussed in detail in Section 2B, and suggestions for preparation of an HDE IV infusion are found in Section 2C.

If pressor therapy is successful in improving hemody-namic status, every effort should be made to reduce the rate of infusion to the lowest level possible needed to sus-tain the desired clinical response.

If There Is ASYSTOLE

Although the prognosis for asystole is never good, the ultimate outcome associated with development of this ar-rhythmia is not necessarily as bleak when it occurs in the hospital as when asystole is the primary mechanism of cardiac arrest occurring *outside* of the hospital.

Asystole that occurs in association with out-of-hospital car-diac arrest is most often a *preterminal* rhythm that develops from deterioration of ventricular fibrillation. In contrast, asys-tole that develops in a hospital setting may at times be the direct result of a massive parasympathetic discharge. It may therefore be surprisingly responsive to atropine therapy on some occasions. This phenomenon is most likely to be asso-ciated with certain operative procedures (i.e., endoscopy, car-diac catheterization), induction of anesthesia, toxic drug re-actions, vasovagal episodes, and/or AV block from acute *in-ferior* infarction. Another factor accounting for a less uniformly dismal prognosis for asystole that occurs within the hospital is that the time elapsed from the onset of this arrhythmia until discovery of the patient by trained personnel tends to be much less than when the rhythm occurs on the outside (i.e., "irre-versibility" may not yet have set in).

Regardless of the setting in which it occurs, treatment considerations for asystole are similar. They include the following:

1) RESUMING CPR

Obviously there is no perfusion with asystole. CPR must therefore be continued while resuscitation is in progress.

2) EPINEPHRINE

Because epinephrine is the *KEY* pharmacologic agent for favoring blood flow to the arrested heart and brain, the drug should be used *liberally* in the treatment of asystole. SDE (i.e., 1 mg by IV or ET) may be tried initially, but the dose should be increased rapidly (to HDE) if the patient fails to respond.

3) ATROPINE

As mentioned above, asystole may occasionally be the direct result of a massive parasympathetic discharge. Consequently, treatment with atropine should always be tried. We favor an initial dose of 1 mg for treatment of asystole, which may be repeated in *several* minutes if there is no response.

4) PACEMAKER THERAPY

In general, pacemaker therapy is *not* effective in the treatment of bradyarrhythmias unless myocardial function has been preserved. As a result, it will usually *not* be helpful in the treatment of asystole. Nevertheless, a trial of pacing may be warranted for the asystolic patient who has not responded to any of the above measures.

> Although data on the use of pacing for treatment of asystole are not encouraging, most studies in the literature attempted to implement pacemaker therapy only after all other measures had failed. *Pacemaker therapy is most likely to be effective if attempted EARLY in the process* (i.e., *as soon as* it becomes apparent that the patient will not respond to atropine and epinephrine—*if not sooner*). Because of its completely noninvasive nature, an *external pacemaker* might best be applied as soon as the device is available.

5) CONSIDER SODIUM BICARBONATE

Because of its questionable benefit (and a potential to be counterproductive), sodium bicarbonate should probably *not* be administered for asystole unless the period of arrest has been extended and/or the patient is strongly suspected of having a severe underlying acidosis that may have precipitated the arrest.

Questions to Further Understanding

WHY SHOULD THE USE OF ATROPINE BE RESERVED FOR TREATMENT OF PATIENTS WITH EVIDENCE OF HEMODYNAMIC COMPROMISE?

Treatment with atropine is not benign. Adverse effects that may at least occasionally occur from the use of this parasympatholytic agent include:

1. An "unmasking" of previously opposed (and underlying) sympathetic hyperactivity that could result in excessive tachycardia and/or precipitate ventricular arrhythmias
2. Acceleration of the supraventricular response—which could paradoxically exacerbate the degree of AV block (since the AV node may not be able to conduct as many impulses at the faster rate).

As a result, *unless* the patient is symptomatic, it may be best to withhold administration of atropine.

IS USE OF AN EXTERNAL PACEMAKER PREFERABLE TO ATROPINE FOR TREATMENT OF HEMODYNAMICALLY SIGNIFICANT BRADYARRHYTHMIAS?

Cardiac pacing is the treatment of choice for hemodynamically significant bradyarrhythmias that occur in the setting of cardiac arrest. The problem with *transvenous pacing* is that the insertion procedure is invasive, takes time, and requires the presence of a skilled operator. Advantages of *external pacing* are that it is easy to apply, takes only seconds, and is completely noninvasive.

As noted above, treatment with atropine is not benign. As a result, use of an external pacemaker may be preferred to atropine therapy if the device is immediately available.

> Practically speaking, the external pacemaker may not always be immediately available when the need arises. Because of the rapidity with which a dose of atropine may be administered, it is reasonable to try this treatment first (if the patient is symptomatic) while sending for the pacemaker.

WHY IS IT PREFERABLE TO ADMINISTER EPINEPHRINE AS AN IV INFUSION WHEN USING THIS DRUG TO TREAT HEMODYNAMICALLY SIGNIFICANT BRADYARRHYTHMIAS?

The drawback of bolus administration is that once a dose of drug has been given, it cannot be "taken back." Hemodynamic effects persist until the action of the drug wears off. In contrast, use of a continuous IV infusion allows moment-to-moment titration of the dose of drug according to its clinical effect.

With respect to epinephrine, the potent chronotropic and inotropic effects of the drug are potentially quite arrhythmogenic when administered to a patient with a spontaneous circulation. Use of a continuous IV infusion allows much more careful dose titration, and the ability to immediately *turn off* the infusion in the event of an adverse hemodynamic effect.

IS IT WORTH TREATING ASYSTOLE?

Admittedly, prognosis for asystole is never good. However, the outlook for this arrhythmia when it develops during cardiac arrest that occurs *IN* the hospital is *not* necessarily as bleak as when asystole is the primary mechanism of a cardiac arrest occurring outside of the hospital. Asystole in this latter setting is most often a preterminal rhythm that arises after ventricular fibrillation deteriorates. In contrast, asystole occurring in a hospital setting may occasionally result from massive parasympathetic discharge—and, consequently, may be surprisingly responsive to atropine therapy. In addition, time until discovery is usually much less for in-hopsital asystole—so that the rhythm may occasionally respond to epinephrine or early institution of pacing!

WHAT IS THE MAXIMAL DOSE OF EPINEPHRINE FOR TREATMENT OF ASYSTOLE?

There is no maximal dose of epinephrine for this indication. Epinephrine is the *ONE (only?)* drug that will favor perfusion to the heart and brain in the setting of cardiac arrest. There is really *nothing to lose* from use of HDE in this situation, and some patients might respond only to higher doses of the drug. Thus, we feel there should be little reservation against HDE administration early in the course of managing asystole if the rhythm fails to respond promptly to other measures.

SHOULD ASYSTOLE EVER BE SHOCKED?

Some clinicians routinely shock asystole on the grounds that the rhythm may be "masquerading" as fine ventricular fibrillation. *We prefer not to do this.*

If the predominant vector of ventricular fibrillation is *perpendicular* to the lead being used to monitor the patient, the rhythm may appear as a flat-line recording (and "masquerade" as asystole) in that particular lead. However, *defibrillation is not benign.* Shocking asystole can produce further damage to

the conduction system and make the rhythm even more resistant to subsequent attempts at therapy.

It is usually easy to determine the true etiology of a flat-line recording. If a monitor is being used, be sure that the gain has not been turned all the way down. Verify that none of the leads have become loose (or have fallen off). Then check the rhythm in multiple leads (which can be done in a matter of seconds if the patient is hooked up to a 12-lead ECG machine). If a flat-line recording is present in all leads, then the rhythm is truly asystole (and countershock will do nothing). Finally, be sure that the battery of the defibrillator is sufficiently charged, since false signals may be produced when the battery is low. Practically speaking, *technical problems appear to be a more common cause of a flat-line recording than the phenomenon of fine ventricular fibrillation masquerading as asystole* (Cummins and Austin, 1988).

IS CALCIUM CHLORIDE EVER INDICATED ANY MORE?

In the past, calcium chloride had been recommended for treatment of asystole and EMD. Studies suggesting an excessive mortality rate from use of this agent for these indications have led to a discontinuation of this practice.

Currently, the *ONLY* indications for the use of calcium chloride in the setting of cardiac arrest and emergency cardiac care are:

1. Hypocalcemia
2. Hyperkalemia
3. Asystole that develops following administration of a calcium channel blocker (such as verapamil)—as may occur during the treatment of a supraventricular tachyarrhythmia
4. As pretreatment and/or posttreatment of hypotension that occurs in association with SVT when use of verapamil is contemplated

WHAT ARE THE KEY PRIORITIES FOR TREATMENT OF EMD?

The three *KEY* priorities for treatment of EMD are to: (1) promptly *resume CPR* (since by definition, EMD is a *nonperfusing* rhythm); (2) administer *epinephrine* (rapidly increasing to HDE if there is no response to lower doses); and (3) look for a potentially reversible cause of the disorder.

The most common potentially treatable causes of EMD to consider are the result of:

- **Inadequate ventilation**—e.g., intubation of the right mainstem bronchus, tension pneumothorax
- **Inadequate perfusion**—e.g., pericardial tamponade, and especially *hypovolemia* (from any of a number of causes including dehydration, blood loss, or other forms of shock)
- **Metabolic abnormalities**—e.g., persistent severe acidosis, hyperkalemia

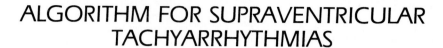

SECTION E

ALGORITHM FOR SUPRAVENTRICULAR TACHYARRHYTHMIAS

Identification of SVT: *Assessment of Hemodynamic Status*

As for ventricular tachycardia, the *MOST* important facet of evaluation and management to assess—even *BEFORE* the emergency care provider beings to *think* about the cause of a particular arrhythmia—is the patient's *hemodynamic status*. If a patient with a tachyarrhythmia becomes acutely symptomatic (as indicated by hypotension, development of chest pain, dyspnea, and/or altered mental status), diagnosis of the specific type of arrhythmia clearly takes on a *secondary role* compared to the urgent need for stabilization *(Figure 1E-1)*.

> The *FIRST* parameters to check in assessing the patient's hemodynamic status are *level of consciousness* and the presence of a *pulse*. If a pulse is present and the patient is conscious, the *blood pressure* should be checked and other parameters evaluated (e.g., presence of chest pain, shortness of breath, mentation ability). Based on this information, the emergency care provider can formulate a plan for proceeding with a better appreciation of the *relative urgency* and need for treatment.

If the Patient IS (or at ANY Time Becomes) Hemodynamically UNSTABLE

Development of *hemodyamic instability* AT ANY TIME during the treatment process is an indication for *immediate* synchronized cardioversion. Antiarrhythmic therapy is relegated to a secondary role in this setting, since delay for the several minutes needed to draw up and administer medications is unacceptable in an acutely unstable situation.

> Judgment is needed in determination of the degree of "hemodynamic instability" associated with a particular arrhythmia. Thus, relatively minor symptoms (such as palpitations) and/or a minimal drop in blood pressure (i.e., to a systolic reading of 80 mm Hg) might not necessarily mandate immediate intervention if the patient was alert and otherwise uncompromised. On the other hand, acute development of a more severe degree of hypotension and/or symptomatology (i.e., loss of consciousness) as a *direct result* of the tachyarrhythmia is a clear indication of the urgent need for immediate cardioversion.

It should be emphasized that if the patient is acutely unstable, diagnosis of the specific type of tachyarrhythmia *no longer matters* with regard to acute treatment. That is, *immediate synchronized cardioversion* is indicated *regardless* of whether the etiology of the rhythm is atrial fibrillation, atrial flutter, PSVT (or ventricular tachycardia)!

1) SYNCHRONIZED CARDIOVERSION

Factors to consider in selecting the amount of energy to use for synchronized cardioversion are the type of arrhythmia and the perceived urgency of the situation. In general, we favor use of relatively higher energies (of *at least* 100 to 200 joules) for emergency cardioversion of a *hemodynamically compromised* patient in the hope that this will maximize the chance for successful conversion of the rhythm on the first attempt. Lower energies might be tried first under more controlled circumstances.

> Certain supraventricular tachyarrhythmias such as atrial flutter are exquisitely sensitive to synchronized cardioversion, and conversion to sinus rhythm can often be achieved with energy levels as low as 10 to 20 joules. Other arrhythmias such as atrial fibrillation are much more resistant to the effects of cardioversion, and usually require much higher energy levels (of at least 200 joules) for success. Intermediate energy levels (of between 50 and 100 joules) are usually recommended for initial treatment of PSVT. MAT does not respond to cardioversion.

If the Patient Is STABLE Hemodynamically

If the patient with a supraventricular tachyarrhythmia is hemodynamically stable (i.e., alert, relatively comfortable, and with an acceptable blood pressure), diagnosis of the specific type of arrhythmia becomes the *KEY* determinant for guiding therapy.

> Diagnostic measures to consider for determining the etiology of the arrhythmia include evaluation of additional leads (and *ideally*, obtaining a 12-lead ECG), application of vagal maneuvers, comparison with previous tracings recorded on the patient, and review of the clinical history.

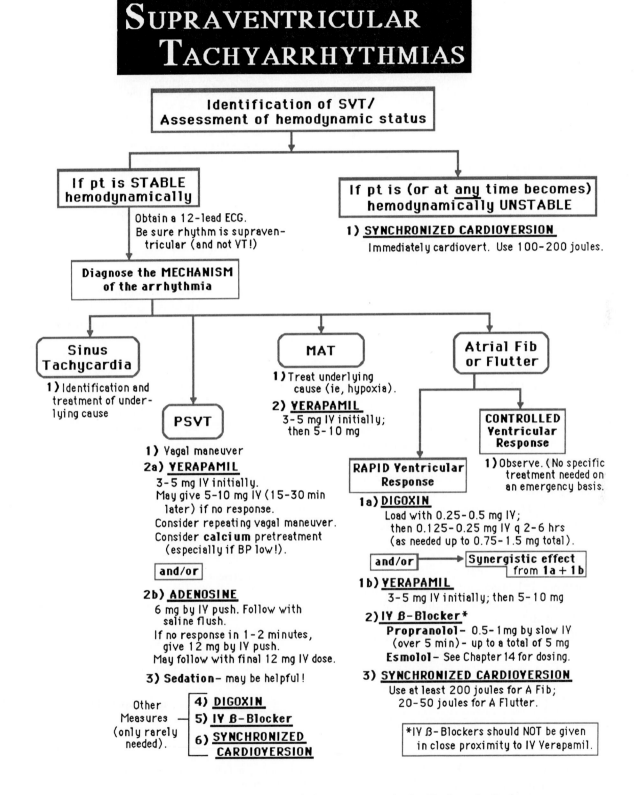

SUPRAVENTRICULAR TACHYARRHYTHMIAS

Identification of SVT/ Assessment of hemodynamic status

If pt is STABLE hemodynamically

Obtain a 12-lead ECG.
Be sure rhythm is supraventricular (and not VT!)

Diagnose the MECHANISM of the arrhythmia

If pt is (or at any time becomes) hemodynamically UNSTABLE

1) **SYNCHRONIZED CARDIOVERSION**
Immediately cardiovert. Use 100-200 joules.

Sinus Tachycardia

1) Identification and
treatment of under-
lying cause

PSVT

1) Vagal maneuver
2a) **VERAPAMIL**
   3-5 mg IV initially.
   May give 5-10 mg IV (15-30 min
   later) if no response.
   Consider repeating vagal maneuver.
   Consider **calcium** pretreatment
   (especially if BP low!).

   [and/or]

2b) **ADENOSINE**
   6 mg by IV push. Follow with
   saline flush.
   If no response in 1-2 minutes,
   give 12 mg by IV push.
   May follow with final 12 mg IV dose.

3) **Sedation**– may be helpful!

Other
Measures
(only rarely
needed).

4) **DIGOXIN**
5) **IV β-Blocker**
6) **SYNCHRONIZED CARDIOVERSION**

MAT

1) Treat underlying
   cause (ie, hypoxia).
2) **VERAPAMIL**
   3-5 mg IV initially;
   then 5-10 mg

Atrial Fib or Flutter

RAPID Ventricular Response

1a) **DIGOXIN**
   Load with 0.25-0.5 mg IV;
   then 0.125-0.25 mg IV q 2-6 hrs
   (as needed up to 0.75-1.5 mg total).

[and/or] → **Synergistic effect from 1a + 1b**

1b) **VERAPAMIL**
   3-5 mg IV initially; then 5-10 mg

2) **IV β-Blocker***
   Propranolol– 0.5-1 mg by slow IV
   (over 5 min)– up to a total of 5 mg
   Esmolol– See Chapter 14 for dosing.

3) **SYNCHRONIZED CARDIOVERSION**
   Use at least 200 joules for A Fib;
   20-50 joules for A Flutter.

*IV β-Blockers should NOT be given
in close proximity to IV Verapamil.

CONTROLLED Ventricular Response

1) Observe. (No specific
   treatment needed on
   an emergency basis.

Figure 1E-1.   Algorithm for treatment of **Supraventricular Tachyarrhythmias.**

> The reason for the importance of examining the arrhythmia in more than one lead is to be absolutely certain that the QRS complex is narrow (and that the rhythm is truly *supraventricular*). If a portion of the QRS complex happened to lie on the baseline in the only lead that was being monitored, ventricular tachycardia could be mistaken for a supraventricular tachyarrhythmia.

Suggestions for management of the principal types of *supraventricular tachyarrhythmias* follow below:

Sinus Tachycardia

No specific treatment is indicated for sinus tachycardia per se. Instead, the approach to management should focus on identification and correction of any underlying conditions that may be causing the arrhythmia.

> Common causes of sinus tachycardia to consider in the setting of emergency cardiac care include congestive heart failure, hypovolemia, shock, and excessive sympathetic tone.

Paroxysmal Supraventricular Tachycardia (PSVT)

The mechanism of PSVT in adults is almost always one of *reentry* into the AV node after the supraventricular impulse has been conducted to the ventricles. A reentry circuit is set up, whereby the impulse is caught returning (in retrograde fashion) to the AV node before being conducted back down again to the ventricles in what becomes a perpetual cycle. *The goal of therapy is simply to interrupt this cycle—* in the hope that a normal rhythm may then take over.

1) VAGAL MANEUVERS

Vagal maneuvers act by transiently increasing parasympathetic tone. This slows conduction through supraventricular and AV nodal tissues. One hopes to delay AV nodal conduction just long enough to interrupt the reentry circuit of PSVT and terminate the arrhythmia.

> Vagal maneuvers include carotid sinus massage, Valsalva, activation of the gag reflex, facial submersion in ice water, eyeball pressure (which is no longer recommended), digital rectal massage, and squatting. Patients with recurrent episodes of PSVT have often instinctively learned how to perform one or more of these maneuvers on their own to terminate their arrhythmia.

In an emergency care setting, carotid sinus massage (CSM) is the vagal maneuver performed most often for treatment. *Under constant ECG monitoring,* the patient's head is turned to the left and the area of the right carotid bifurcation (near the angle of the jaw) is gently but *firmly*

massaged for 3 to 5 seconds at a time. If right carotid massage is ineffective, the left side may be tried. (One should *never* massage both sides simultaneously!)

> In addition to its role in treatment, CSM may also be helpful as a diagnostic maneuver for distinguishing between PSVT, sinus tachycardia, and atrial flutter. When CSM is applied to a patient in PSVT, the rhythm will either be converted by the maneuver, or nothing will happen. In contrast, with sinus tachycardia or atrial flutter, transient slowing of the ventricular response during massage often allows telltale atrial activity to become apparent.
>
> It should be emphasized that CSM is *not* a totally benign maneuver, particularly in older individuals. It has been associated with syncope, stroke, sinus arrest, high-grade AV block, prolonged asystole, and ventricular tachyarrhythmias in patients with digitalis intoxication. As a result, it should probably *not* be attempted in patients with a history of sick sinus syndrome, cervical bruits, or cerebrovascular disease, or when the possibility of digitalis intoxication exists.

2a) VERAPAMIL*

Until recently, verapamil had been the pharmacologic agent of choice for acute treatment of PSVT. When used appropriately, the drug is usually well tolerated and effective in converting this reentry tachyarrhythmia in more than 90% of cases.

> Additional advantages of verapamil include the duration of action of its antiarrhythmic effect (which lasts for up to 30 minutes), availability of an oral formulation of the drug (which facilitates long-term antiarrhythmic control), and its efficacy in treating other supraventricular tachyarrhythmias (including atrial fibrillation or flutter, and MAT).

The recommended initial dose of verapamil is 5 mg IV, administered over a 1- to 2-minute period. Use of a lower initial dose (i.e., 3 mg), and administration over a somewhat *longer* period of time (i.e., over 3 to 4 minutes) may be preferable for the treatment of elderly patients and those with borderline hemodynamic status. Cautious dosing in this manner may help to minimize the incidence of hypotension and excessive heart rate slowing.

> **Pretreatment** with IV infusion of **calcium chloride** (infusing 500 to 1,000 mg over a 5- to 10-minute period) has also been shown to minimize the hypotensive response of verapamil *without* diminishing the drug's efficacy in converting or controlling the ventricular response of patients with supraventricular tachyarrhythmias. Such pretreatment might be considered particularly for patients with a borderline hemodynamic status (i.e., systolic blood pressure of *less* than 100 mm Hg).

If there is no response to verapamil after 15 minutes, a second dose (of 5 to 10 mg) may be given. This can be

---

*IV diltiazem has been approved for treatment of supraventricular tachyarrhythmias, and offers an alternative to IV verapamil. Advantages of IV diltiazem include its availability as an approved formulaion for continuous IV infusion, and the fact that it appears to be less likely to cause excessive hypotension or left ventricular decompensation. Further discussion on the use of this new agent follows in the *"Questions to Further Understanding"* portion of this section—and in Chapter 14.

followed in several minutes by another attempt at a vagal maneuver, since the effect of the drug and the maneuver are often synergistic.

> The principal concern regarding verapamil is the need to be sure that the drug is not given to a patient who has ventricular tachycardia. If this were to happen, the vasodilatory and negative inotropic effects of the drug are likely to precipitate deterioration of the rhythm to ventricular fibrillation. Thus, verapamil should *NEVER* be used as a diagnostic/therapeutic trial for treatment of a wide complex tachycardia of uncertain etiology.

As suggested above, a decided advantage of verapamil is that if IV use of the drug successfully converts the arrhythmia, the antiarrhythmic effect can be maintained (and the chance of recurrence minimized) by continuing the patient on an oral regimen of the drug. Thus, one might administer 80 mg (PO) of verapamil shortly after the last IV dose was given (and repeat this oral dose at 8-hour intervals).

2b) ADENOSINE

One of the most exciting advances in antiarrhythmic therapy has been development of adenosine for treatment of PSVT. The drug is equally effective as IV verapamil for this indication, and is a suitable alternative first-line agent for initial treatment of this arrhythmia.

> The most remarkable pharmacologic features of adenosine are its rapid onset of action and exceedingly short half-life (which is estimated to be *less* than 10 seconds in duration!). One advantage arising from these features is that the clinician will know within a very short perod of time whether or not the drug will be effective. Side effects such as cough, flushing, and excessive bradycardia may occur—but even if they do, they are likely to be extremely short-lived.

The recommended dose of adenosine is to initially administer 6 mg by IV push. This dose should be immediately followed by a saline flush to ensure that none of the drug gets caught in the IV tubing (where it rapidly breaks down). If there is no response within 1 to 2 minutes, a *second* dose (of 12 mg) may be tried—and followed with a *final* (third) dose (of 12 mg) 1 to 2 minutes later (for a total dose of 6 + 12 + 12 = 30 mg). If this is ineffective, it is unlikely that adenosine will work—and alternative therapy (i.e., IV verapamil) should be tried.

> The principal drawbacks of adenosine also result from its short half-life. They are that the drug is ineffective for treatment of other supraventricular tachyarrhythmias (since slowing of the ventricular response with atrial fibrillation and atrial flutter is so transient)—and that recurrence of PSVT is likely to occur in many patients after the effect of the drug wears off.

3) SEDATION

In addition to relieving the anxiety that so often accompanies PSVT, sedation lowers sympathetic tone. Because the degree of autonomic tone exerts a direct influence on

AV nodal reentry pathways, sedation may significantly contribute to conversion of the arrhythmia.

4) OTHER MEASURES

Although *digoxin, propranolol,* and *synchronized cardioversion* were frequently used in the past to treat PSVT, the tremendous success of verapamil and adenosine have dramatically reduced the need for these therapies in the acute care setting.

> The newer IV β-blocking agent *esmolol* demonstrates almost comparable efficacy as IV verapamil and adenosine in the acute treatment of PSVT. However, because the protocol for administration of this agent is relatively complex, use of the other two drugs seems to be preferred by most clinicians. Moreover, IV β-blockers should *never* be administered in close proximity (i.e., within 20 to 30 minutes) of IV verapamil because the combination of these agents could lead to marked bradycardia (and even asystole!).

As is the case for treatment of other tachyarrhythmias, immediate synchronized cardioversion is indicated if hemodynamic instability develops *at any time* during the treatment process. Clinically, this is a relatively uncommon occurrence with PSVT.

Multifocal Atrial Tachycardia (MAT)

MAT is most often seen in the setting of chronic obstructive pulmonary disease (COPD), and is associated with hypoxemia. It is important not to confuse this arrhythmia with atrial fibrillation, since treatment of these two conditions may be very different.

> Digoxin has traditionally been used as a treatment of choice for achieving control of the ventricular response with atrial fibrillation. Although digoxin can also be used for treatment of MAT, extra caution is urged because such patients are exquisitely sensitive to this medication (and susceptible to developing digitalis toxicity).

1) TREAT THE UNDERLYING CAUSE OF MAT

Far better than pharmacologic therapy of MAT is identification and treatment of the underlying cause of the rhythm disorder. For patients with COPD, this generally entails correction of hypoxemia (i.e., oxygen therapy and use of bronchodilators).

> MAT may also occur in acutely ill patients with multisystem disease (e.g., shock, sepsis, pneumonia). Treatment priorities in this setting are the same as for the patient who develops MAT in association with COPD: *Try to correct the underlying disorder(s).* Thus, the arrhythmia will usually resolve if the patient's underlying medical condition can be improved.

2) VERAPAMIL

If pharmacologic therapy is needed to control the ventricular rate with MAT, verapamil is the drug of choice. Dosing recommendations are similar to those suggested for use of the drug to treat PSVT.

> Small doses of digoxin may be tried for treatment of MAT, and when combined with verapamil a synergistic effect may be noted. However, as emphasized above, large doses of digoxin should definitely be avoided with this rhythm disturbance since they readily lead to toxicity.

Atrial Fibrillation or Flutter

IF THE VENTRICULAR RESPONSE IS CONTROLLED

Atrial fibrillation with a controlled ventricular response is often a very stable rhythm. In an emergency care setting, *no specific antiarrhythmic treatment is needed in the asymptomatic patient.* Although atrial flutter is a somewhat less stable rhythm, it need not be treated either if the patient is asymptomatic and the ventricular response is controlled.

IF THERE IS A RAPID VENTRICULAR RESPONSE

Treatment is indicated when the ventricular response to atrial fibrillation and atrial flutter is rapid. If the patient is tolerating the rapid rate, pharmacologic therapy may be tried first. However, if the patient becomes hemodynamically compromised *at any time* during the treatment process, immediate cardioversion is in order.

> Although the medications used to treat atrial fibrillation and atrial flutter are similar, the clinical response of these two arrhythmias to treatment is often quite different. In general, it is usually much easier to achieve rate control of the ventricular response with atrial fibrillation than it is for atrial flutter. In contrast, atrial flutter is decidedly more responsive to synchronized cardioversion than atrial fibrillation.

1a) Digoxin

Until recently, digoxin had been the pharmacologic agent favored by most clinicans for initial treatment of atrial fibrillation and atrial flutter. Contrary to popular belief, the drug per se is *not* extremely effective in converting these tachyarrhythmias to sinus rhythm. However, it is helpful in slowing the ventricular response—and this is the principal rationale for its use in an emergency setting.

When treating a patient who has not previously received digoxin, one usually begins with an initial IV loading dose (of 0.25 to 0.5 mg). This may be followed with additional incremental doses (of 0.125 to 0.25 mg IV) every 2 to 6 hours as needed (i.e., depending on the ventricular response), until a total loading dose of 0.75 to 1.5 mg of drug has been given.

In the absence of hyperthyroidism, hypoxemia, acute myocardial infarction, and electrolyte disturbance, the ventricular rate response to the above therapy has been used as an indicator of the adequacy of digitalization. According to this practice, persistence of a rapid rate after administration of several boluses suggests that additional digoxin may still be needed to achieve adequate control of the ventricular response. In the presence of any of the above conditions, however, increased sensitivity to the effects of digitalis (and a correspondingly increased risk of developing toxicity) augurs for much greater caution (and use of lower doses) in administering the drug.

An additional caveat to beware of is that dependence on the ventricular rate response per se for determination of the dose of digoxin to administer may *not* be reliable in clinical settings in which underlying sympathetic tone is increased. This is because the principal mechanism for the rate slowing effect of digoxin results from enhancement of vagal tone. Conditions that lead to an increase in endogenous catecholamine secretion (i.e., stress states, shock, acute illness, and especially cardiac arrest) may therefore be relatively resistant to even high doses of the drug. *This is the reason that many clinicians have begun to select verapamil as their initial drug of choice for achieving control of the ventricular response with rapid atrial fibrillation* (Falk and Leavitt, 1991).

1b) Verapamil

As implied above, use of IV verapamil has become increasingly popular for emergency treatment of rapid atrial fibrillation and flutter. Although the drug is *not* very effective in converting these tachyarrhythmias to sinus rhythm, the AV nodal blocking effect reliably slows the ventricular response. Dosing considerations are similar to those presented in the section for treatment of PSVT.*

A useful clinical point to remember is that *combined* use of digoxin and IV verapamil may produce a **synergistic effect** in controlling the ventricular response. Combination therapy will also often allow use of lower doses of each agent for achieving adequate rate control than if either of the drugs were used independently.

---

2) IV β-Blockers

Mechanistically, β-blockers would seem to be ideal antiarrhythmic agents for emergency treatment of patients with supraventricular tachyarrhythmias (provided there is no overt heart failure or severe bronchospasm). And, although these drugs are extremely effective in clinical practice for this indication, they appear to be used much

---

*IV diltiazem has been approved for treatment of supraventricular tachyarrhythmias, and offers an alternative to IV verapamil. Advantages of IV diltiazem include its availability as an approved formulation for continuous IV infusion, and the fact that it appears to be less likely to cause excessive hypotension or left ventricular decompensation. Further discussion on the use of this new agent follows in the *"Questions to Further Understanding"* portion of this section—and in Chapter 14.

less frequently than in the past. This can probably be attributed to a preference toward using IV verapamil (and/or digoxin) in this situation. Nevertheless, use of an IV β-blocker (either propranolol or esmolol) should not be forgotten as a potentially effective alternative treatment modality.

> Dosing considerations for the use of IV propranolol are discussed in detail in Section 2D, and those for esmolol in Chapter 14. As noted previously, IV β-blockers should *never* be administered in close proximity (i.e., within 20 to 30 minutes) of IV verapamil because the combination of these agents could lead to marked bradycardia (and even asystole!).

3) Synchronized Cardioversion

As suggested above, pharmacologic therapy (i.e., with digoxin and/or IV verapamil) is often preferred for the initial treatment of rapid atrial fibrillation or flutter when the patient is not acutely unstable. If medical therapy is not effective, and/or the patient becomes hemodynamically unstable *at any time* during the treatment process, *immediate* cardioversion is in order.

> In general, atrial flutter is much more responsive to synchronized cardioversion than atrial fibrillation. Thus, low energy levels (of between 20 to 50 joules) are often all that is needed for successful conversion to sinus rhythm. In contrast, significantly higher energy levels (of 200 joules) are often required for cardioversion of atrial fibrillation—and even then the procedure may not be successful.
>
> It should be noted that although synchronized cardioversion is best avoided (if at all possible!) when excessive doses of digitalis have been administered, the procedure can almost always be performed safely if digitalis toxicity is not present.

Questions to Further Understanding

IS IT LIKELY THAT ADENOSINE WILL REPLACE VERAPAMIL FOR THE TREATMENT OF PSVT?

No. Despite comparable efficacy for initial conversion rates of PSVT, individual characteristics of adenosine and verapamil are likely to preserve a niche for each of these agents.

> The principal advantages of adenosine result from its rapid onset of action and ultrashort half-life. These features allow expeditious control of the arrhythmia in most cases. Adverse effects are usually of minimal clinical significance because they so rapidly resolve.
>
> Administration of adenosine may also be used as a diagnostic maneuver. Thus, the transient slowing of AV conduction produced by the drug may serve as a "medical Valsalva" to facilitate identification of atrial activity that was not readily apparent on the initial tracing.
>
> The principal disadvantages of adenosine are its cost and the high rate of PSVT recurrence after initial conversion to sinus rhythm. Verapamil is far more economical. The longer

half-life of verapamil's IV preparation lessens the chance of immediate recurrence, and availability of an oral formulation of verapamil facilitates long-term antiarrhythmic control. Verapamil offers the additional advantage of efficacy in the treatment of other supraventricular tachyarrhythmias (such as atrial fibrillation, atrial flutter, and MAT).

A final point to consider is that although both adenosine and verapamil are more than 90% effective in initial conversion of PSVT, *the drugs won't always work*. Failure to respond to one of these agents is an indication to try the other (which may then be successful!).

IS ADENOSINE EFFECTIVE FOR TREATMENT OF ATRIAL FIBRILLATION? ATRIAL FLUTTER?

No. Adenosine is effective in terminating *reentry* tachyarrhythmias. Although it may transiently reduce the ventricular response of a patient in atrial fibrillation, it does nothing to convert this rhythm. Rapidity of the ventricular response resumes as soon as the effect of the drug wears off.

Similarly, adenosine is not effective in the treatment of atrial flutter. Transient slowing of the ventricular response is seen, but quickly resolves as the effect of the drug wears off.

UNDER WHAT CONDITIONS IS VERAPAMIL LIKELY TO BE MORE EFFECTIVE THAN DIGOXIN FOR TREATMENT OF ATRIAL FIBRILLATION?

The principal mechanism by which digoxin slows the ventricular response in atrial fibrillation is enhancement of vagal tone. As a result, digoxin is likely to be much less effective in achieving adequate rate control in a setting in which the primary reason for the rapid ventricular response is catecholamine excess from increased sympathetic activity.

> Conditions leading to increased sympathetic activity are common in emergency care situations, and include sepsis, shock, stress states, and cardiac arrest. Under such circumstances, either verapamil (which *directly* slows AV nodal conduction) and/or β-blockers (which counteract sympathetic nervous system activity) are more likely to be effective in controlling the ventricular response of atrial fibrillation than is digoxin.

WHICH SUPRAVENTRICULAR TACHYARRHYTHMIA IS MOST LIKELY TO RESPOND TO SYNCHRONIZED CARDIOVERSION? WHICH IS LEAST LIKELY TO RESPOND?

Atrial flutter is the supraventricular tachyarrhythmia most amenable to the effects of synchronized cardioversion. Use of as little as 20 to 50 joules is likely to be successful in converting atrial flutter to sinus rhythm in the vast majority of cases.

In contrast, atrial fibrillation is much more resistant to cardioversion, and will not always respond to this treatment modality. Use of higher initial energy levels (of 200 joules) is suggested when trying to convert this arrhythmia.

PSVT usually responds to synchronized cardioversion, although higher energy levels (of between 50 to 100 joules) may be needed than for treatment of atrial flutter.

MAT does not respond to cardioversion.

> Interestingly, ventricular tachycardia usually responds to relatively low energy levels (of between 50 to 100 joules)—although higher energy levels are often selected when attempting to cardiovert an acutely unstable patient.

OTHER THAN MEDICATION AND CARDIOVERSION, WHAT FACTOR IS <u>KEY</u> TO TREATMENT OF ATRIAL FIBRILLATION?

Identification and treatment of the *precipitating (underlying) cause* of the arrhythmia! Outside of the setting of cardiac arrest, the most important underlying conditions to consider in a patient who presents with atrial fibrillation include:

1. Heart failure
2. Ischemic heart disease (especially acute myocardial infarction)
3. Valvular heart disease (especially mitral stenosis)
4. Hyperthyroidism
5. Alcohol use (i.e., the "holiday heart syndrome"—although on occasion a *single* episode of drinking in a non-alcoholic patient may precipitate the arrhythmia!)
6. Acute pulmonary embolus
7. Sick sinus syndrome (i.e., "tachycardia-bradycardia syndrome"—especialy in elderly patients)
8. Acute systemic illness (i.e., pneumonia, sepsis, shock)
9. Atrial myxoma (admittedly rare—but important because it is potentially curable if found)
10. "Lone" atrial fibrillation (i.e., atrial fibrillation that occurs in the *absence* of an underlying disorder)

Practically speaking, use of medication and/or cardioversion tends to be much less effective in successfully converting the patient to sinus rhythm (and especially in *maintaining* sinus rhythm) if the underlying condition persists. Clinically then, acute care efforts should also focus on correcting heart failure (if present); optimizing the metabolic profile (i.e., being sure that serum electrolytes are normal and that the patient is not hypoxemic); and addressing all potentially treatable medical conditions (e.g., sepsis, shock, etc.). Additional concerns in evaluation of the *less acutely ill* patient who presents with new onset atrial fibrillation might be addressed by obtaining an echocardiogram and thryoid function studies.

WHY IS NEW-ONSET RAPID ATRIAL FIBRILLATION LIKELY TO PRECIPITATE/ AGGRAVATE HEART FAILURE?

There are two principal reasons why sudden development of rapid atrial fibrillation is likely to precipitate/ aggravate heart failure:

1. *Loss of the atrial kick*—which accounts for between 5% to 40% of cardiac output
2. *Decreased filling time*—since the rapid rate of the arrhythmia results in a shortening of the R-R interval (and encroaches most on the period of diastole). Because the ventricular filling phase occurs during diastole, cardiac output may be significantly reduced by the fast rate. Slowing the ventricular response to atrial fibrillation (i.e., with digoxin) may therefore improve cardiac output *even if the atrial fibrillation persists.*

WHAT WILL BE THE LIKELY ROLE OF IV DILTIAZEM IN THE MANAGEMENT OF SUPRAVENTRICULAR ARRHYTHMIAS?

Recent approval of an IV formulation of the calcium channel-blocking agent diltiazem is an exciting development that may have potentially important clinical implications. Although its precise role remains to be determined, the drug has a number of attractive features.

> IV diltiazem offers the following advantages compared to IV verapamil (Ellenbogen, 1992):
> • Less risk of producing significant hypotension
> • Less risk of precipitating/exacerbating heart failure
> • Less potential for drug interaction with concomitant digitalis use
> • Availability of an approved formulation for use as a continuous IV infusion for maintenance of antiarrhythmic effect

Onset of action following administration of an IV bolus of diltiazem is rapid (i.e., usually *within* 3 minutes—with peak effect usually occurring by 7 minutes). Effects of the bolus last 1 to 3 hours. Availability for use as a continuous IV infusion allows for continued antiarrhythmic effect over the ensuing 24 hours.

> One might expect the anticipated impact of IV diltiazem on the treatment approach of reentry tachyarrhythmias (such as PSVT) to be relatively modest. Clinical experience with IV verapamil and adenosine is considerable, and both of these agents are rapidly acting and highly effective for treatment of this disorder.
> On the other hand, administration of a continuous IV infusion of the drug appears to offer a decided advantage compared to other antiarrhythmic agents (such as digoxin or ve-

rapamil). This is particularly true for *maintaining* heart rate control over a period of hours in the treatment of atrial fibrillation or flutter when the ventricular response is rapid and not readily controlled by bolus therapy.

HOW SHOULD IV DILTIAZEM BE DOSED?

The *initial* recommended dose for IV use of diltiazem in an average-sized adult is administration of an **IV bolus** of approximately **20 mg** (i.e., 0.25 mg/kg) given over a 2-minute period. If this fails to produce the desired clinical response within 15 minutes, the dose may be increased with a *second* IV bolus of approximately **25 mg** (i.e., 0.35 mg/kg).

If continued antiarrhythmic effect is desired, an IV infusion may be started after bolus administration.

The recommended *initial* infusion rate for IV diltiazem is **10 mg/hr.** If this is not effective, the rate of infusion may be increased to **15 mg/hr.** Lower rates of infusion (i.e., 5 mg/hr) suffice for some patients. IV infusion should generally not be continued for more than 24 hours. *(See Chapter 14 for additional details and recommendations regarding the use of IV diltiazem.)*

ALGORITHM FOR USE OF THE AUTOMATIC EXTERNAL DEFIBRILLATOR (AED)

Development of the **automatic external defibrillator (AED)** is one of the most exciting advances in the field of cardiopulmonary resuscitation. The KEY feature of the device is its automaticity, which significantly reduces the time period from discovery of a victim in cardiac arrest until delivery of electrical countershock. *Minimizing this time interval is clearly the single most important factor for improving survival from cardiac arrest.* Additional benefits derived from automaticity of the AED are that it facilitates the process of defibrillation by less experienced medical personnel, and even enables lay individuals with no prior medical training to deliver a countershock to a family member in the event that a cardiac arrest occurs in the home.

> Surprisingly, use of an AED will reduce the time interval from arrival at the scene of a cardiac arrest until countshock delivery by an average of *at least* 1 minute—*even for highly skilled paramedic teams!* Thus, regardless of the clinical experience of the operator, incorporation of an AED into the protocol for defibrillation will save invaluable seconds that may prove to be the difference for determining whether a patient will recover (and if so, whether neurologic function will be intact).

Procedure for Use of the AED

Although many different AED brands are available on the market, they share many common features, and all work essentially in the same manner. Basic operation is relatively simple by design (to facilitate use by lay individuals). Allowing for minor differences in certain features among the various brands, the basic procedure for operation of any AED can be summarized by the framework of the following four sequential steps (Chapter 20 of the AHA ACLS Text): (1) Power on; (2) Cable attachment; (3) Rhythm analysis; and (4) Defibrillation (if indicated).

Application of these sequential steps for operation is incorporated into a suggested algorithm for use of the AED *(Figure 1F-1).*

Identification of Cardiopulmonary Arrest and Initial Patient Assessment

Initial assessment and management of the patient with cardiovascular collapse is similar *regardless* of the therapeutic modalities that happen to be available (and *regardless* of whether initial rescue personnel are lay individuals or a skilled medical team). Thus, initial priorities consist of:

1. Establishing unresponsiveness (i.e., *identification* of cardiopulmonary arrest)
2. Calling for help
3. Positioning the victim (and opening the **A**irway)
4. Assessing **B**reathing (and beginning *rescue breathing* if the victim is breathless)
5. Assessing **C**irculation (and considering delivery of a **precordial thump** if the victim is pulseless)

It is at this point that the process will differ—depending on which treatment modalities are available and the skill of the rescue team. Clearly, once the diagnosis of *pulseless* cardiac arrest has been confirmed (and respiratory obstruction has been ruled out), *immediate defibrillation* becomes *THE* most important intervention to implement. Performance of CPR is of secondary importance compared to the urgent need for immediate defibrillation.

> Practically speaking, intervention by the lay rescuer has been limited to performing CPR (and awaiting arrival of EMS personnel). Development of the AED has added an extra dimension to the treatment approach.

AED Available; ACLS *cannot* YET Be Provided—There Is Still NO PULSE

If ACLS cannot yet be provided and an AED is available, all efforts should be directed to immediate activation of the device. Thus, if only one rescuer is present, he/she should STOP CPR in favor of activating the AED. If more than one rescuer is present, CPR may be continued by additional personnel while the initial rescuer activates the AED.

> The initial step in operation of the AED is to *turn power* on. This activates the recording of all events that transpire during the code (in the form of a tape recording and/or printed record, that will then be available for subsequent review of the resuscitation effort).
>
> All AEDs are equipped with *patient (defibrillatory) cables* and *adhesive defibrillator pads.* The two defibrillator pads must be attached to the defibrillatory cables, which are in turn connected to the AED unit. The pads are then placed on the patient's chest in two positions (at the right upper sternal border and on the left side of the chest over the apex). These pads serve the dual function of sensing the rhythm and conducting the current that will defibrillate the patient.
>
> At this point, CPR is stopped and the *rhythm analysis control* is activated. The reason for stopping CPR during the 5 to 15 seconds required for rhythm analysis is to prevent introduction of artifact (i.e., from chest compression) that could theoretically affect the validity of AED rhythm interpretation. For similar reasons, the device should not be operated in a moving

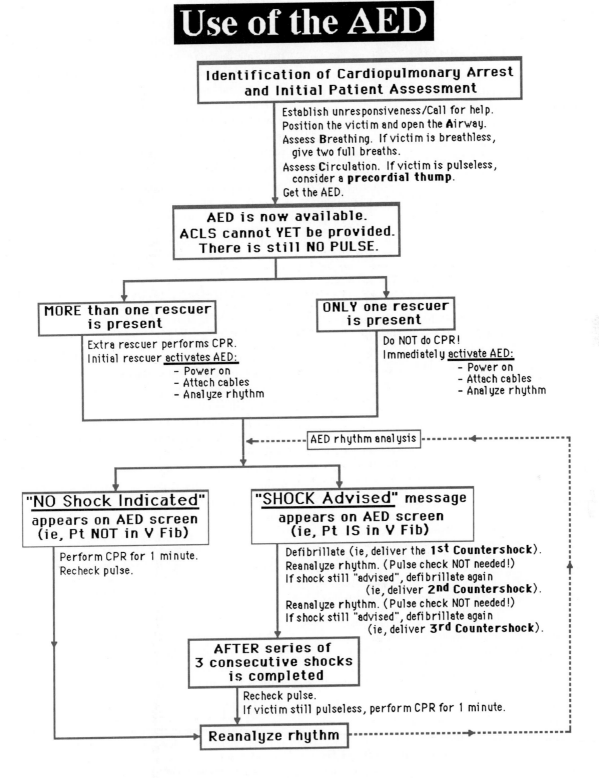

Use of the AED

Identification of Cardiopulmonary Arrest and Initial Patient Assessment

Establish unresponsiveness/Call for help.
Position the victim and open the **A**irway.
Assess **B**reathing. If victim is breathless,
    give two full breaths.
Assess **C**irculation. If victim is pulseless,
    consider a **precordial thump**.
Get the AED.

AED is now available. ACLS cannot YET be provided. There is still NO PULSE.

MORE than one rescuer is present

Extra rescuer performs CPR.
Initial rescuer <u>activates AED</u>:
    - Power on
    - Attach cables
    - Analyze rhythm

ONLY one rescuer is present

Do NOT do CPR!
Immediately <u>activate AED</u>:
    - Power on
    - Attach cables
    - Analyze rhythm

AED rhythm analysis

"NO Shock Indicated" appears on AED screen (ie, Pt NOT in V Fib)

Perform CPR for 1 minute.
Recheck pulse.

"SHOCK Advised" message appears on AED screen (ie, Pt IS in V Fib)

Defibrillate (ie, deliver the **1st Counckershock**).
Reanalyze rhythm. (Pulse check NOT needed!)
If shock still "advised", defibrillate again
    (ie, deliver **2nd Counckershock**).
Reanalyze rhythm. (Pulse check NOT needed!)
If shock still "advised", defibrillate again
    (ie, deliver **3rd Counckershock**).

AFTER series of 3 consecutive shocks is completed

Recheck pulse.
If victim still pulseless, perform CPR for 1 minute.

Reanalyze rhythm

Figure 1F-1.   Algorithm for use of the **AED** in evaluation and treatment of the victim of cardiac arrest. *(The algorithm is applicable both for lay person use of the AED, as well as for use by EMS personnel.)*

ambulance. Practically speaking, however, even abrupt patient movements (such as seizure activity and/or agonal respirations) will usually not result in delivery of an inappropriate shock.

AED Rhythm Analysis

AED rhythm analysis is performed by a highly sophisticated microprocessor, and is based on assessment of ECG signal characteristics such as amplitude, frequency, and slope of the waveform. Incorporation of additional safety features into the rhythm analysis program (to detect false signals from 60-cycle interference and/or loose electrode leads)—as well as *cessation of CPR* (and elimination of other potential sources of patient movement while rhythm analysis is occurring)—all contribute to the extremely high level of accuracy achieved by most of these devices in clinical practice.

> The AED can be counted on to reliably deliver a shock when it determines that the rhythm is ventricular fibrillation. It will also shock cases of ventricular tachycardia in which the ventricular rate exceeds a certain preset value. The AED will *not* shock asystole.

In general, it is rare for the AED to make an *error of commission* (i.e., shocking a rhythm that is not ventricular fibrillation). *Errors of omission* (i.e., failure to shock a rhythm that should be shocked) are more likely to occur, and are usually the result of the machine not distinguishing between very fine ventricular fibrillation and a flat-line recording. Fortunately, this type of error tends to be of little clinical significance because realistic chances for survival are almost as poor when the initial mechanism of cardiac arrest is *fine* ventricular fibrillation as when it is asystole.

An additional "check" against delivery of an inappropriate shock automatically results from the protocol recommended for use of the AED, since rescuers are taught to apply the device ONLY to unresponsive patients who are breathless and pulseless. Practically speaking, administration of countershock is a reasonable therapeutic option for almost any arrhythmia that occurs in this situation (such as ventricular fibrillation, ventricular tachycardia, and/or supraventricular tachycardia).

The degree of *automaticity* incorporated into the operation of an AED is variable. There are two basic types of devices: (1) "fully automatic" models; and (2) partially (or "semi-") automatic models. **Fully automatic AEDs** are ideal devices for lay person use because they do not depend on the operator to make any decisions. Instead, they simply require the operator to turn power on and attach the patient cables. *The device does the rest.* If the AED interprets the patient's rhythm as ventricular fibrillation

(or ventricular tachycardia at an exceedingly fast rate), it automatically charges the machine and defibrillates. *The operator NEVER sees the rhythm that is analyzed.*

Semiautomatic AEDs (i.e., **SAEDs** or "shock-advisory" defibrillators) differ from fully automatic devices in that one or more additional operator steps are required for defibrillation to occur. More than simply turning power on and attaching the patient cables, the operator must also activate the rhythm analysis control and physically depress a switch to discharge the electrical energy if defibrillation is indicated. This extra measure of operator control is the reason trained medical personnel generally prefer semiautomatic devices.

Theoretically, one might expect semiautomatic AEDs to be safer than fully automatic devices (since the operator retains control of the final step in the decision-making process). Surprisingly, this expectation has not been borne out in practice. Clinical performance of both types of AEDs is comparable—and highly accurate (Stults and Commins, 1987).

The Shock Advisory Message: "NO Shock Indicated"

All AEDs inform the operator of the decision they reach from analysis of the patient's rhythm. This **advisory message** is then conveyed to the operator in one or more ways, such as a statement in writing (that may appear on the AED oscilloscope screen), a visual or auditory alarm, and/or a voice synthesized phrase. If the message conveyed is, **"NO Shock Indicated"**—the operator will be advised to perform (resume) CPR for 1 min. At the end of this time the patient's pulse is rechecked and their rhythm reanalyzed to determine if defibrillation may now be needed. If not, CPR is continued until ACLS can be provided.

As suggested by the broken line loop in the algorithm, as long as the **"NO Shock Indicated"** message appears on the AED screen, the rescuer should *continue* to check the patient (for return of a pulse) and reanalyze the rhythm at *1-minute intervals* in between performance of CPR to be sure that nothing has changed (and that a "shockable rhythm" such as ventricular fibrillation is not now present).

Practically speaking, if the patient remains pulseless and unresponsive after three successive *"NO Shock Indicated"* messages, the rhythm is likely to be asystole, and realistic chances for ultimate survival are minimal.

It is important to emphasize that persistent display of the *"NO Shock Indicated"* message does not necessarily mean persistance of a nonshockable, pulseless rhythm of cardiac arrest (such as asystole). *Return Of Spontaneous Circulation (ROSC) could have occurred in the interim (despite the fact that the patient may still be unresponsive).* Early recognition of ROSC if (and when) it occurs, is the purpose of inserting *periodic* **pulse checks** after each minute's performance of CPR (and after completion of each series of consecutive shocks). Return of a pulse clearly negates the need for subsequent countershock (assuming the pulse persists).

"SHOCK Advised"

Instead of a *"NO Shock Indicated"* message, rhythm analysis of the AED may result in a ***"SHOCK Advised"*** message. In this case, *immediate defibrillation is in order*. Depending on the type of AED used, charging of the defibrillator and discharge of the electrical energy will either occur *automatically*—or *on command* from the operator. As a safety precaution, a visual and/or auditory warning will be issued to rescuers to stop CPR and stand clear while the machine is charging and defibrillating.

> The amount of energy delivered with defibrillation by AED devices varies. Virtually all models begin with 200 joules for the initial countershock attempt. Some automatically increase energy to 300 to 360 joules for subsequent attempts. Others maintain a constant energy level for all defibrillation attempts—or allow preprogramming of the amount of energy to be used. Finally, some semiautomatic AEDs provide the operator with the option of determining the amount of energy to be used at the time defibrillation is ordered.

Defibrillatory shocks should be "stacked" in groups of three. *Pulse checks need NOT be performed after each countershock attempt in a series.* However, the *rhythm* MUST be analyzed after each countershock attempt to verify persistence of ventricular fibrillation.

> Fully automatic AEDs *automatically* verify continued ventricular fibrillation before each countershock that they deliver. Thus, once these devices are activated, three successive countershocks will be automatically delivered if ventricular fibrillation persists.
>
> In contrast, semiautomatic AEDs require the operator to reactivate the rhythm analysis control after each countershock attempt. If a shock is still "advised," the operator then activates the control to defibrillate the patient.

The reason pulse checks are not required with the AED after each countershock attempt is that the sensor system of this device is specifically designed to detect loose leads and other artifactual causes of "false" ventricular fibrillation. Elimination of pulse checks does not adversely affect the accuracy of these devices for determining whether a particular rhythm is "shockable." It offers the distinct advantage of saving time and minimizing the chance of operator error by allowing the defibrillation cycle (of delivering three successive countershocks) to proceed in an uninterrupted manner.

AFTER Series of 3 Consecutive Shocks Is Completed

After each series of three successive countershocks is completed, the patient should be rechecked. If there is still no pulse, CPR should be performed for 1 minute, and the rhythm reanalyzed. Subsequent management is then determined by the ***Shock Advisory Message.***

> Practically speaking, the chance for ultimate recovery is exceedingly small if the patient fails to respond after 9 shocks

(i.e., after completion of three series of 3 successive countershocks).

If the patient regains a perfusing rhythm, but later refibrillates, the treatment sequence should be restarted. Thus, the *"Shock Advised"* message will appear on the screen, and the patient should receive another series of consecutive countershocks.

Questions to Further Understanding

HOW DOES AVAILABILITY OF AN AED ALTER THE RECOMMENDED PROTOCOL FOR DEFIBRILLATION?

In the absence of an AED, a single rescuer is advised to perform CPR for approximately 1 minute after arrival on the scene. If the victim is still breathless and pulseless at the end of this time, help (i.e., activation of the EMS system) should be called for.*

Priorities change when there is access to an AED. As soon as breathlessness and pulselessness are confirmed (and airway obstruction is ruled out), *defibrillation* becomes the single *most* important intervention to implement. Consequently, activation of the AED and immediate delivery of successive countershocks take precedence over all other resuscitative actions (i.e., performance of CPR and summoning help). Activation of the EMS system should be deferred until either a second rescuer arrives, the patient is no longer in ventricular fibrillation, and/or the patient is resistant to multiple series of successive countershocks.

> Because delivery of successive countershocks assumes highest priority when an AED is available, CPR cessation for a much longer period of time (of up to 90 seconds!) becomes acceptable to implement defibrillation. The drawback of stopping CPR for this much time is more than outweighed by the potential benefit of early countershock delivery.

The other major difference in the protocol for defibrillation when the AED is available is that precious time need not be spent checking for a pulse after each countershock attempt. Instead, successive countershocks are "stacked" in groups of three.

---

*New guidelines now advise foregoing this initial minute of rescue support in favor of immediate EMS activation for adult victims of out-of-hospital cardiac arrest.

WHY ARE PULSE CHECKS UNNECESSARY AFTER EACH COUNTERSHOCK ATTEMPT WITH AN AED?

The reason pulse checks are an essential part of conventional defibrillation protocols is to ensure that the patient is truly in ventricular fibrillation *before* delivery of each countershock. Leads may loosen and/or other sources of artifact may produce an ECG tracing that simulates ventricular fibrillation, when in fact a spontaneous rhythm has returned.

This precaution is generally unnecessary for the AED because its sensor system is specifically designed to detect loose leads and differentiate between artifact and true ventricular fibrillation.

> Elimination of routine pulse checks from the AED protocol for defibrillation not only saves time, but also minimizes the chance of operator error by allowing the defibrillation sequence to proceed in an uninterrupted manner.

HOW DOES THE PROTOCOL FOR CARE CHANGE ONCE ACLS PROVIDERS ARRIVE ON THE SCENE?

Once ACLS providers arrive on the scene, they should take over care. Ideally, this will be done in a coordinated manner with the AED operators already present who had initiated the resuscitation effort.

> Shocks already delivered by AED operators count as part of the ACLS protocol. Initially, ACLS providers should continue to use the AED for rhythm monitoring and delivery of any additional shocks that may be needed. Changeover to a conventional defibrillator should only be made if (after) the patient regains a spontaneous rhythm, at the time of transport, and/or if the ACLS provider suspects AED malfunction.

WHY ARE AEDS NOT RECOMMENDED FOR TREATMENT OF PEDIATRIC CARDIAC ARREST?

The reason is simple—*ventricular fibrillation is an extremely uncommon cause of cardiopulmonary arrest in children*. Because respiratory arrest is a far more common precipitating mechanism in this age group, primary attention should focus on airway control and optimizing ventilation rather than defibrillation.

> An additional limitation that prevents use of the AED for pediatric resuscitation is that most devices cannot be programmed to deliver less than 200 joules—an amount that far exceeds recommendations for pediatric resuscitation.

References

American Heart Association: Chapter 20—Automated external defibrillation. In AHA Textbook of ACLS, Dallas, 1990.

Callaham M, Barton C: Prediction of outcome of cardiopulmonary resuscitation from end-tidal carbon-dioxide concentration, *Crit Care Med* 18:358-362, 1990.

Cummins RO, Austin D: The frequency of "occult" ventricular fibrillation masquerading as a flat line in prehospital cardiac arrest, *Ann Emerg Med* 17:813-817, 1988.

Ellenbogen KA: Role of calcium antagonists for heart rate control in atrial fibrillation, *Am J Cardiol* 69:36B-40B, 1992.

Falk RH, Leavitt JI: Digoxin for atrial fibrillation: A drug whose time has gone? *Ann Int Med* 114:573-575, 1991.

Kerber RE, Martins JB, Kienzle MG, Constantin L, Olshansky B, Hopson R, Charbonnier F: Energy, current, and success in defibrillation and cardioversion: Clinical studies using an automated impedance-based method of energy adjustment, *Circulation* 77:1038-1046, 1988.

Martin TG, Hawkins NS, Weigel JA, Rider DE, Buckingham BD: Initial treatment of ventricular fibrillation: Defibrillation or drug therapy? *Am J Emerg Med* 6:113-119, 1986.

Paradis NA, Martin GB, Goetting MG, Rivers EP, Feingold M, Nowak RM: Aortic pressure during human cardiac arrest: Identification of pseudo-electromechanical dissociation, *Chest* 101:123-128, 1992.

Stueven HA, Alfderheide TP, Thakur RK, Hargarten K, Vanags B: Defining electromechanical dissociation: Morphologic presentation, *Resuscitation* 17:195-203, 1989.

Stults KR, Cummins RO: Fully automatic vs shock advisory defibrillators: What are the issues? *J Emerg Med Serv* 12:71-73, 1987.

Wang Y, Scheinmann MM, Chien WW, Cohen TJ, Lesh MD, Griffen JC: Patients with supraventricular tachycardia presenting with aborted sudden death: Incidence, mechanism, and long-term follow-up, *J Am Coll Cardiol* 18:1711-1719, 1991.

Weaver WD, Cobb LA, Compass MK, Hallstrom AP: Ventricular defibrillation: A comparative trial using 175-J and 320-J shocks, *N Engl J Med* 307:1101-1106, 1982.

Williams ML, Woelfel A, Casco WE, Simpson RJ, Gettes LS, Foster JR: Intravenous amiodarone during prolonged resuscitation from cardiac arrest, *Ann Int Med* 110:839-842, 1989.

CHAPTER 2

ESSENTIAL DRUGS AND TREATMENT MODALITIES

Ken Grauer
John Gums
Dan Cavallaro

SECTION A

OVERVIEW

The armamentarium of drugs and treatment modalities for cardiopulmonary resuscitation and emergency cardiac care is continually expanding. This situation could easily be overwhelming, especially for the ACLS provider who does not work with these drugs and modalities on a daily basis. In view of this and considering that the reader's need (and/or desire) to know about this material is likely to vary greatly, we have organized our presentation of the subject in as practical a format as possible. In this introductory section, we address the importance of the autonomic nervous system, adrenergic receptors, determinants of cardiac performance, and considerations that go into choosing a pressor agent. Although this material may be basic and/or review for some readers, we have included it in the hope that it may lay the groundwork for understanding the description of the drugs and treatment modalities to follow.

For each drug that is covered, we include dispensing and dosing information, indications for current use, and changes that have been made since the previous guidelines were published. Fortunately, the number of truly *essential* medications that one must be thoroughly familiar with to effectively manage a cardiac arrest is limited. These **"Key Drugs"** (the ones you need to master to pass the ACLS course) are discussed in Section B of this chapter. In Section C, we present an easy-to-learn method for **Simplified Calculation of IV Infusions** for the commonly used medications in emergency cardiac care. This is followed in Section D by a brief discussion of the basic **Key Treatment Modalities** (e.g., defibrillation, cardioversion, and pacing).

The 1986 guidelines facilitated our task by deemphasizing or eliminating a number of agents that were previously recommended for use. These include sodium bicarbonate, isoproterenol, calcium chloride, and bretylium tosylate. Although there are still some indications for the use of each of these agents, these **Deemphasized Drugs** (discussed in Section E) are no longer viewed as *essential* in the management of cardiopulmonary arrest. Familiarity with their use may therefore be looked on as *optional*, particularly for the reader with only a limited amount of time to prepare for the ACLS course. Similarly, drugs discussed in Chapter 14 comprise material "beyond the core" of what one needs to know to pass the course. It may be useful for those exposed to cardiology and acute care medicine on a regular basis and helpful as a reference to those who are not.

The Autonomic Nervous System

The **autonomic nervous system** is the *involuntary* nervous system of the body. It is made up of a series of reflex arcs that regulate functions of the body not under conscious control. Such functions include modulation of heart rate, control of blood pressure, intestinal motility, bladder function, and release of glandular secretions. Because it innervates the viscera, the autonomic nervous system is sometimes referred to as the *visceral* nervous system. Fibers from the autonomic nervous system are distributed to smooth muscles in all parts of the body. In contrast, the central nervous system per se supplies areas of the body that are under conscious control (or everything except the viscera).

The autonomic nervous system is divided into two major branches: the **sympathetic nervous system (SNS)** and the **parasympathetic nervous system (PNS).** A series of intricate interconnections exists between the central nervous system, efferent nerve fibers of the SNS and the PNS, autonomic ganglia, and the various target tissues and organs innervated by the autonomic nervous system.

> *Preganglionic* fibers of the autonomic nervous system transmit nerve signals from the central nervous system to the autonomic ganglia. Preganglionic fibers of both the SNS and the PNS stimulate nerve cells in these ganglia by releasing acetylcholine and therefore are said to be *cholinergic*.

Postganglionic fibers of the autonomic system emanate from the ganglia and continue on to innervate their respective target organs. Postganglionic fibers of the SNS are **adrenergic** (with the exception of those nerves stimulating sweat glands and portions of skeletal muscle). They are so called because they mediate their effects on target organs by releasing *norepinephrine*. In contrast, postganglionic fibers of the PNS are cholinergic. Like preganglionic fibers of both branches of the autonomic system, they mediate their effects by releasing acetylcholine.

Generalized activation of the SNS results in a "fight or flight" reaction. In addition to adrenergic stimulation and release of the neurotransmitter norepinephrine, the adrenal gland is stimulated to release endogenous epinephrine. Heart rate and blood pressure increase, the pupils dilate, the individual perspires, bronchodilation occurs, intestinal peristalsis and glandular secretion are inhibited, and the anal sphincter contracts. In contrast, the PNS is the "repose and repair" system. Its activation results in slowing of the heart rate, a fall in blood pressure, and resumption of glandular secretion and peristalsis.

Adrenergic Receptors of the Autonomic Nervous System

The autonomic nervous system exerts an extremely important influence on cardiac function. Similar to other internal organs of the body, the heart is doubly innervated by both sympathetic and parasympathetic nerve fibers. (In contrast, blood vessels have only sympathetic innervation.)

Impulses from the PNS are transmitted to the heart via the **vagus nerve.** The vagus innervates the sinoatrial and atrioventricular nodes and primarily exerts an *inhibitory* effect on the heart. Its stimulation therefore results in slowing of the heart rate and delay in atrioventricular (AV) conduction. As a result of optimal conditioning, young athletes often exhibit significant vagal tone at rest. Therefore they may demonstrate a fairly marked sinus bradycardia and/or arrhythmia, first-degree AV block, and/or second-degree AV block Mobitz type I as *normal phenomena* that simply reflect the presence of marked vagotonia. On the other hand, excessive vagal discharge may also be commonly noted in association with acute inferior myocardial infarction. In this latter setting, the accompanying bradycardia, hypotension, and AV conduction disturbances are clearly pathologic.

Adrenergic fibers of the SNS innervate the myocardium and primarily exert an *excitatory* effect. This results in acceleration of the heart rate (enhanced *chronotropy*) and increased contractility (positive *inotropic* effect). Adrenergic innervation is also present in the respiratory system and in vascular smooth muscle. Stimulation of these fibers may result in bronchodilation or changes in vasomotor tone (vasoconstriction or vasodilation, depending on the predominant type of adrenergic receptor activity).

Adrenergic activation is mediated by **alpha- (α)** and **beta (β)-adrenergic receptors** that are located on cellular surfaces. These receptors are of two subtypes: α-1 and α-2, and β-1 and β-2, respectively.

β-1 receptors are predominantly located in the myocardium. Adrenergic stimulation of these receptors is responsible for enhanced chronotropy and positive inotropy of the heart.

β-2 receptors are predominantly located in respiratory and vascular smooth muscle. Stimulation of these receptors results in bronchodilation and vasodilation.

As an aid to remembering what each β-adrenergic receptor does, you may find it helpful to think of "**one** heart, **two** lungs":
- *β-1* receptors act on the **heart**
- *β-2* receptors act on the **lungs**

Thus selective β-2 agonists (activators) such as terbutaline are very useful in the treatment of asthma because of the bronchodilation they produce. On the other hand, an adverse effect of β-blockers is that they may precipitate bronchospasm. Theoretically, "selective" β-blockers should be less likely to precipitate bronchospasm because they primarily affect β-1 receptors, whereas "non-selective" β-blockers inhibit *both* β-1 and β-2 activity. Practically speaking, however, "β-selectivity" is probably lost at therapeutic doses.

α-1 receptors are primarily *postsynaptic* in location. That is, they are found on the effector cell (i.e., vascular smooth muscle) *after* the synapse between the nerve that is stimulated and the target organ.

α-1 receptors respond preferentially to neurotransmitter catecholamines that are released by presynaptic nerve endings. Stimulation of α-1 receptors results in potent vasoconstriction.

α-2 receptors are presynaptic *and* postsynaptic in location (and *not* just presynaptic as was previously thought).

Stimulation of α-2 receptors also results in vasoconstriction. In addition, α-2 receptors participate in a feedback loop in conjunction with α-1 receptors that acts to prevent further release of neurotransmitter catecholamines. As opposed to postsynaptic α-1 receptors (that respond preferentially to neurotransmitter norepinephrine), *α-2 receptors respond preferentially to circulating catecholamines.*

With respect to cardiac resuscitation, *vasoconstriction* is the α-adrenergic receptor activity with which we are most concerned because that is the property that favors coronary and cerebral blood flow when CPR is performed in the arrested heart. For simplicity (and unless otherwise specified) we use the general term *α-adrenergic stimulation* to refer to stimulation of *α-1* adrenergic receptors.

Technically, the differential responsiveness of α-1 and α-2 receptors explains why epinephrine (which stimulates *both* types of α-receptors) is a more effective agent in the setting of cardiopulmonary resuscitation than pure α-1 stimulating drugs (such as methoxamine and phenylephrine). Low-flow states such as cardiac arrest result in a down-regulation of α-1 receptor activity and an up-regulation of α-2 receptor activity (Gonzalez and Ornato, 1991). This effect enhances responsiveness to vasoactive agents that stimulate α-2 receptors (such as epinephrine and norepinephrine). In contrast, pure α-1 stimulating agents are far less likely to produce effective vasoconstriction in the setting of cardiac arrest because of the down-regulation of these receptors in this situation. As a result, methoxamine and phenylephrine generally exert little effect on aortic diastolic pressure, and therefore do not significantly augment coronary perfusion during CPR (Gonzalez and Ornato, 1991).

In our subsequent discussion of vasoactive drugs, note will be made of their relative degree of α- and β-adrenergic receptor activity. For example, *isoproterenol* is a pure β-adrenergic receptor stimulator. It therefore exerts a potent chronotropic and inotropic effect on the heart (β-1 action), as well as causing bronchodilation and peripheral vasodilation (β-2 effect).

In contrast to isoproterenol, *epinephrine* possesses *both* α- and β-adrenergic activity. Its β-1 effects produce enhanced chronotropy and inotropy in a similar manner as does isoproterenol. Its vasoactive action, however, will be somewhat dose dependent. At low doses, the β-2 effects of epinephrine predominate, and the result is vasodilation. With higher doses (as are used in the treatment of cardiac arrest), the α-adrenergic (vasoconstrictor) effect of epinephrine overrides the β-2 (vasodilatory) action of the drug. It is this vasoconstrictor effect of epinephrine that becomes so vitally important in maintaining coronary blood flow during cardiopulmonary resuscitation.

Under normal circumstances, *circulating* catecholamines (principally endogenous epinephrine, and to a lesser extent norepinephrine) exert little influence on cardiac function. Instead, cardiac tone and function are mediated by the autonomic nervous system. However, with chronic stress-inducing conditions (such as congestive heart failure), myocardial catecholamine stores may become depleted. In such situations, circulating catecholamines probably assume a much more important role.

Administered medication with adrenergic stimulating properties may exert profound chronotropic and inotropic effects on the heart. In contrast, administration of a β-blocking agent (such as propranolol) may dramatically depress myocardial function in patients who become dependent on circulating catecholamines to stimulate cardiac contraction. Thus β-blocking agents may depress cardiac function (and worsen heart failure) in a number of ways: (1) heart rate reduction; (2) blood pressure reduction; (3) direct negative inotropic effect; and (4) catecholamine inhibition. As noted, the latter effect may be particularly important in acutely ill patients who are dependent on catecholamine secretion as their principal mechanism of compensation.

On the other hand, the sympatholytic and negative chronotropic and inotropic effect of β-blockers may prove invaluable as a therapeutic measure in the treatment of patients with acute anterior infarction in which tachycardia, hypertension,

and excessive sympathetic tone combine to increase myocardial oxygen consumption and exacerbate ischemia.

Determinants of Cardiac Performance

The principal parameter for assessing cardiac performance is **cardiac output (CO).** This is simply a measurement of the volume of blood pumped out by the heart each minute. It is equal to stroke volume **(SV)** times heart rate **(HR)** as expressed by the following equation:

$$CO = HR \times SV$$

where **SV** reflects the average amount of blood ejected from the heart with each contraction.

Heart rate is a reflection of the interaction between *sympathetic* and *parasympathetic* tone of the autonomic nervous system. It is important to remember that the resting heart is normally under the influence of *both* of these divisions of the autonomic nervous system. Parasympathetic tone usually predominates. This is especially true for the case of the young well-trained athlete who, as was mentioned earlier, frequently manifests sinus bradycardia as the result of marked vagotonia. A certain amount of resting sympathetic tone is *also* usually present in most individuals. This is evidenced by experiments that demonstrate an increase in heart rate following parasympathetic denervation that far exceeds the original resting heart rate.

Clinically, this becomes important when atropine is administered for treatment of hemodynamically significant bradyarrhythmias. Especially when a large dose of the drug (such as 1 mg at a time) is given, blockade of parasympathetic discharge may unmask underlying sympathetic hyperactivity (that previously had been held in check), with potentially deleterious effects including tachycardia, increased myocardial oxygen consumption, and/or tachyarrhythmias.

The second determinant of cardiac output in the above equation is **stroke volume.** The amount of blood ejected from the heart with each contraction depends on the interplay between three factors:

1. **Preload:** the amount of passive "stretch" placed on myocardial fibers before the onset of contraction
2. **Afterload:** the force (or resistance) against which the heart must pump
3. **Contractility:** the force with which contraction takes place

Clinically, *preload* is determined by left ventricular end diastolic volume (LVEDP). Under normal circumstances, the greater the LVEDP, the more the heart will be "stretched," and the stronger it will contract. Physiologically, this relationship is reflected by the **Frank-Starling** principle. This concept explains why a failing heart requires a higher left ventricular filling pressure to perform the same amount of work as a normal ventricle. *Unless adequate myocardial "stretch" occurs, the heart will simply not contract forcefully enough to adequately eject blood.* As a result, one frequently tries to achieve slightly higher than normal filling pressures in patients with acute myocardial infarction in an attempt to improve cardiac function. However, because excessive filling pressures may precipitate cardiac decompensation (as the heart will be unable to contract when there is too much "stretch"), hemodynamic monitoring (with a Swan-Ganz catheter) may be needed to assist in making manipulations when adjusting preload.

The other principal manner of improving cardiac output with acute infarction is to reduce *afterload*. Blood pressure control becomes vitally important in this setting. What would normally be a mild-to-moderate elevation in blood pressure (i.e., a blood pressure of 150 to 160 mm Hg systolic and 90 to 100 mm Hg diastolic) might severely overload an infarcting ventricle and precipitate overt cardiac decompensation. An agent such as IV nitroglycerin is ideal in this situation because it improves cardiac function *both* by decreasing preload *as well as* by reducing afterload in a patient in whom LVEDP is too high.

> A very fine balance must be sought to maximize cardiac function without adversely affecting hemodynamics. Producing too potent an inotropic effect may disproportionately increase myocardial oxygen consumption and become deleterious. For this reason, agents that increase *contractility* (such as isoproterenol) are usually avoided in acute infarction. On the other hand, agents that produce too great an increase in peripheral vascular resistance (increasing afterload) may place too great a strain on the heart and also result in a reduction of cardiac output. Thus to select the optimal agent for a given patient in a particular situation, a host of factors must be keep in mind.

Selection of a Pressor Agent

The cardiovascular drugs used in emergency cardiac care each affect one or more of the above determinants of myocardial performance. Adrenergic receptor agents with β-1 stimulating properties (i.e., isoproterenol, epinephrine, dopamine, dobutamine) increase heart rate and myocardial contractility. Those that also possess β-2 stimulating properties (isoproterenol, low-dose epinephrine) vasodilate. Finally, those with α-adrenergic stimulating properties (moderate-to-high doses of epinephrine and dopamine, norepinephrine) vasoconstrict.

Collectively such drugs are frequently referred to as ***"pressor agents."*** However, in light of the fact that isoproterenol and dobutamine produce little vasoconstriction per se, this is probably *not* the most appropriate term. Instead it may be better to think of these agents with regard to whether they provide *chronotropic* and / or *inotropic support* (i.e., act to improve cardiac output by increasing rate and force of contraction) or *pressor support* (i.e., increase peripheral vascular resistance and blood pressure).

> Drugs such as dopamine may affect all of the above parameters, depending on the dose of administration. At low-to-moderate infusion rates, dopamine increases cardiac output by its predominant β-adrenergic effect, often with little change in blood pressure. At higher infusion rates, the vasoconstrictor effect of the drug (α-adrenergic effect) predominates and the pressor effect takes over. At this higher dose range, dopamine acts very much like epinephrine or norepinephrine.

Which drug is selected for a particular situation depends principally on the needs of that situation. In the case of cardiac arrest, the primary concern is to restart the heart and maintain adequate coronary and cerebral flow until a spontaneously perfusing rhythm takes over *(Table 2A-1)*. The drug of choice in this situation is *epinephrine*. Its α-adrenergic action favors coronary flow (by raising aortic diastolic blood pressure) and the cerebral circulation (by shunting blood from the external to the internal carotid artery), while its β-adrenergic effect stimulates contractility. High-dose *dopamine* will probably provide similar success. In contrast, isoproterenol will not.

> Although *isoproterenol* provides potent chronotropic and inotropic activity, the pure β-adrenergic stimulation it produces results in vasodilation. This leads to a lowering of peripheral vascular resistance and aortic diastolic pressure, with a corresponding reduction in coronary blood flow. Isoproterenol is therefore contraindicated in the arrested heart.

Table 2A-1

	IN THE ARRESTED HEART (e.g., ventricular fibrillation, asystole)	ONCE THE HEART HAS BEEN RESTARTED
Selection of a Pressor Agent in the *Arrested Heart* and the Period Immediately Thereafter		
Needs of therapy	To restart the heart To maintain coronary and cerebral perfusion	To improve cardiac output and peripheral perfusion
Drug of choice	**Epinephrine** by bolus or infusion. *Use high-dose epinephrine (HDE) if there is no response to standard dose epinephrine (SDE)*	**Dopamine** infusion (at low-to-moderate doses)
Alternative agent(s)	**Dopamine** infusion (at moderate-to-high doses)	**Epinephrine** by infusion (for a slow idioventricular rhythm with a low blood pressure) **Isoproterenol** (if *only* chronotropic support is needed and blood pressure is adequate)
Drugs that are contraindicated	Isoproterenol	**Epinephrine** by *bolus* (since it is difficult to judge how much drug is needed)

As indicated in Table 2A-1, once the heart has been restarted and a *perfusing* rhythm is restored, priorities change. Achievement of a high aortic diastolic pressure is no longer essential for maintaining coronary flow. Instead, the goal of therapy after restarting the heart becomes improvement of cardiac output and peripheral perfusion.

Once the heart has been restarted, *dopamine* (at low-to-moderate infusion rates) is probably the drug of choice.

Epinephrine by bolus is contraindicated because of the difficulty in determining the appropriate dose when the drug is administered by this route to a patient with a pulse. If too much epinephrine is given, there is no way to rescind the dose. In contrast, *epinephrine by infusion* may be an effective method to administer the drug for treatment of a slow idioventricular rhythm with associated hypotension. Caution is advised in using epinephrine infusion in a patient with a supraventricular rhythm and less marked hypotension because the drug may be deleterious if it increases afterload to a greater extent than it improves cardiac output.

Isoproterenol may be effective for the treatment of hemodynamically significant bradyarrhythmias if *chronotropic support* is the primary need (i.e., if the heart rate is slow but the blood pressure is adequate). However, if hypotension accompanies the bradycardia (as is usually the case), use of isoproterenol runs the risk of exacerbating the situation by producing further vasodilation.

Use of other "pressor" agents (i.e., dobutamine, norepinephrine, and amrinone) is much less frequent in the setting of cardiac arrest or in the immediate postarrest period. We have therefore reserved our discussion of these drugs for the specific section under each agent.

SECTION B

KEY DRUGS

Epinephrine

How Dispensed:

As a 1:10,000 solution of Epinephrine: 1 mg per 10 ml syringe (i.e., 0.1 mg/ml).

As a 1:1,000 solution of Epinephrine: 30 mg per 30 ml vial (i.e., 1 mg/ml).

Indications: Ventricular fibrillation (that has not responded to countershock); asystole; EMD; hemodynamically significant bradyarrhythmias (that have not responded to atropine/pacemaker therapy).

DOSE AND ROUTE OF ADMINISTRATION

Initial Dose: 1 mg by IV bolus (10 ml of a 1:10,000 solution).

Subsequent Dosing: May repeat initial dose in several minutes and/or increase the dose as needed until the desired clinical response is obtained.

> The effect of an IV bolus of epinephrine peaks within 2 to 3 minutes, and dissipates 1 to 3 minutes later (Gonzalez et al, 1989; Paradis and Koscove, 1990). Thus *5 minutes may be too long to wait between IV boluses of the drug.*

The optimal dose of epinephrine remains unknown (Med Letter, 1992). At the present time (and until definitive studies can be performed), we favor administration of **S**tandard-**D**ose **E**pinephrine (= **SDE**) initially (i.e., 1 mg by IV bolus)—repetition of this dose in several minutes—and then *rapid escalation* to **H**igh-**D**ose **E**pinephrine (= **HDE**) with IV boluses of 3, 5, and 10 to 15 mg—and/or administration of HDE by IV infusion.

> For patients with out-of-hospital cardiac arrest in whom the duration of time from patient collapse until arrival of EMS personnel is thought to be more than a few minutes, *more rapid escalation* to HDE may be preferable (i.e., within 2 to 3 minutes) if there has been no response after the initial dose of SDE. Alternatively, *immediate* use of HDE may be reasonable in this situation.

IV Infusion (Standard Dosing = SDE): Mix 1 mg of a **1:10,000** solution of epinephrine in 250 ml of D5W, and begin the infusion at a rate of between at 15 to 30 drops/min (= 1 to 2 μg/min). *Titrate the rate of infusion upward as needed.*

IV Infusion (High-Dose Epinephrine = HDE): Mix **50 mg** of a **1:1,000** solution of epinephrine in 250 ml of D5W, and begin the infusion at a rate of between 30 to 60 drops/min (= 100 to 200 μg/min).

> Initiation of an IV infusion of epinephrine at a rate of 200 μg/min provides 1,000 μg (= 1 mg) of drug every 5 minutes. This rate would not appear to be excessive for a patient in refractory ventricular fibrillation who has not responded to initial attempts at defibrillation and SDE. The rate of the infusion can then be titrated upward as needed.

IV infusion of epinephrine is an effective alternative to IV bolus administration of the drug. Potential indications for IV infusion of epinephrine include *pressor treatment* (as an alternative agent to dopamine or isoproterenol) for patients with hemodynamically significant bradyarrhythmias that have not responded to atropine—and/or as a pharmacologic treatment of ventricular fibrillation, asystole, or EMD.

> The advantage of using an IV infusion of the drug (as opposed to IV bolus therapy) is that it allows *moment-to-moment* titration of the dose given. Thus, if the initial rate of infusion is unsuccessful, it can be gradually and progressively increased as needed until the desired effect is achieved. Once the optimal clinical response is obtained, the rate of infusion may either be continued at this level (if needed), and/or tapered at the earliest opportunity.
>
> In general, it may be easier (and more practical) to initially go with IV bolus therapy for treatment of ventricular fibrillation, asystole, and EMD. In practice, most emergency care providers appear to choose this route. However, the titratability of IV infusion therapy provides a definite advantage when epinephrine is used for treatment of a spontaneously perfusing rhythm (such as a slow idioventricular rhythm with associated hypotension). In this situation, IV administration of a bolus of drug runs the risk of producing a potentially *irreversible* adverse hemodynamic reaction. IV infusion therapy is also warranted as an alternative (albeit harder to quantitate) method for administering HDE after IV boluses of SDE have failed.

Endotracheal (ET) Instillation: Inject the contents of 1 ampule (1 mg diluted in 10 ml) down the endotracheal tube, and follow by several forceful insufflations of the Ambu bag.

> Epinephrine is effectively absorbed across bronchotracheal structures. Thus ET administration of epinephrine appears to be an adequate alternative route for drug delivery if a central line or large-bore IV is not available. It is probably superior to giving the drug through a small-bore peripheral IV from a distal site (such as the dorsum of the wrist or foot). However, blood levels following endotracheal administration of epinephrine are significantly lower than after IV administration of a comparable dose (Paradis and Koscove, 1990; Crespo et al, 1991). As a result, *higher* doses of the drug (2 to 3 times the peripheral IV dose—*or more!*) may be needed with subsequent ET administration if IV access is still unavailable and the patient has not responded to the initial 1-mg ET dose.

Intracardiac Injection: Essentially contraindicated.

Intracardiac injection is fraught with hazard and is contraindicated under most circumstances. It should be resorted to *only* when all else fails.

COMMENTS

The importance of epinephrine in the management of cardiac arrest has been known since 1896. Nearly a century later the drug is still regarded as the most useful agent in the pharmacologic treatment of cardiovascular collapse.

Epinephrine is an endogenous catecholamine with both α- and β-adrenergic stimulating properties. The latter are responsible for the drug's potent *chronotropic* and *inotropic* effects, acting to increase the rate and force of myocardial contraction.

Theoretically, epinephrine may facilitate conversion of ventricular fibrillation by countershock because it increases conduction velocity and shortens repolarization. This results in a reduction of *dispersion* for the refractory periods of individual myocardial cells. With greater uniformity during repolarization, the impetus for perpetuating ventricular fibrillation (persistence of multiple disorganized reentry circuits) is less, enhancing the chance of sustaining sinus rhythm following defibrillation.

It is now generally accepted that the *α-adrenergic* effect of epinephrine is its most important attribute in the setting of cardiac arrest. It is this effect that promotes the peripheral vasoconstriction that results in an increase in aortic diastolic pressure. In the arrested heart, **aortic diastolic pressure** determines the gradient for blood flow to the coronary arteries.

Under the best of circumstances, cardiac output produced by basic life support during cardiac arrest is no more than 20% to 30% of cardiac output during spontaneous circulation. Without the use of medication, however, only a fraction of this output is delivered to the heart and brain.

The coronary arteries are perfused during diastole. As a result, the *gradient* for blood flow to the coronary arteries (i.e., **coronary perfusion pressure [= CPP]**) is determined by the *difference* in pressure between the aorta and the right atrium during the phase of diastole. That is:

$$CPP = \frac{\text{Aortic diastolic}}{\text{pressure}} - \frac{\text{Right atrial diastolic}}{\text{pressure}}$$

Achieving an adequate aortic diastolic pressure during cardiac arrest appears to be the single most important determinant of survival. In human subjects, **return of spontaneous circulation (= ROSC)** is unlikely in patients whose maximal coronary perfusion pressure remains below 15 mm Hg. For there to be a realistic chance for survival (i.e., of ROSC), mean CPP must *exceed* 20 mm Hg (Paradis et al, 1990). To attain CPP values of this level, it appears necessary to achieve an aortic diastolic pressure of *at least* 30 mm Hg (Gonzalez and Ornato, 1991).

Practically speaking, performance of basic life support during cardiac arrest does little to favor coronary blood flow. This is because the pressure generated by external chest compression is primarily *systolic* in nature. Although generation of an appreciable aortic systolic pressure may produce a pulse during external chest compression, this *in no way* ensures that coronary flow will be adequate.

To emphasize the point that CPP may be inadequate *despite* generation of a palpable pulse with cardiac compression, consider the following example. Imagine that cardiac compression performed on a patient in cardiac arrest is able to generate an **aortic systolic pressure** of **80** mm Hg. Imagine that such compression results in an **aortic *diastolic* pressure** of **30** mm Hg and a **right atrial diastolic pressure** of **20** mm Hg. If this were the case, although you would probably be able to palpate a pulse with each compression, *it is unlikely that CPP would be high enough to ensure adequate coronary flow.*

Detection of a palpable pulse (during CPR or with spontaneous circulation) *depends on* **pulse pressure** (i.e., the *difference* between systolic and diastolic pressure readings). One would therefore expect a pulse to be palpable with each compression in this example because of the significant difference between aortic systolic and aortic diastolic pressure readings (i.e., 80 − 30 = 50 mm Hg). However, despite the presence of a palpable pulse during CPR *(and despite a seemingly adequate aortic diastolic pressure reading of 30!)*, the gradient for coronary flow in this particular case (= aortic − right atrial diastolic pressure) will still be too low (i.e., 30 − 20 = 10 mm Hg) to ensure adequate coronary perfusion. Thus, *the presence of a palpable pulse with chest compression during CPR says nothing about the adequacy of coronary perfusion.*

In the past pure β-adrenergic agents (such as isoproterenol) were recommended for treatment of cardiac arrest in the hope that potent chronotropic and inotropic stimulation might facilitate restoration of spontaneous cardiac activity. However, *pure β-adrenergic stimulation* also produces peripheral *vasodilatation*. This results in a reduction of peripheral vascular resistance and aortic diastolic pressure. Because of this latter effect, isoproterenol is no longer indicated in the setting of cardiac arrest. The reduction in aortic diastolic pressure that isoproterenol produces leads to a corresponding reduction in CPP, and tends to counteract any beneficial effect that might have been obtained from the positive chronotropic and inotropic action of the drug.

In contrast to the vasodilatory effect of isoproterenol, the vasoconstrictor (α-adrenergic) effect of epinephrine acts to increase aortic diastolic pressure, and therefore enhances the gradient for coronary flow during CPR.

Vasoactive effects of epinephrine appear to be dose dependent (Gonzalez et al., 1989). Whereas use of the drug at lower doses favors the β-adrenergic stimulating actions, use of the drug at higher doses results in a more pronounced α-adrenergic (vasoconstrictor) effect. This may explain why certain patients fail to respond to resuscitation attempts with SDE, and are only able to achieve a meaningful gradient for coronary flow when the dose of epinephrine is increased (Koscove and Paradis, 1988; Martin et al, 1990; Barton and Callaham, 1991; Gonzalez and Ornato, 1991).

Epinephrine may also help to preserve blood flow to the brain. When CPR is performed in the absence of pharmacologic therapy, flow from the common carotid artery is primarily directed *away* from the internal branch of the carotid artery and *toward* the external branch of this artery. As a result, cerebral perfusion is minimal during basic life support, whereas blood flow to areas served by the external carotid artery (i.e., the face, neck, and tongue) is preserved (i.e., "*the tongue lives forever, but the brain dies*").

Epinephrine acts to *redistribute* flow from the common carotid artery. This results in a shunting of blood from the external to the internal branch of the carotid artery, and leads to a significant increase in the amount of cerebral flow (Michael et al, 1984; Koehler et al, 1985; Paradis and Koscove, 1990).

> The actions of epinephrine may also produce a redistribution of flow in the systemic circulation. Epinephrine-induced vasoconstriction leads to an increase in systemic vascular resistance and an increase in afterload. As a result, overall cardiac output is reduced. However, despite any net reduction in cardiac output that may occur from the use of epinephrine, vital organ perfusion (to the heart and brain) is selectively *increased* as a result of preferential shunting to the vascular beds that supply these areas (Paradis and Koscove, 1990). Thus, *redistribution* of flow may be the explanation for why noninvasive indicators of cardiac output during CPR (such as **End-Tidal CO₂** recordings) tend to *decrease* following administration of epinephrine despite the beneficial effect of this drug on the coronary circulation (Martin et al., 1990).

Epinephrine is not unique in its actions. Other pressors with an α-adrenergic (vasoconstrictor) effect will also act to increase aortic diastolic pressure and therefore enhance coronary flow. This is particularly true for the nonselective, predominantly α-adrenergic stimulating agents such as *norepinephrine*—and probably also for high-dose infusion of *dopamine*. In contrast, *selective* α-1 adrenergic stimulating agents (i.e., *methoxamine* and *phenylephrine*) appear to be much less likely to produce an overall beneficial effect on coronary flow because of the down-regulation in responsiveness to α-1 receptor activity that typically occurs in the setting of cardiac arrest (Brown et al, 1988; Gonzalez and Ornato, 1991). Whether the component of β-adrenergic stimulation that epinephrine possesses is in some way essential for optimizing the distribution of flow to vital organ tissue beds, or whether similar effects could be obtained with norepinephrine or high-dose dopamine is not yet entirely clear. Until such time as this information is known, *epinephrine remains the pressor agent of choice for resuscitation of the arrested heart* (Gonzalez et al, 1989; Callaham, 1990).

> β-adrenergic stimulation appears to lower the defibrillation threshold (i.e., facilitate defibrillation), whereas β-blockade appears to raise it (Paradis and Koscove, 1990). This finding provides at least a theoretical advantage in favor of epinephrine (with its *combined* α- and β-adrenergic effect) over the predominantly α-adrenergic action of norepinephrine for the treatment of ventricular fibrillation.

Epinephrine Dosing: How Much Is Enough?

The ideal dose of epinephrine for the treatment of cardiac arrest remains unknown. Until recently, the recommended dose for IV bolus administration in adults had been 0.5 to 1 mg, to be repeated at an interval of *at least* every 5 minutes as needed (AHA Text, 1986). Recommendations for initiating an IV infusion of the drug have been to start at 1 to 2 µg/min, and to titrate the rate of the infusion upward as needed. An increasing body of evidence suggests that these previous recommendations substantially *underdosed* many patients with cardiac arrest.

> Doses of epinephrine routinely used in the laboratory for resuscitation of animals are proportionately much greater when consideration is given to the much lighter body weight of such animals (Brown et al, 1986; Brown et al, 1987). Adjusting recommendations for epinephrine dosing in humans to correct for their significantly greater body weight would require IV bolus doses of 10 to 14 mg to achieve a comparable effect.
>
> On a milligram per kilogram basis, a dose of 0.5 to 1 mg of epinephrine only provides 0.0075 to 0.015 mg/kg of drug for a 70-kg adult. In studies on laboratory animals, administration of a comparable amount of epinephrine has generally not been sufficient to achieve and maintain an aortic diastolic pressure high enough to ensure coronary perfusion during CPR. From such studies, it appears that significantly higher doses of epinephrine (on the order of **0.2 mg/kg**)* may be needed to ensure adequate coronary flow during CPR (Gonzalez and Ornato, 1991; Paradis et al, 1991; Barton and Callaham, 1991).

Unfortunately, outcome studies are few on the role of HDE in the resuscitation of human subjects.† A major problem in this regard is that achievement of ROSC does not necessarily guarantee intact neurologic recovery. On the contrary, because most reports on the use of epinephrine during cardiopulmonary resuscitation reserve the use of higher doses of the drug until a relatively late point in the code (until after standard measures have failed), a bias will automatically be built into the results. Paradoxical findings may therefore be reported in which HDE improves survival (i.e., succeeds in restoring the spontaneous circulation), but with a much higher rate of irreversible neurologic injury because of the necessarily prolonged nature of such resuscitation attempts. That is, those patients failing to respond to repeated attempts at defibrillation and SDE, and who *only* respond to HDE (given as a treatment of last resort) are the very patients most likely to be left with permanent neurologic sequelae (Ornato, 1991; Stiell, 1992).

---

*For a 70-kg adult, a dose of 0.2 mg/kg corresponds to bolus administration of 14 mg of drug.

†Recently several studies have been completed comparing the use of HDE and SDE in patients with cardiac arrest who have not responded to defibrillation. None have shown improved outcome with the use of HDE (Brown et al, 1992; Stiell et al, 1992).

Designing protocols to specifically examine the effect of HDE on survival from cardiopulmonary resuscitation is no simple task. *Time* (rather than drugs!) is by far the most important determinant of outcome from ventricular fibrillation. The most critical time parameters are the period from patient collapse until discovery (and documentation of ventricular fibrillation), and the period from such discovery until the actual application of defibrillation. Practically speaking, time until discovery is an incredibly difficult parameter to control for in a randomized, prospective manner. Furthermore, the overwhelming majority of patients who can be resuscitated from ventricular fibrillation will be saved by initial attempts at defibrillation. Thus, the *percentage* of patients with cardiac arrest who might *potentially* benefit from the use of HDE (with improved long-term survival and preservation of intact neurologic function) is likely to be exceedingly small (Paradis and Koscove, 1990; Ornato, 1991). As a result, any trial hoping to demonstrate a beneficial effect on the quality of life with long-term outcome from the use of HDE would have to include an extremely large number of patients. Performance of smaller trials might easily overlook a beneficial effect because of inadequate sample size.

Complicating the determination of the "ideal" dose of epinephrine is the finding of a nonlinear relationship between the dose of epinephrine administered and the effect of this dose on the serum epinephrine level. Thus administration of a more than 10-fold increased amount of epinephrine has been found to increase the serum epinephrine level *less* than 3-fold (Paradis and Koscove, 1990; Paradis et al, 1991). This suggests that, as epinephrine begins to exert its physiologic redistribution effects (i.e., to open tissue capillary beds and improve organ perfusion), the *volume of distribution* of the drug may change (i.e., increase) markedly. Appreciation of this phenomenon helps to explain why much higher doses of epinephrine are sometimes needed to achieve and maintain hemodynamic effects in the arrested heart.

Another factor to consider is the effect of stress on *endogenous* catecholamine secretion. Cardiac arrest is clearly the "ultimate state" of *maximal biologic stress*. Even without exogenous (i.e., IV) administration of epinephrine, serum catecholamine levels may increase 10-fold to 100-fold in the setting of cardiac arrest (Paradis and Koscove, 1990). In view of this tremendous spontaneous surge in the body's intrinsic catecholamine response, the question obviously raised is whether a relatively small dose of epinephrine (i.e., 0.5 to 1 mg) will be enough to further increase serum catecholamine levels sufficiently to exert a clinically important effect.

Alternatively, it may be that *tolerance* to adrenergic stimulation develops when catecholamine levels (from endogenous secretion) are high (Gonzalez et al, 1989). This may be the result of either *down-regulation* of receptors (i.e., a decrease in the number and activity of available receptors) and/or a decrease in receptor affinity (Gonzalez et al, 1989).

Finally, determination of the optimal dose of epinephrine during cardiac arrest should include consideration of the condition being treated. Previous guidelines failed to differentiate between pharmacologic recommendations for dosing of epinephrine in the treatment of ventricular fibrillation, asystole, and EMD. In view of the obvious pathophysiologic differences between these conditions, one might anticipate that pharmacologic treatment requirements will also differ. Thus resuscitation of a patient in asystole (in which there is no spontaneous cardiac activity at all) may require a different dose of epinephrine than for treatment of ventricular fibrillation (in which some cardiac activity is present, albeit totally chaotic and ineffective). Practically speaking, it would seem impossible to "overdose" on epinephrine in a patient with asystole (Grauer, Cavallaro, Gums, 1991). In contrast, relatively lower doses of epinephrine may be needed for certain cases of EMD in view of recent echocardiographic evidence of *purposeful* (albeit insufficient) cardiac contractility in some patients with this condition (Paradis and Koscove, 1990; Barton and Callaham, 1991). One might also expect lower doses of epinephrine to be needed when the drug is administered at a relatively early stage of resuscitation, compared to a later point in the process (when vascular tone and responsiveness is more likely to be lost).

It is important to emphasize that SDE may be *more than adequate* to produce effective vasoconstriction (and the necessary increase in aortic diastolic pressure to ensure coronary perfusion) *IF it is administered promptly* after the onset of cardiac arrest (Ornato, 1991). However, when administration of SDE fails to produce the desired response, increasing the dose of epinephrine appears to be warranted. In this case, the rapidity and extent of dose escalation should be a function of the condition being treated, the estimated duration of vascular collapse, patient responsiveness to the treatment administered, local practice, and/or the practice beliefs of the treating health care team.

In general, IV bolus administration of HDE to victims of cardiac arrest (at doses as high as 15 mg at a time!) does *not* produce residual adverse effects in those patients who ultimately survive the resuscitation (Callaham et al, 1991). In contrast, administration of HDE to a patient with a spontaneously perfusing rhythm may be harmful and could even be lethal. Adverse effects that may be produced by administration of excessive amounts of epinephrine to patients with spontaneous rhythms include tachycardia, hypertension, ventricular irritability, exacerbation of ischemia, and depression of cardiac output (in response to the increase in afterload). As a result, the dose of epinephrine should be reduced as soon as possible if (after) ROSC is achieved. A dopamine infusion is preferable in this situation if pressor treatment is needed.

In summary, it is clear that epinephrine is the most important pharmacologic agent in the treatment of cardiac arrest. Optimal dosing of the drug is still uncertain. A reasonable approach may be as follows:

1. SDE (i.e., 1 mg by IV bolus) for the initial dose.
2. Repetition of this dose in several minutes if there has been no response—followed by *rapid escalation* to HDE (with IV boluses of 3, 5, and 10 to 15 mg, and/or IV infusion of epinephrine

at as rapid a rate as is needed to produce the desired response).

3. Consideration of escalation to HDE at an even *earlier* point in the process if there has been no response to SDE after 2 to 3 minutes (and/or immediate use of HDE if the period of vascular collapse is likely to have been long).
4. Endotracheal administration of epinephrine to patients without reliable IV access.
5. Use of an IV infusion of epinephrine (instead of bolus therapy!) when the drug is used for treatment of a spontaenously perfusing rhythm.
6. Rapid reduction in the rate of infusion *at the earliest opportunity* as soon as the desired hemodynamic response is achieved (and/or consideration of switching to a dopamine infusion if a pressor agent is still needed).

Lidocaine

How Dispensed:
IV Bolus: 100 mg per 10 ml syringe
IV Infusion: 1 g per 25 ml syringe

Indications: New-onset ventricular ectopy in association with acute ischemic heart disease; ventricular tachycardia; ventricular fibrillation; as a *prophylactic* measure (for *selected* patients with suspected AMI or in those receiving thrombolytic therapy).

DOSE AND ROUTE OF ADMINISTRATION

IV Bolus: Give ≈1 mg/kg (50 to 100 mg) for the initial IV bolus (to be administered over 1 to 2 minutes). Repeat boluses of 50 to 75 mg may be given every 5 to 10 minutes up to a total loading dose of 225 mg.

IV Infusion: Mix 1 g in 250-ml D5W and begin drip at 30 drops/min (2 mg/min). Usual range of infusion = 0.5 to 4 mg/min.

ET Tube: Administer 100 mg (the contents of a 10-ml syringe), followed by several forceful insufflations of the Ambu bag.

COMMENTS

Lidocaine is the most commonly used antiarrhythmic agent for the emergency treatment of ventricular arrhythmias. It is the drug of choice for new onset PVCs associated with acute ischemic heart disease (i.e., AMI or suspected AMI), as well as for acute management of precipitating rhythms of cardiac arrest (i.e., sustained ventricular tachy-

cardia or ventricular fibrillation). Lidocaine has also been used in selected patients as a *prophylactic* measure to prevent primary ventricular fibrillation in patients with suspected AMI and in those with AMI who receive thrombolytic therapy.

There is no indication for antiarrhythmic therapy of *long-standing* (i.e., chronic) ventricular ectopy in asymptomatic individuals who do not have underlying heart disease. Long-term treatment is expensive, necessitates close monitoring and follow-up, and is associated with a significant incidence of adverse effects (including at least a 5% to 10% chance of *exacerbating* the very arrhythmia one is trying to treat). Moreover, long-term treatment of such individuals has never been shown to improve prognosis.

Long-term antiarrhythmic treatment may be indicated for *selected* individuals with ventricular ectopy who are *symptomatic*, and/or who have underlying heart disease. The most tangible potential benefit of such treatment is symptom relief—a clear justification for therapy as long as significant adverse effects are not produced by the antiarrhythmic drug. Benefits from treatment of long-term ventricular ectopy in asymptomatic individuals with underlying heart disease are less clear. Although such individuals are at increased risk of sudden cardiac death, antiarrhythmic therapy has not been shown to prolong survival. In contrast, survival may be improved by comprehensive evaluation and treatment of survivors of out-of-hospital cardiac arrest not associated with AMI *(see Section 11E, Survivors of Cardiac Arrest: Options for Management).*

Clinical concerns regarding the management of patients with *new-onset* PVCs that occur in association with acute ischemic heart disease are very different than the concerns posed by long-standing ventricular ectopy. Because the risk of developing malignant ventricular arrhythmias (i.e., sustained ventricular tachycardia or ventricular fibrillation) is much greater in the acute setting, much greater consideration should be given to active antiarrhythmic therapy. If the decision is made to treat, IV lidocaine is the drug of choice.

Patients who are at the greatest risk for developing malignant ventricular arrhythmias with AMI are those who are seen within the first few hours of the onset of symptoms. Consequently, patients with new onset chest pain in whom there is a high index of suspicion for acute infarction would seem to be the group most suited for consideration of lidocaine prophylaxis, especially if they are seen within the first 6 hrs of the onset of symptoms. However, because the incidence of primary ventricular fibrillation is less in patients over 70 years of age (and the risk for developing lidocaine toxicity is significantly greater), antiarrhythmic prophylaxis is less likely to be beneficial in elderly subjects—and may not be worth the risk. Overall, the issue remains controversial. Therapeutic decisions—on whether to initiate lidocaine prophylaxis and/or treatment—must therefore be *individualized*, and are usually based on clinical circumstances and the judgment/beliefs of the health care team.

Detailed discussion on the use of lidocaine for patients with suspected AMI (including the rationale for treatment and dosing recommendations) is covered in Sections 12B and 12E, and summarized in *Table 12B-2*. We limit discussion here to emphasis of several key points in management:

1. *IV lidocaine should NOT be used to treat chronic PVCs that occur in an asymptomatic patient who is not having an acute ischemic syndrome.* In most instances, this general rule should be followed even if PVCs are frequent and short runs of repetitive forms are present.

2. When used *prophylactically* (i.e., in the absence of PVCs), aggressive loading with IV lidocaine is probably not needed and may unnecessarily increase the risk for drug toxicity. In most cases, 1 to 2 boluses of lidocaine and constant infusion at a rate of 2 mg/min is perfectly adequate to ensure the drug's protective effect. Even if some ventricular ectopy persists, additional boluses and higher infusion rates may still not be needed as long as repetitive forms (i.e., ventricular couplets or salvos) are infrequent. *Elimination of every PVC is NOT essential for protection against ventricular fibrillation.*

3. Lidocaine toxicity is prone to develop in patients with congestive heart failure or shock (who are likely to have difficulty clearing the drug), the elderly, patients with lower body weights, and with concomitant use of propranolol or cimetidine. Use of lower infusion rates (i.e., 0.5 to 1 mg/min) and monitoring with lidocaine levels (if available) should be considered for such patients.

4. Although still the subject of controversy, lidocaine has been recommended as a drug of choice for treatment of refractory ventricular fibrillation. Studies to date have not demonstrated a significant difference in clinical efficacy between this drug and bretylium in this situation. Because lidocaine may be a safer agent, and most emergency care providers are more comfortable with its use, this drug is favored over bretylium for treatment of refractory ventricular fibrillation.

   Because of the markedly decreased clearance of lidocaine during cardiac arrest, 1 to 2 boluses of the drug (with or without initiation of a maintenance infusion) is usually all that is needed to achieve therapeutic levels during this low-flow state. Once the patient has been converted out of ventricular fibrillation, however, clearance of the drug markedly increases. Resumption of a normal dosing schedule (i.e., rebolus and institution of a maintenance infusion) is essential at this time to minimize the chance that ventricular fibrillation will recur. Practically speaking, it may be far simpler to *always* initiate a maintenance infusion (at 2 mg/min) *at the same time* the decision is made to administer IV loading boluses—even during the low-flow state of cardiac arrest *(see Section 12E).*

5. Although lidocaine may be administered by the endotracheal route, absorption of the drug is unreliable during cardiac arrest. Peak concentrations of lidocaine may be delayed for up to 10 minutes following intratracheal instillation. Therefore, if IV access is available, this route is definitely preferred for administration of lidocaine.

6. Lidocaine will not always be successful in terminating sustained ventricular tachycardia. However, because the drug is rapidly administered, well tolerated by most patients, associated with relatively few adverse effects, and does not impair the ability to subsequently give other drugs—lidocaine remains the first-line agent for *medical* treatment of this arrhythmia. If at any time the patient becomes hemodynamically unstable, *immediate* cardioversion becomes the treatment of choice.

7. Lidocaine is most likely to be effective in the treatment of acute ventricular arrhythmias that develop as a result of *ischemia.* It appears to be much less effective in the treatment of long-standing arrhythmias that arise from a fixed anatomic substrate such as commonly occurs under *nonischemic* conditions (Wesley et al, 1991). If such nonischemic-related arrhythmias are to be treated at all, other antiarrhythmic agents (such as procainamide) are more likely to be effective than lidocaine.

Atropine Sulfate

How Dispensed: 1 mg per 10 ml syringe.
Indications: *Hemodynamically significant* bradyarrhythmias; asystole.
Precautions: Hemodynamically significant 2° AV block of the Mobitz II type (because atropine may paradoxically *reduce* the ventricular response of this conduction disturbance).

DOSE AND ROUTE OF ADMINISTRATION

IV Bolus: 0.5 mg IV every 5 minutes up to the usual maximum dose of 2 mg. It should be emphasized that *1 mg of atropine may be given at a time for marked bradycardia and/or hypotension.*
ET Tube: 1.0 mg at a time, followed by several forceful insufflations of the Ambu bag.

COMMENTS

Atropine is a parasympathetic (anticholinergic) blocking agent that has been recommended for use in the treatment of bradyarrhythmias. However, the drug is *not* without adverse effects. Because it also enhances the rate of discharge from the sinus node, atropine may precipitate atrial tachyarrhythmias. Moreover, by blocking parasympathetic output, it may unmask underlying enhanced sympathetic activity that had previously been contained and thus lead to development of ventricular arrhythmias. Myocardial oxygen consumption is increased and angina may result. Case reports of ventricular tachycardia and ventricular fibrillation following atropine administration have been noted (Massumi et al, 1977; Scheinman et al, 1975).

Because of the potentially deleterious responses that may result from IV administration of atropine, use of the drug is only recommended for treatment of *hemodynamically significant* bradyarrhythmias or frequent ventricular ectopy in which development of PVCs is felt to be *directly* attributed to the slow heart rate.

In addition to the vagolytic effect of atropine, the drug also improves conduction through the AV node. This explains its beneficial effect in the treatment of 2° and 3° AV block *during the early hours* of acute inferior infarction at a time when these conduction defects are most likely to reflect excessive vagal tone. The drug should not be expected to work nearly as well *after* the first 6 to 8 hours of inferior infarction, or with anterior infarction because excessive parasympathetic tone is much less of a causative factor under these circumstances (ACC/AHA Task Force, 1990).

It is important to emphasize that the effects of atropine sometimes act as a double-edged sword (ACC/AHA Task Force, 1990). The fact that the drug enhances the rate of sinus node discharge may actually *counteract* its beneficial action on AV nodal conduction. For example, in the setting of acute inferior infarction, the AV node may be able to conduct every sinus impulse to the ventricles at a heart rate of 50 beats/min. However, acceleration of the rate (i.e., to 80 beats/min, such as may occur following atropine administration) could result in a heart rate that is simply too rapid for an ischemic AV node to continue conducting with a 1:1 AV ratio. If at this faster rate the AV node was only able to conduct every *other* sinus impulse, then for an atrial rate of 80 the ventricular response might only be 40 beats/min (2:1 AV conduction). *In this theoretical example, administration of atropine would actually have made the patient's condition worse by decreasing the ventricular response from 50 to 40 beats/min.*

This phenomenon—in which administration of atropine paradoxically *reduces* the ventricular response—is particularly likely to occur in a patient with 2° AV block of the Mobitz II type. This is because atropine is unlikely to improve AV nodal conduction for this rhythm disturbance (ACC/AHA Task Force, 1990).

Thus, atropine is most likely to be effective for treatment of hemodynamically significant bradyarrhythmias that result from excessive parasympathetic tone (i.e., 2° AV block of the Mobitz I type, or 3° AV block with a narrow QRS complex escape rhythm—especially when either of these conduction disturbances occurs during the *early* hours of inferior AMI).

On the other hand, atropine must be used with great caution (if at all) for treatment of hemodynamically significant 2° AV block of the Mobitz II type (because acceleration of the atrial rate in this setting may result in paradoxical *slowing* of the ventricular response). If the decision is made to use atropine to treat this bradyarrhythmia, it would be prudent to have an external pacemaker readily available.

Atropine has also been recommended for treatment of asystole. The rationale for its use in this setting stems from the finding that certain individuals demonstrate at least some parasympathetic innervation of the ventricles.

Although the prognosis for asystole is never good, it is important to emphasize that the outlook for this condition is not nearly as poor when it occurs *inside* the hospital as when it occurs *outside* the hospital (McGrath, 1987; Tortolani et al, 1989). Asystole in this latter setting is most often a preterminal event that results after prolonged cardiopulmonary arrest, and that follows deterioration of ventricular fibrillation. On a cellular level, this type of asystole is associated with tissue hypoxia, acidosis, and cellular disruption (Coon et al, 1981; Niemann et al, 1985). Response to treatment is dismal (Stueven et al, 1984; Myerburg et al, 1982).

In contrast, asystole that occurs within the hospital can sometimes be due to massive parasympathetic discharge. This may occur in association with certain operative or diagnostic procedures, anesthesia, toxic drug reactions, vasovagal episodes, or heart block from acute inferior infarction. In addition, the time from the onset of asystole until discovery by trained personnel will usually be significantly less in the hospital than when the condition occurs on the outside. As a result, asystole that occurs in a hospital setting may respond surprisingly well for a "prelethal" arrhythmia to atropine therapy (Coon et al, 1981).

The recommended dose of atropine has been 0.5 mg IV every 5 minutes until a total dose of 2 mg is given. However, this dosing schedule may not be practical for treatment of conduction disorders when the heart rate is extremely slow (i.e., under 40 beats/min) and the blood pressure very low (i.e., less than 80 mm Hg systolic) because it takes no less than *15 minutes* to administer the full 2 mg dose of drug! Moreover, peak drug effects are usually observed within 3 minutes of IV administration (ACC/AHA Task Force, 1990). It may therefore be preferable under the circumstances of a severe conduction disturbance to administer 1 mg of atropine at a time, repeating the dose in 2 to 3 minutes if the desired clinical response has not been observed.

On the other hand, when symptoms produced by the bradyarrhythmia are less severe (i.e., for mild bradycardia associated with minimal signs of hemodynamic compromise), increments of 0.5 mg of IV atropine should be given at the recommended 5-minute intervals because larger doses may be associated with an unacceptable incidence of adverse effects (Scheinman et al, 1975).

- The reason doses less than 0.5 mg should *not* be used in adults is that paradoxic slowing of the heart rate may result (caused by either a central reflex stimulation of the vagus or a peripheral parasympathomimetic effect on the heart).
- Although in most individuals, 2 mg is the full atropinization dose, up to **0.04 mg/kg** (i.e., up to **3 mg** or more) of the drug may occasionally be needed to obtain maximal effect (Jose et al, 1969). However, *most emergency care providers tend to turn to a pressor agent if a symptomatic bradyarrhythmia does not respond to the usual 2-mg dose of atropine.*

An additional beneficial effect of atropine is that it may reduce nausea and vomiting that occurs as a result of morphine administration (ACC/AHA Task Force, 1990).

Cardiovascular effects of atropine last an estimated 2 to 4 hours. Other systemic effects (including pupillary dilation) may persist much longer (Kaiser et al, 1970; Thomas and Woodgate, 1966).

A common problem in the management of patients with cardiac arrest is deciding at what point to terminate efforts at resuscitation. Pupillary size and responsiveness have traditionally been regarded by emergency care providers as important clinical clues that help in making this determination. Widespread belief exists that administration of atropine (which is so frequently used for treatment of bradycardic/asystolic cardiac arrest) precludes use of the pupillary size parameter. *This may not be the case!* A recent study by Goetting (1991) suggests that, despite producing a small (but definite) amount of pupillary dilatation, *atropine administration in conventional doses during cardiopulmonary resuscitation will usually NOT abolish pupillary reactivity to light.* Thus, the presence of fixed and dilated pupils in a patient who has failed to respond to resuscitation efforts is likely to indicate severe neurologic (hypoxic-ischemic) injury, and should not be attributed to atropine administration.

A final clinical concern that occasionally arises is whether use of a topical cycloplegic agent could be responsible for pupillary dilation and unresponsiveness. Topical application of **1% pilocarpine** may help resolve this question because it tends to reverse pupillary dilation caused by neurologic injury but not affect pharmacologically induced pupillary dilation (Goetting, 1991).

Atropine may also be given by the ET route. Although there is much less experience in administering the drug by this method than there is for epinephrine, absorption across tracheobronchial structures appears to be good and substantial atropine levels are achieved within 10 minutes of dosing (Greenberg, 1982). A dose of at least 1 mg at a time is advised when using atropine by the ET route.

In summary, enhanced appreciation of the potentially deleterious effects of atropine, and the ever increasing availability of external pacemakers have led to a change in the approach to management of bradyarrhythmias. Asymptomatic patients with a heart rate of over 40 beats/minute need *not* be treated. Pacemaker therapy—rather than atropine—is generally preferred as initial treatment of bradyarrhythmias that are (and/or become) hemodynamically significant.

Dopamine (Intropin)

How Dispensed: 200 mg per 5 ml ampule.
Indications: Hemodynamically significant bradyarrhythmias; medical treatment of cardiogenic shock.

DOSE AND ROUTE OF ADMINISTRATION

IV infusion: Mix 1 ampule (200 mg) in 250-ml D5W and begin drip at 15 to 30 drops/min ($\approx$ 2 to 5 μg/kg/

min in an average-sized person). Titrate drip upward and adjust for the lowest infusion rate that maintains the desired clinical response.

Dopamine is a chemical precursor of norepinephrine with dopaminergic, α- and β-adrenergic receptor stimulating properties. Which of these pharmacologic actions predominates depends primarily on the *rate of infusion* of the drug:

At Low Infusion Rates (0.5 to 2 μg/kg/min)—the *dopaminergic* effect prevails. This produces dilation of renal and mesenteric blood vessels. Heart rate and blood pressure may not be greatly affected at this low infusion rate.

At Moderate Infusion Rates (2 to 10 μg/kg/min)—the β-adrenergic receptor stimulating action prevails. *β-1 adrenergic receptors* (rather than β-2) are primarily affected. The result is an increase in cardiac output without necessarily raising the blood pressure.

At High Infusion Rates (>10 μg/kg/min)—the *α-adrenergic receptor* stimulating effect predominates. Peripheral vasoconstriction results. There is usually no further increase in cardiac output as blood pressure increases. The initial dilation of the renal and mesenteric vasculature reverses itself at higher doses.

At moderate-to-high doses the actions of dopamine resemble those of epinephrine. As the infusion rate of dopamine is increased even further (i.e., to 15 to 20 μg/kg/min), the drug becomes more and more like norepinephrine in its effects (i.e., predominant vasoconstriction).*

As with all pressor agents, dopamine may precipitate ventricular ectopy and/or tachyarrhythmias, necessitating a reduction in the infusion rate. However, the arrhythmogenic effect of the drug is generally much less marked than for isoproterenol.

Dopamine is indicated for the medical treatment of hemodynamically significant bradyarrhythmias and cardiogenic shock. *It is probably the most commonly used pressor agent for this purpose.* It also has been used to maintain coronary perfusion in the arrested heart. A large part of the appeal of dopamine appears to lie in its flexibility, which allows this one drug to be used not only for management of car-

---

*Although the relative degree of dopaminergic, α- and β-adrenergic receptor activity can be anticipated for most patients from the rate of infusion (as suggested above), variations may occur for any given individual (Chatterjee, 1990). Surprisingly, in addition to nearly doubling renal blood flow, low-dose dopamine (i.e., 1 to 2 μg/kg/min) significantly increases cardiac output (by up to 40%) in many patients (Dasta, 1991). In others, the dopaminergic effect is almost abolished with β-1 adrenergic activity predominating at infusion rates of 2 μg/kg/min. Still in others, α-adrenergic activity may predominate at relatively low infusion rates (i.e., <5 μg/kg/min). *Dose titration of dopamine infusion must always be individualized and carefully adjusted according to each patient's response.*

diac arrest, but also for blood pressure support and maintenance of vital organ perfusion during the immediate post-resuscitation period.

The dopaminergic (renal vasodilatory) effect of *low-dose* dopamine is an extremely attractive feature of the drug—especially for management of hypotensive patients with oliguria. As an extension of this principle, **combined pressor treatment** is sometimes tried in which a potent vasoconstrictor (such as norepinephrine) is used to increase blood pressure *together with* low-dose dopamine (for its dopaminergic effect) in an attempt to maintain adequate renal perfusion and urine output. It should be emphasized that the dopaminergic effect of dopamine will be lost as the rate of infusion is increased (i.e., usually at levels of more than 2 to 5 μg/kg/min).

Another pressor combination that is sometimes tried is dobutamine and dopamine. The goal of the joint use of these drugs is to enhance cardiac output (from the positive inotropic effect of dobutamine), while maintaining arterial blood pressure (with the α-adrenergic effect of dopamine). Combining pressor agents in this manner may allow lower doses of each drug to be used, thus minimizing the potential for adverse effects. Invasive monitoring will often be needed to optimize hemodynamic parameters when joint pressor therapy is used.

When dopamine is being used for its *pressor* effect (i.e., at infusion rates ≥5 μg/kg/min), it is important not to abruptly discontinue the infusion after achieving the desired blood pressure level; otherwise the patient may become hypotensive.

In summary, dopamine is a favored agent for medical treatment of hypotensive states that are not the result of hypovolemia. Although the drug may be used at high doses (>10 to 20 μg/kg/min) to improve coronary perfusion in the arrested heart, epinephrine (by bolus or infusion) is usually preferred for this purpose. The drug may also be used at somewhat lower doses as treatment of hemodynamically significant bradyarrhythmias that have not responded to atropine during the period until pacemaker therapy can be initiated.

Oxygen

Indications: Suspected hypoxemia of any cause (including cardiopulmonary arrest, acute ischemic chest pain, AMI, etc.)

Contraindications: Virtually none in the acute care setting!

DOSE AND ROUTE OF ADMINISTRATION

Nasal Canula: 24% to 40% O_2 can be delivered with flow rates of 6 L/min.

Face Mask: Up to 50% O_2 can be delivered with flow rates of 10 L/min.

Venturi Mask: Fixed O_2 concentrations of 24%, 28%, 35%, and 40% may be delivered with flow rates of 4 to 8 L/min.

Pocket Mask: 50% O_2 can be delivered with flow rates of 10 L/min.

Bag-Valve Mask Devices: May deliver room air or up to 90% O_2 with a high-flow oxygen source and attached reservoir.

Non-Rebreathing Oxygen Mask: A superior device for delivering high oxygen concentrations of up to 90%.

COMMENTS

Oxygen is one of the truly essential drugs in cardiopulmonary resuscitation and emergency cardiac care. It is the treatment of choice for suspected hypoxemia of any cause (including cardiopulmonary arrest, acute ischemic chest pain, and AMI), and should *not* be withheld for fear of causing carbon dioxide retention in emergency situations. *(Delivery systems for oxygen are discussed in detail in Chapter 7 on Airway Management.)*

Morphine Sulfate

How Dispensed: 5, 10, or 15 mg per ampule.

Indications: Acute ischemic chest pain (as well as the anxiety that so often accompanies it); pulmonary edema.

DOSE AND ROUTE OF ADMINISTRATION

IV Dose: 2- to 5-mg increments, which may be repeated every 5 to 30 minutes as needed.

COMMENTS

Morphine sulfate is a drug that has withstood the test of time. Even today it remains an ideal agent for treatment of acute ischemic chest pain and pulmonary edema.

Morphine works in a number of different ways. In addition to its extremely potent analgesic effect, it also allays anxiety in patients with acute chest pain or air hunger from pulmonary edema. Hemodynamically, the drug markedly increases venous capacitance. This significantly reduces preload (by decreasing venous return) and relieves symptoms of pulmonary congestion. Morphine also induces mild arterial vasodilatation, which improves cardiac performance by lowering afterload. Finally, the drug *indirectly* reduces the level of circulating catecholamines (and the tendency toward arrhythmias) by its analgesic and antianxiety effect.

Caution has been urged when using morphine sulfate for treatment of acute inferior infarction because of concern that the drug might induce heart block, excessive bradycardia, or hypotension. Many authorities have even advocated substituting another analgesic agent (such as IV meperidine) for use in this setting rather than risk an adverse reaction to morphine. This degree of concern may *not* be necessary. A relatively large study by Semenkovich and Jaffe (1985) evaluated 184 patients who presented with chest pain and suspected AMI. All patients were treated with morphine sulfate. Eighty-five percent of study subjects went on to develop a documented infarction. Adverse effects from morphine sulfate administration occurred in only four patients (*less* than 3% of the study group). These consisted of hypotension and heart rate slowing, suggesting a vasovagal influence contributed to the reaction. Three of the patients responded promptly to atropine and/or fluid administration, and hypotension spontaneously resolved within 1 minute in the other. *Each of the four patients went on to receive an additional 8 to 31 mg of IV morphine over the next 12 to 48 hours WITHOUT additional sequelae.*

Thus, it appears that adverse reactions to morphine sulfate administered for acute ischemic chest pain have been overemphasized in the past, and probably are much *less* common than is generally thought. When they do occur, they most often follow administration of the first dose *and in no way preclude cautious additional use of the drug.*

In the study by Semenkovich and Jaffe, the adverse reactions encountered in the four patients consisted of hypotension and/or heart rate slowing. Conduction system defects were *not* seen. Adverse reactions promptly resolved with treatment (atropine and/or fluid administration) or spontaneously. Moreover, only *one* of the four patients had inferior or posterior infarction, which contradicts the previous notion that the adverse effects from morphine are more common with inferior AMI.

Optimal use of IV morphine sulfate entails incremental dosing in small amounts (i.e., 2 to 5 mg) repeated at frequent intervals (q 5 to 30 minutes) according to the patient's symptoms and clinical response. In addition to occasional bradycardia and hypotension, the drug may cause oversedation, nausea, and respiratory depression. Fortunately, the latter effect may be quickly reversed with 0.4-mg IV **naloxone (Narcan).** As noted above, vagotonic actions of the drug are easily reversed in most cases by either atropine or saline infusion.

Some clinicians choose to withhold morphine from patients with AMI who are treated with thrombolytic therapy because they believe it may "mask" the principal clinical sign of reperfusion (relief of chest pain). Considering the adverse pathophysiologic effects of continued chest pain on an ischemic myocardium, this practice is not advised. *Instead, chest pain associated with AMI should ALWAYS be treated (and relieved) as soon as possible.* Incremental dosing with IV morphine sulfate is an excellent way to accomplish this goal.

(See Section 12B for additional information on the use of morphine sulfate in the management of AMI.)

Verapamil (Calan, Isoptin)

How Dispensed: 5 mg per ml ampule.
Indications: Superventricular tachyarrhythmias (including PSVT, rapid atrial fibrillation, atrial flutter, MAT).

Contraindications: Wide complex tachyarrhythmias of unknown etiology; rapid atrial fibrillation in patients with WPW.

DOSE AND ROUTE OF ADMINISTRATION

IV Dosing: 3 to 5 mg to be given IV over a 1 to 2 minute period (or over 3 to 4 minutes in the elderly). May give up to 10 mg in a dose and repeat once in 30 minutes if needed.

COMMENTS

Verapamil is an extremely effective pharmacologic agent for treatment of the *supraventricular tachyarrhythmias* that are most commonly seen in emergency cardiac care. In particular, IV verapamil is a drug of choice (along with adenosine) for the *acute* treatment of PSVT; a drug of choice (along with IV digoxin) for acute treatment of rapid atrial fibrillation; *the* drug of choice for MAT (when medical therapy is indicated); and an effective *adjunctive* agent for rate control of rapid atrial flutter.

Verapamil exerts its primary physiologic effect on AV nodal tissue, slowing conduction and prolonging the effective refractory period within the AV node. As a result, this calcium channel-blocking agent is able to alter conduction properties in one or both arms of the reentrant pathway of patients with PSVT—an action that will usually serve to interrupt the cycle and terminate the arrhythmia.

PSVT should first be treated by attempting to increase vagal tone with either carotid sinus massage (provided there is no history of carotid disease or neck bruits on examination) or a Valsalva maneuver. If these vagal maneuvers are not effective, a trial of *either* IV verapamil or adenosine is indicated. The usual adult dose of verapamil is 5 mg, which should be given IV over a 1 to 2 minute period. Lower doses (3 mg) given more slowly (over 3 to 4 minutes) are advised in the elderly.

Verapamil usually works within minutes. It successfully converts more than 90% of cases of PSVT. There may be gradual slowing of the tachyarrhythmia, and then sudden conversion to sinus rhythm. If the initial dose of the drug does not produce the desired effect, a second dose (of 5 to 10 mg IV) may be given 15 to 30 minutes later.

Either verapamil *or* adenosine may be used as acute treatment of PSVT. Comparative features of these two agents are summarized in *Table 2B-1*, which appears in our discussion on adenosine.

In patients with frequent episodes of PSVT, long-term maintenance on oral verapamil may reduce (or even eliminate) the number of recurrences. In many patients, episodes of

PSVT are intermittent—sometimes occurring as infrequently as once every 3 to 6 months. In such individuals, use of an **"antiarrhythmic cocktail"** that the patient may take *at home* on a "prn" basis may be far preferable (in terms of cost-efficacy and minimization of long-term side effects) to daily prescription of a drug for prevention of a relatively benign disorder that only occurs once every few months (Margolis et al, 1980; Rose et al, 1986).

> The contents of an **antiarrhythmic "cocktail"** may be individualized to fit patient needs—and might consist of oral **verapamil** (80 to 120 mg PO)— together with a dose of a *benzodiazepine* to allay anxiety and reduce sympathetic tone that may be contributing to perpetuation of the arrhythmia. Alternatively, a *β-blocker* (i.e., 10 to 80 mg of propranolol) may be used in the cocktail instead of/in addition to verapamil.
>
> Conversion of the arrhythmia is likely to occur within 30 to 90 minutes of taking the cocktail. If it persists, and/or the patient develops significant symptoms, formal medical attention should be sought.

Verapamil is also a very useful agent for acute treatment of atrial fibrillation and flutter. Although conversion to sinus rhythm occurs *less* than a third of the time, the AV nodal depressant effect of the drug reliably slows the ventricular response to both of these tachyarrhythmias.

> Despite the efficacy of verapamil for treatment of rapid atrial fibrillation in the usual patient, the drug should *not* be used to treat this arrhythmia if Wolff-Parkinson-White syndrome is present. This is because verapamil may accelerate antegrade (i.e., forward) conduction down the accessory pathway in such cases—an effect that may lead to deterioration of the rhythm and precipitation of ventricular fibrillation (McGovern et al, 1986).

Combining small doses of IV digoxin with IV verapamil may produce a *synergistic* effect when treating atrial fibrillation or flutter with a rapid ventricular response. For patients whose condition is controlled by this regimen in the acute phase, maintenance therapy with oral verapamil is often effective for long-term maintenance.

> Surprisingly, maintenance therapy with a calcium channel blocker (*either* verapamil or diltiazem) is more effective for long-term rate control of atrial fibrillation than maintenance digoxin (Lang et al, 1983; Singh and Nademanee, 1987). Combination therapy (i.e., use of digoxin *and* one of these calcium channel blockers) results in even better heart rate control than the use of any agent alone (Roth et al, 1986; Steinberg et al, 1987).

Verapamil has become the drug of choice for treatment of MAT when rate control is needed (i.e., for patients who remain symptomatic despite improved oxygenation and electrolyte correction).*

> Although the precise mechanism of MAT remains unclear, it appears that increased atrial automaticity, due in part to intracellular calcium overload, plays a contributing role. Verapamil acts to improve intracellular homeostasis. Thus, in addition to slowing the ventricular response by its effect on the AV node, verapamil also exerts a direct depressant effect on atrial automaticity that reduces the number of ectopic atrial impulses (Levine et al, 1985; Kastor, 1991). Use of verapamil is clearly preferable to digoxin for treatment of MAT.

Several words of caution regarding the use of verapamil are in order. The drug should never be used to slow the heart rate of a patient in sinus tachycardia for whom the rapid heart rate may be needed to sustain cardiac output. Instead, treatment of sinus tachycardia must be directed toward the underlying cause. Because of verapamil's depressant effect on sinoatrial (SA) and atrioventricular (AV) conduction, it should be used very cautiously in patients with evidence of sinus node disease (i.e., sick sinus syndrome) or in connection with digitalis, which also slows AV nodal conduction. For the same reason, verapamil should probably not be given within 30 minutes of administering an IV β-blocker. Because of its negative inotropic effects, the drug is relatively contraindicated for use in patients with congestive heart failure. Finally, the vasodilatory action of verapamil may produce hypotension, especially if the drug is injected too rapidly or given to overly sensitive elderly individuals. Slower administration and use of lower doses may help to avoid this problem.

> **Pretreatment** with **calcium chloride** has become increasingly popular as a technique for minimizing (and often eliminating) the hypotensive response of verapamil without diminishing its efficacy for converting or controlling the ventricular rate of patients with supraventricular tachyarrhythmias (Haft and Habbab, 1986; Barnett and Touchon, 1990). A dose of between 500 to 1,000 mg of calcium chloride (i.e., 5 to 10 ml of a 10-ml ampule of 10% calcium chloride) is infused IV over 5 to 10 minutes.† Too rapid infusion may produce a generalized sensation of heat in the patient. Conversion of the rhythm or slowing of the ventricular response occasionally results from calcium infusion alone even before

---

*Recently, IV β-blockers have been shown to be at least equally (if not more) effective as IV verapamil for treatment of MAT (Kastor, 1991). However, because bronchospasm and/or heart failure are so commonly seen in patients who present with this arrhythmia, the use of IV β-blockers for this indication would seem to be quite limited.

---

†NOTE: There is three times as much *elemental calcium* in one 10-ml ampule of **10% calcium chloride** (270 mg) as in one 10-ml ampule of **10% calcium gluconate** (90 mg). Thus, it is essential to specify which salt of calcium you desire! Lower doses of calcium chloride (i.e., 5 ml—*or perhaps even less!*) may be adequate when use is for prophylactic pretreatment of PSVT to prevent hypotension (Dolan, 1991).

In view of the fact that the optimal dose of calcium for pretreatment use is not yet known, and that excessive administration of this cation could potentially produce adverse effects (such as marked bradycardia), we share the concern urged by Jameson and Hargarten (1992) to at least initially consider use of a lower dose (i.e., no more than half an ampule of calcium chloride).

verapamil is administered. This probably reflects the blood pressure raising effect of calcium infusion, and resultant stimulation of carotid baroreceptors (Schoen et al, 1991).

Consideration of pretreatment calcium infusion would seem to be most suitable for patients with supraventricular tachyarrhythmias when the hemodynamic status is borderline (i.e., systolic blood pressure <90 to 100 mm Hg). In patients with supraventricular tachyarrhythmias who are given verapamil without such pretreatment, one should not forget that IV infusion of calcium chloride may help to reverse hypotension should it occur.

Practically speaking, verapamil does *not* have any role in the acute treatment of ventricular arrhythmias.* This point *cannot* be emphasized too strongly! Thus, *verapamil should never be given indiscriminately as a diagnostic and/or therapeutic trial to patients with regular, wide QRS complex tachyarrhythmias of uncertain etiology.*

Illustration of the potentially disastrous consequences that may result from empiric use of verapamil in this setting has been borne out in a study performed by Stewart et al (1986). Thirty-nine percent of the patients in the study presented with a wide-complex tachycardia that was misdiagnosed as PSVT, when in fact the rhythm was ventricular tachycardia. Hemodynamic deterioration occurred in *all* of the patients presumptively treated with IV verapamil.

Considering that verapamil is a vasodilator with negative inotropic properties, it should not be surprising that inadvertent administration of this drug to a patient with hemodynamically stable ventricular tachycardia commonly precipitates acute decompensation. That is, the vasodilatory effect of verapamil counteracts the principle compensatory mechanism (i.e., vasoconstriction) that the patient had been using to maintain perfusion and preserve consciousness. Rather than reflexive administration of verapamil when the etiology of a wide-complex tachyarrhythmia is unclear, it would seem far more prudent to thoroughly search the 12-lead ECG for subtle clues to the etiology of the arrhythmia, and/or to consider IV pro-

---

*There are two special forms of ventricular tachycardia that DO respond to treatment with verapamil. *Both of these forms are rare*—and we mention them *only* for completeness. In one of the forms, the site of origin of the ventricular tachycardia is the right ventricular outflow tract. As a result, a 12-lead ECG demonstrates a wide-complex tachycardia with a LBBB configuration and an inferior frontal plane axis (Buxton et al, 1987). The other form appears to originate from the midinferior septum, and manifests as a wide-complex tachycardia with a RBBB and LAHB configuration on the 12-lead ECG (Lin et al, 1983; Miller and Josephson, 1990). When these unusual forms of ventricular tachycardia are seen, they usually occur in relatively young adults *without* other evidence of underlying organic heart disease. Hemodynamic stability is the general rule. Exercise commonly precipitates the arrhythmia, and treatment with either β-blockers or verapamil is often effective. Long-term prognosis is usually excellent.

A final situation in which IV verapamil may be used acutely to terminate an episode of ventricular tachycardia is for patients who develop this arrhythmia as a *direct result* of coronary spasm (Singh and Nademanee, 1987).

It should be emphasized that *all three of these types of ventricular tachycardia are rare*—and that practically speaking, **IV verapamil has NO place in the acute treatment of a wide-complex tachycardia of uncertain etiology.**

cainamide—a drug that may work for either supraventricular or ventricular tachycardia (Wellens, 1986).

Adenosine (Adenocard)

How Dispensed: 6 mg are contained in a 2-ml vial (= 3 mg/ml).

Indications:

- Supraventricular tachyarrhythmias such as PSVT in which a portion of the reentrant loop involves the AV node.
- As a diagnostic maneuver to help determine the etiology of supraventricular tachyarrhythmias in which atrial activity is not evident.

DOSE AND ROUTE OF ADMINISTRATION

IV Bolus: 6 mg by *IV push*. If there is no response after 1 to 2 minutes, give 12 mg by IV push—which may be repeated a final time (1 to 2 minutes later) for a total dose of 6 + 12 + 12 = 30 mg. *If there is still no response, it is unlikely that adenosine will work—and alternative therapy should be tried.*

Because of the ultrashort half-life of adenosine, administration should be by **IV push**—*with the drug injected as fast as possible*—followed immediately by a **saline flush** to prevent any of the drug from getting caught in the IV tubing where it rapidly breaks down (Medical Letter, 1990).

- Therapeutic effects from a dose of IV adenosine are almost always seen within 10 to 40 seconds. As a result, one need *not* wait more than 1 to 2 minutes between repeat doses.
- Alteration in the degree of underlying adrenergic or vagal tone may affect individual patient susceptibility to the drug, and account for at least some of the variation in the therapeutic dose range. Patients with a higher degree of underlying sympathetic tone are more likely to require a higher dose of the drug.
- Higher doses of adenosine are also likely to be needed for patients receiving theophylline or consuming large quantities of caffeine because adenosine is competitively antagonized by methylxanthines (Medical Letter, 1990).
- Lower than usual doses (i.e., 3 mg or less) should be used in patients receiving dipyridamole (persantine) because this drug inhibits adenosine transport and greatly potentiates its effect (Medical Letter, 1990). Extra caution (and lower than usual doses) should also be used in patients receiving carbamezepine (tegretol) because this drug may potentiate the degree of AV block produced by adenosine (Medical Letter, 1990; Mader, 1992).

Pediatric Dosing: 0.05 mg/kg by IV push initially, increasing each dose by 0.05 mg/kg (up to a maximal pediatric dose of 0.25 mg/kg).

COMMENTS

One of the most exciting advances in antiarrhythmic therapy is the development of adenosine for treatment of PSVT. Although the antiarrhythmic effect of the drug has been known for more than 50 years, and adenosine was considered along with verapamil in the early 1980s as a treatment for PSVT, it has only recently been approved for general use in this country.

Adenosine is a naturally occurring endogenous nucleoside that is found in all cells of the body in the form of ATP. Its primary effect is to slow conduction through the AV node (Belhassen and Pelleg, 1984; Munoz et al, 1984). It also depresses SA node automaticity and alters repolarization characteristics of atrial tissue (DiMarco et al, 1983). Actions of the drug are thought to be mediated by depression of calcium-dependent slow conduction channels, increased potassium conduction, and possibly indirect adrenergic effects (DiMarco et al, 1985).

By far, the most intriguing clinical characteristics of adenosine are its rapid onset of action and ultrashort half-life, which is estimated to be *less than* 10 seconds (Crankin et al, 1989; Garratt et al, 1989). As a result, both beneficial and adverse effects of the drug are extremely short-lived. Although a definite drawback of the short half-life is that recurrence of the arrhythmia may be seen in the immediate post-conversion period, the advantages of an *almost immediate* therapeutic effect and minimal *duration* of any adverse effects that do occur seem to far outweigh this drawback.

> It is important to appreciate that adenosine will *not* be useful in the treatment of either atrial fibrillation or MAT. This is because reduction in the rate of the ventricular response to these arrhythmias will last only as long as the duration of action of the drug. Because the principle site of action of adenosine is the AV node, the drug does little to convert the disorganized atrial activity inherent in both atrial fibrillation and MAT.
>
> For the same reason, adenosine will usually *not* convert atrial flutter to sinus rhythm. However, by transiently increasing the degree of AV block, it typically produces a momentary reduction in the ventricular response—similar to the effect produced by application of a vagal maneuver (i.e., **"medical Valsalva"**). As a result, administration of IV adenosine may be invaluable as a *diagnostic aid* for revealing atrial activity that was not readily apparent on the initial ECG (Crankin et al, 1989).

Adenosine is most effective in terminating *reentry* tachyarrhythmias such as PSVT, especially when a portion of the reentry circuit involves the AV node. Alteration of conduction properties in at least one arm of the reentry loop—even if it is of only *momentary* duration—is usually all that is needed to interrupt the cycle and restore sinus rhythm. Thus, clinical reports in the literature for acute termination of the *initial* episode of PSVT generally exceed 90% when full doses of adenosine are used (Crankin et al, 1989; Garratt et al, 1989; DiMarco et al, 1990).

> An interesting observation to be made from the literature is that most reported studies on the use of adenosine for treatment of PSVT have been performed in the electrophysiologic laboratory. Immediate recurrence of PSVT after treatment is less common in this type of setting in which the arrhythmia often has to be *induced* (by programmed delivery of one or more electrical stimuli at a critical point in the cardiac cycle) in order to be studied.
>
> In contrast, one might anticipate recurrence of the arrhythmia to be much more common when PSVT is studied as it occurs in its "natural setting." A recent trial by Cairns and Niemann (1991) suggests this to be the case. In their review of a series of patients who presented to the emergency department with acute onset of PSVT, administration of IV adenosine was highly (>90%) effective in converting the initial episode to sinus rhythm. However, *more than half of the patients had recurrence of their arrhythmia within 5 minutes after initial conversion!*
>
> In all cases, recurrence of the arrhythmia was preceded by the presence of frequent PACs—which presumably altered conduction properties in one or both arms of the reentrant circuit—and ultimately led to arrhythmia recurrence. Although repeat administration of adenosine was uniformly successful in terminating the recurrent episode, *all patients required additional therapy with another (i.e., longer-acting) antiarrhythmic agent to maintain sinus rhythm!*

Important points to take away from the study by Cairns and Niemann are that:
1. Adenosine is extremely effective in *initial* conversion of reentrant supraventricular tachyarrhythmias such as PSVT that involve the AV node as part of the reentrant loop.
2. Recurrence of the arrhythmia (within *minutes* after initial conversion) is common—and should not be unexpected considering the extremely short half-life of the drug.
3. Although repeat doses of adenosine are usually equally effective in converting the recurrent episode, use of another (longer-acting) antiarrhythmic agent will often be needed to maintain sinus rhythm.

The actions of IV adenosine are most commonly compared to the actions of IV verapamil. Although both drugs are similar in their efficacy in the acute treatment of PSVT, there are important clinical differences between these two agents *(Table 2B-1)*.

> In addition to the treatment of PSVT, IV verapamil is a drug of choice for acute treatment of rapid atrial fibrillation and MAT (when heart rate control is needed). Verapamil is also useful as an adjunctive treatment measure for slowing the ventricular response to atrial flutter. Long-term antiarrhyth-

mic control can then be maintained by the use of oral vera-pamil.

Practically speaking, the much shorter duration of action of adenosine limits its use to *acute conversion* of PSVT. Despite the drawback of a relatively high recurrence rate of PSVT, the almost immediate onset of action and rapid disappearance of drug from the circulation provide distinct advantages compared to verapamil that allow more rapid determination of whether the drug will work, a shorter duration of any adverse effects that do occur, and the use of adenosine as a diagnostic aid for uncovering the mechanism of certain complex cardiac arrhythmias.

Adenosine may be of *diagnostic assistance* in a number of ways. As already noted, transient increase in the degree of AV block may unmask hidden atrial activity (especially atrial flutter) in a manner similar to that which occurs with application of vagal maneuvers (i.e. "medical Valsalva"). Reduction in the ventricular response of a wide-complex tachyarrhythmia (as a result of adenosine-induced AV block) may facilitate confirmation of a supraventricular etiology with aberrant conduction (Camm and Garratt, 1991). The drug may also facilitate diagnosis of ventricular tachycardia in some patients who demonstrate retrograde atrial activation by producing transient ventriculoatrial (i.e. V-A) dissociation (Crankin et al, 1989). Finally, adenosine may have special utility in uncovering a previously unsuspected (i.e., "latent") accessory pathway in some patients with PSVT by allowing conduction of occasional preexcited complexes at the time of termination of the arrhythmia (Carratt et al, 1989). This may occur as a result of the block in AV conduction (leaving the accessory pathway as the only available avenue for transmission of the impulse) and/or from the reduction in accessory pathway antegrade refractoriness that adenosine produces (Camm and Garratt, 1991).

Discussion of adverse effects and precautions for using IV verapamil were included in our review of that drug. Adenosine is a mild cutaneous vasodilator and bronchoconstrictor. As a result, it may produce transient flushing and/or cough (especially in patients with a history of bronchospasm). In addition, it occasionally produces chest discomfort and/or *marked* slowing of the heart rate (including sinus pauses of up to several seconds in duration!). Although adverse effects are relatively common, they are almost always short-lived and are usually not of clinical significance (Medical Letter, 1990; DiMarco et al, 1990; Camm and Garratt, 1991). Caution is advised, however, in using this drug for treatment of patients with a history of asthma (Camm and Garratt, 1990).

IV verapamil is *contraindicated* for treatment of a wide-complex tachycardia when the etiology of the arrhythmia is unclear. Although we do not advocate routine use of adenosine in this situation, the drug appears to be much less likely to precipitate ventricular fibrillation than verapamil if inadvertently given to a patient who turns out to have ventricular tachycardia (Sharma et al, 1990; Camm and Garratt, 1991). Similarly, the risk of precipitating ventricular fibrillation from administration of adenosine to a patient with a wide-complex tachycardia from atrial fibrillation or flutter in the presence of WPW appears to be exceedingly small (Camm and Garratt, 1991). Adenosine may therefore be a preferable (i.e., *safer*) agent to use if empiric medical treatment of a *presumed* supraventricular tachycardia is *emergently* needed in a prehospital setting (McCabe et al, 1992). Like verapamil, adenosine may also be effective in treating the rare form of ventricular tachycardia that arises from the right ventricular outflow tract, and that is usually seen in younger adults without significant underlying heart disease (Camm and Garratt, 1991).

A final advantage of adenosine is that it is the preferred agent for medical treatment of PSVT in infants and children (Till et al, 1989; Rossi and Burton, 1989). Experience in treatment of PSVT during pregnancy with both verapamil and adenosine is extremely limited. Both drugs appear to be effective in this situation (Podolsky and Varon, 1991; Byerly et al, 1991; Propp, 1992). However, verapamil crosses the placenta, and there have been isolated case reports of the drug causing intrauterine fetal death (Podolsky and Varon, 1991; Gianopoulos, 1989). Moreover, the markedly shorter half-life of adenosine as compared with verapamil, minimizes the duration of fetal exposure (Mariani, 1992). Thus, until additional prospective studies are performed, adenosine is probably the preferred agent to use if a pregnant patient with PSVT is in need of treatment.

Table 2B-1

Comparative Features of Verapamil and Adenosine*		
	VERAPAMIL	**ADENOSINE**
Efficacy for initial conversion of PSVT to sinus rhythm	≥90% efficacy. (Adenosine may work if verapamil is ineffective!)	≥90% efficacy. (Verapamil may work if adenosine is ineffective)
NOTE: As discussed in detail in Chapter 14, recent release of IV diltiazem (for bolus and infusion administration) offers yet another alternative treatment for supraventricular tachyarrhythmias.		

Table 2B-1

Comparative Features of Verapamil and Adenosine*—cont'd		
	VERAPAMIL	**ADENOSINE**
Likelihood of PSVT recurrence	Variable. (Follow-up use of IV and/or oral verapamil may help to maintain sinus rhythm)	High (because of the ultrashort half-life of the drug). Another antiarrhythmic agent will often be needed to maintain sinus rhythm
Efficacy for diagnosis or treatment of other supraventricular arrhythmias	Also effective in conversion and/or helpful in rate control of: • Rapid atrial fibrillation • Atrial flutter • MAT	Antiarrhythmic use is essentially limited to *acute* conversion of reentrant tachyarrhythmias such as PSVT May have diagnostic utility (i.e., "medical Valsalva," detection of a previously latent accessory pathway)
Additional beneficial features	Antiarrhythmic effect from IV formulation lasts longer (up to 30 minutes) Available in an oral formulation (facilitates long-term antiarrhythmic control) Less expensive May be used *synergistically* with digoxin in selected cases to optimize control of the ventricular response (although caution is needed because verapamil may significantly increase serum digoxin levels).	Less likely to precipitate ventricular fibrillation if inadvertently given to a patient with ventricular tachycardia or atrial fibrillation/flutter with WPW Adverse effects are extremely short-lived (usually *less* than a minute) Does not interfere with digitalis, quinidine, or other cardioactive agents Almost immediate onset of action allows rapid determination of whether the drug will be effective. If not, rapid elimination allows subsequent use of IV verapamil or IV β-blocker therapy Agent of choice for medical treatment of PSVT in infants and children May be preferable to verapamil for treatment of PSVT during pregnancy
Contraindications and precautions to use	Should *never* be used if the etiology of a wide-complex tachycardia is unclear May precipitate ventricular fibrillation if given to a patient with WPW and rapid atrial fibrillation Avoid use in patients with sick sinus syndrome, heart failure, or AV block	Use cautiously (if at all) in patients with a history of bronchospasm/asthma Avoid use in patients with sick sinus syndrome, AV block

Table 2B-1

Comparative Features of Verapamil and Adenosine*—cont'd		
	VERAPAMIL	**ADENOSINE**
Adverse effects	Negative inotropic effect Bradyarrhythmias Hypotension	Facial flushing Dyspnea Chest discomfort Bradyarrhythmias Hypotension

Magnesium Sulfate

How Dispensed: 5 g/10 ml:

10% solution—10-ml ampules (5 g) and 20-ml ampules (10 g)

50% solution—2-ml ampules (1 g) and 10-ml ampules (5 g)

Indications:

- Selected cardiac arrhythmias in the acute care setting (i.e., PVCs, MAT, PSVT) that occur in patients who are (or who are likely to be) hypomagnesemic—*especially if conventional measures have failed.*
- *Torsade de pointes* (regardless of whether serum magnesium levels are low).
- Ventricular arrhythmias associated with *digitalis toxicity* (especially if serum magnesium or potassium levels are low or in the low normal range).
- *Possibly* in acute myocardial infarction as an antiarrhythmic treatment/prophylactic measure.
- *Possibly* in cardiac arrest (from refractory ventricular tachycardia/ventricular fibrillation) when other measures have failed (*regardless* of whether prearrest serum magnesium levels were known to be low).

> We emphasize that there is little (i.e., virtually nothing) to lose from empiric administration of IV magnesium to a patient in *refractory* cardiac arrest—and potentially everything to gain.

DOSE AND ROUTE OF ADMINISTRATION

For life-threatening arrhythmias: Give 1 to 2 g (8 to 16 mEq of MgSO$_4$) of the 10% solution IV over 1 to 2 minutes. This dose may be repeated in 5 to 15 minutes if there is no response.

- If time permits, it may be safer to administer the 2 to 4 g of magnesium sulfate as an IV infusion over 20 to 60 minutes. The rate of infusion should be slowed (or temporarily stopped) if hypotension develops.

- A short-lasting flushing sensation is commonly seen with rapid administration of IV magnesium. The sensation usually resolves if the rate of infusion is slowed or temporarily stopped.
- It is best not to administer IV magnesium in the presence of AV block. In addition, caution (and reduced dosing) is advised for patients with significantly impaired renal function or preexisting hypotension.
- When giving magnesium IV, 1 ampule of **calcium chloride** (10 ml of a 10% solution) should be available for IV injection in the event that signs of magnesium toxicity (hypotension, hyporeflexia, decreased respirations) occur.

For less urgent magnesium replacement: Consider more gradual IV infusion (i.e., adding 1 to 2 g of the 10% solution to the patient's IV fluids, and infusing over several hours). This may be repeated one or more times daily over several days (or weeks!) until magnesium body stores have been replenished.

> Despite these precautions—and our suggestion to slow the rate of infusion when the clinical need is less urgent—it should be emphasized that IV infusion of magnesium sulfate is generally well tolerated by patients who are *not* hypotensive. *Significant adverse reactions are surprisingly uncommon*—even when higher doses (1 to 2 g) are given relatively rapidly (i.e., over 1 to 2 minutes) to patients whose baseline serum magnesium level is not low.

IM magnesium replacement: Alternatively for less urgent magnesium replacement, one may administer 1 to 2 g (8 to 16 mEq) of 50% MgSO$_4$ daily by IM injection as needed until body stores are replenished.

COMMENTS

Magnesium is "the forgotten cation." Because serum magnesium levels are still not routinely included as part of the automated chemistry profile at most institutions, *hypomagnesemia commonly goes unrecognized* (Whang and Ryder, 1990). It appears to be present much more frequently than is generally appreciated, and has been found in more than 20% of hospitalized patients who have another associated electrolyte disorder (Whang et al, 1984). A number of other clinical settings are also associated with an increased likelihood of developing hypomagnesemia. As a result, we suggest obtaining a **serum magnesium level** *routinely* in patients with any of the conditions listed in *Table 2B-2.*

Table 2B-2

Clinical Conditions Commonly Associated with Hypomagnesemia

We suggest obtaining a serum magnesium level routinely in patients who:

1. have any of the following other electrolyte abnormalities:
   - Hypokalemia
   - Hyponatremia
   - Hypocalcemia
   - Hypophosphatemia

2. are receiving digitalis or diuretics

3. have congestive heart failure, acute myocardial infarction, significant cardiac arrhythmias, or cardiac arrest

4. have a history of alcohol abuse

5. have renal insufficiency

6. have diabetes mellitus

7. are not receiving adequate nutrition

8. are elderly

Adapted from Whang et al: *Arch Intern Med* 144:1794-1796; 1984; Whang et al: *Arch Intern Med* 145:655-656, 1985; Tzivoni D, Karen A: *Am J Cardiol* 65:1397-1399, 1990.

Caution is advised in interpreting serum magnesium levels. Like potassium, magnesium is largely an *intracellular* cation. More than 98% of body magnesium is contained within the intracellular compartment. However, serum magnesium levels reflect *extracellular* magnesium. As a result, *serum magnesium levels may be normal despite significant body depletion of this cation* (Gums, 1987; Kulick et al, 1988; Tzivoni and Keren, 1990).

Clinically, magnesium administration may therefore still be indicated (as antiarrhythmic treatment or as replacement therapy) *despite* serum magnesium levels in the low normal range for selected patients with certain conditions (such as those suggested in Table 2B-2) in which body depletion of this cation is highly likely.

Serial serum magnesium levels (looking for a trend) may be especially helpful in interpreting the clinical significance of borderline values (Gums, 1987). For example, if it were known that a patient's initial serum magnesium level was 2.7 mEq/L, a repeat serum level of 1.9 mEq/L obtained after initiation of diuretic therapy would be likely to reflect a total body magnesium deficiency even though this value still falls within the "normal" range (i.e., ≥ 1.7 mEq/L).

The electrophysiologic consequences of hypomagnesemia produce similar cardiovascular effects (including arrhythmias) as hypokalemia. Magnesium is a *cofactor* of membrane Na-K-ATP-ase,* and as such plays an integral role in maintaining intracellular potassium levels. Magnesium deficiency thus may lead to inadequate intracellular potassium content with disruption of the intra-extracellular potassium gradient responsible for maintaining the resting membrane potential. This may result in a lowering of membrane threshold potential and an increase in cellular and Purkinje fiber excitability (Perticone et al, 1986; Tzivoni and Keren, 1990; Tobey et al, 1992). A natural accompaniment of these changes is an increased potential for arrhythmogenesis.

The essential role of magnesium as a cofactor in the Na-K-ATP-ase enzyme system explains why simple replacement with potassium supplementation is often unable to correct an intracellular (tissue) potassium deficiency in patients who are also deficient in magnesium. Magnesium replacement (i.e., cofactor replenishment) is imperative in such cases to restore electrical membrane potential to normal. For the same reason, **magnesium administration may be an essential component of the treatment of patients with *hypokalemia* and cardiac arrhythmias** (Tzivoni and Keren, 1990).

The mechanism for magnesium's beneficial effect in the treatment of various cardiac arrhythmias remains unclear. Restoration of electrolyte balance and intracellular membrane stability (as described above) may partially explain its action in patients with torsade de pointes or ventricular arrhythmias, especially when the latter are due to digitalis toxicity (Kulick et al, 1988). Digitalis excess inhibits the function of Na-K-ATP-ase, an effect that magnesium supplementation may counteract (Cannon et al, 1987). Magnesium also prolongs AV nodal conduction and refractoriness, and this could account for recent reports describing the beneficial effect of this cation in treatment of certain supraventricular arrhythmias (Kulick et al, 1988; Wesley et al, 1989). Finally, an association has been noted between low serum magnesium levels and the occurrence of frequent ventricular ectopy in the setting of acute myocardial infarction (Rasmussen et al, 1988; Tzivoni and Keren, 1990).

Less is known about the role of magnesium in the setting of cardiac arrest, although an association has been noted between low myocardial magnesium levels and cases of sudden cardiac death (Cannon et al, 1987; Tzivoni and

---

*Sodium potassium adenosine triphosphatase (Na-K-ATP-ase) is the membrane associated enzyme responsible for pumping sodium out of the cell and potassium into the cell.

Keren, 1990). Anecdotal reports suggest that emergency administration of IV magnesium (as a bolus of 2 to 4 g) may successfully resuscitate certain patients in refractory cardiac arrest, even after prolonged efforts with standard measures have failed (Craddock et al, 1991; Tobey et al, 1992).

> Theories on the proposed mechanism for magnesium's beneficial effect in treatment of malignant ventricular arrhythmias are that it may increase resting membrane potential and prolong the effective refractory period of myocardial cells (Iseri et al, 1983). Alternatively, magnesium infusion may blunt the stress-induced fall in serum potassium caused by the catecholamine surge that is seen with acute myocardial infarction (Rasmussen et al, 1988). A final theory for the mechanism of magnesium's beneficial effect in patients with acute myocardial infarction is that the cation exerts a *cardioprotective* rather than antiarrhythmic action (Schechter et al, 1990). Magnesium possesses a degree of calcium channel-blocking activity, and prophylactic magnesium infusion has been shown to limit infarct size, decrease platelet aggregation, reduce peripheral vascular resistance, and produce coronary vasodilatation (Roden, 1989; Schechter et al, 1990; Abraham et al, 1990).

> *No consensus yet exists on the indications for magnesium administration in emergency cardiac situations such as acute myocardial infarction and cardiac arrest.* We feel it reasonable to strongly consider empiric use of this agent in these settings, particularly if:
> - There is reason to suspect magnesium depletion (as suggested by the presence of any of the conditions listed in Table 2B-2), *or*
> - The patient fails to respond to conventional measures.
>
> The amount of magnesium, route of administration, and rapidity of dosing (i.e., IV bolus over 1 to 2 minutes, or more gradual IV infusion) can then be determined depending on the cause and urgency of the clinical situation.
> We anticipate future years may see increased use of this agent in the management of acute cardiac conditions (*possibly* including an indication for prophylactic infusion with suspected AMI).

Additional discussion on the clinical use of magnesium appears in **Section 11B** *(The Role of Electrolytes in Cardiac Arrest),* **Section 12B** *(Treatment of AMI),* **Section 13G** *(Tricyclic Antidepressant Overdose), and* **Section 16C** *(Torsade de Pointes).*

Procainamide (Pronestyl)

How Dispensed:
For IV bolus: 100 mg/ml (10-ml vials) and 500 mg/ml

For IV infusion: 1 g/2-ml vial
For oral use:
> Procainamide or Pronestyl—tablets of 250, 375, 500, and 750 mg
> Sustained-release preparations (Procan SR—250, 375, 500, and 1,000 mg; Pronestyl-SR—500 mg)

Indications: In the acute care setting indications include treatment of potentially life-threatening ventricular arrhythmias (not responding to lidocaine); wide-complex tachyarrhythmias of uncertain etiology; medical treatment of rapid atrial fibrillation in patients with WPW.

> In less acute settings, procainamide (administered IV or orally) may be used in a similar manner as quinidine to attempt medical conversion of atrial fibrillation or flutter.

Precautions: Procainamide is *contraindicated* for treatment of torsade de pointes (i.e., for ventricular tachyarrhythmias associated with QT interval prolongation). The drug should be used cautiously in patients with borderline blood pressure or significant QRS complex widening.

DOSE AND ROUTE OF ADMINISTRATION

IV Loading Dose: Administer the drug in increments of 100 mg IV *slowly* over a 5-minute period until:
1. The arrhythmia is suppressed.
2. Hypotension occurs.
3. The QRS complex widens by ≥50% over its baseline value.
4. A total loading dose of 1,000 mg has been given.

> Alternatively, IV loading may be accomplished by mixing 500 to 1,000 mg of drug in 100 ml of D5W, and infusing this over a period of 30 to 60 minutes.

IV Infusion: Following IV loading, a continuous infusion at a rate of 2 mg/min (1 to 6 mg/min range) is sometimes used to maintain the antiarrhythmic effect.

> Alternatively, oral therapy may be started after IV loading with procainamide (375 to 500 mg PO q 3 to 4 hours) or a sustained release preparation (Procan SR or Pronestyl-SR in a dose of between 500 to 1,000 mg PO q 6 to 8 hours).

COMMENTS

Procainamide is a type IA antiarrhythmic agent with electrophysiologic and clinical properties that are similar to those of quinidine. As a result, it decreases conduction velocity and automaticity, and is effective in the treatment of *both* atrial and ventricular arrhythmias.

In the setting of cardiac arrest, procainamide is the second drug of choice (after lidocaine) for treatment of frequent and complex PVCs (including sustained ventricular tachycardia). On occasion, it may be used together with lidocaine to produce a synergistic antiarrhythmic effect.

A number of features make procainamide an extremely attractive antiarrhythmic agent for use in emergency cardiac care. Like quinidine, the drug is effective for treatment of *both* supraventricular and ventricular tachyarrhythmias. In a non-ischemic setting, IV procainamide appears to be *at least* as effective as lidocaine in the treatment of ventricular arrhythmias including ventricular tachycardia (Armengol et al, 1989; Wesley et al, 1991). Procainamide is also effective for treatment of rapid atrial fibrillation in patients with WPW (because it prolongs the *anterograde* refractory period of the accessory pathway). This is a decided advantage over digoxin and verapamil, which may each facilitate anterograde conduction over the accessory pathway (and potentially precipitate ventricular fibrillation if inadvertently given to a patient with atrial fibrillation and WPW).

A unique feature of IV procainamide is its utility in the setting of a wide-complex tachycardia of uncertain etiology. IV verapamil is contraindicated in this situation because of the high likelihood of precipitating ventricular fibrillation if the rhythm turns out to be ventricular tachycardia. Although some authorities favor empiric use of adenosine, others question the safety of this approach. Adenosine is unlikely to be helpful if the rhythm turns out to be ventricular tachycardia, and it could (at least theoretically) prove harmful. In contrast, empiric use of IV procainamide is likely to produce a beneficial response *regardless* of what the wide-complex tachycardia turns out to be! It may convert PSVT with aberrant conduction or preexisting bundle branch block by altering conduction properties in one (or both) arms of the reentry circuit. If the rhythm is slightly irregular, IV procainamide may help in the medical conversion of atrial fibrillation, and it is a drug of choice for acute treatment of rapid atrial fibrillation in association with WPW. The drug is also likely to be effective if the rhythm turns out to be ventricular tachycardia. Even if IV procainamide fails to convert ventricular tachycardia to sinus rhythm, it will often slow the ventricular response of this arrhythmia. Thus, a patient with persistent ventricular tachycardia is much more likely to be able to tolerate the arrhythmia at a heart rate of 140 beats/min, than at a rate of 180 beats/min.

A final advantage of procainamide is the availability of an oral form of the drug. This greatly facilitates conversion from IV administration to long-term antiarrhythmic maintenance therapy.

In general, administration of IV procainamide is well tolerated as long as the precautions highlighted above are observed.

Adverse effects seen with long-term use of the drug include nausea, vomiting, neutropenia, and drug-induced lupus erythematosus (with fever, malaise, arthralgia or arthritis, and pleural or pericardial effusions). As is the case for other antiarrhythmic agents, there is an approximately 5% to 10% incidence of *proarrhythmia* (i.e., paradoxic worsening of the arrhythmia being treated).

Propranolol (Inderal)

How Dispensed: 1 mg/1-ml vial

Indications: Limited in the acute care setting to refractory ventricular arrhythmias, including ventricular fibrillation (especially if acute ischemia, excessive sympa-

thetic discharge, digitalis toxicity, and/or cocaine overdose are suspected as contributing etiologic factors); supraventricular tachyarrhythmias (as an alternative agent for patients who have not responded to IV verapamil, adenosine, and/or digoxin).

Precautions: Propranolol is contraindicated in patients with acute bronchospasm, congestive heart failure, and/or intraventricular conduction disturbances.

If IV verapamil has been given, IV propranolol is contraindicated for at least the next 30 minutes (because the combination of these agents may result in marked cardiac slowing or even asystole).

DOSE AND ROUTE OF ADMINISTRATION

Administer 0.5 to 1 mg IV *slowly* over at least a 5-minute period *(not to exceed 1 mg/min!)*. Allow several minutes for the drug to work. Repeat increments of 0.5 to 1 mg may be given up to a total dose of 5 mg.

COMMENTS

Propranolol is a nonselective β-blocking agent. The drug decreases automaticity, reduces the sinus rate of discharge, and prolongs AV conduction time. Despite these beneficial actions, it appears that the use of IV propranolol in the acute care setting has greatly decreased in recent years. This is unfortunate because *there are situations when this IV β-blocking agent (or esmolol) becomes the drug of choice for the treatment of life-threatening ventricular tachyarrhythmias!*

The most difficult part about making recommendations for the use of IV β-blockers in the setting of cardiopulmonary arrest is knowing when to administer these drugs. Clearly there are times when all other antiarrhythmic agents will fail, and *only* IV β-blockers may save the patient (Mason et al, 1985).

Situations in which IV β-blockers are most likely to be successful in the treatment of life-threatening ventricular arrhythmias are those in which *excessive sympathetic tone* is implicated as an important etiologic factor. This is most likely to be the case in patients who develop ventricular tachycardia/fibrillation in association with acute *anterior* infarction, especially when the arrhythmia was preceded by a period of sinus tachycardia and/or systolic hypertension. It may also occur when cardiac arrest is precipitated by *cocaine overdose*, or an extremely *stressful/anxiety-producing* event. Another situation in which IV β-blockers are likely to be successful is in the treatment of patients who demonstrate a period of antecedent *ischemia*, as may be suggested by development of ST segment depression on monitoring prior to the arrest. Moreover, administration of empiric IV β-blocker therapy would also be reasonable (if not advisable) for patients with *recurrent cardiac arrest* (especially if other antiarrhythmic agents have failed and/or sinus tachycardia appears to precede each recurrence). The stress of the cardiac arrest itself in this situation may *secondarily* contribute/lead to a hyperadrenergic state with elevated catecholamine levels that might respond favorably to β-blocker therapy (Morisaki et al, 1991). Finally, persistent reflex stimulation of sympathetic tone may result in response to *severe left ventricular dysfunction* and lead to a chronic state of catecholamine excess that predisposes the patient to the development of life-threatening ventricular arrhythmias (Meredith et al, 1991).

We are *not* advocating IV propranolol as a panacea treatment for all ventricular tachyarrythmias that occur in the setting of cardiopulmonary arrest. Clearly, lidocaine remains the drug of choice for treatment of ventricular arrhythmias, and procainamide or bretylium (and perhaps magnesium sulfate?) are next in line. However, in select situations (such as those described above), a trial of IV propranolol may occasionally prove to be lifesaving—especially if other standard measures have failed.

Amiodarone (Cordarone)

How Dispensed: 200 mg scored tablets

NOTE: As of this writing, IV amiodarone remains an *investigational* drug that is *NOT* yet available for general use. We nevertheless have chosen to include it in this "Essential Drug" section because of the potential role it may assume in the near future in the treatment of refractory ventricular fibrillation and other life-threatening ventricular arrhythmias that have not responded to more conventional measures.

Indications:

In the Setting of Cardiac Arrest: Refractory ventricular fibrillation.

In Emergency Cardiac Care: Life-threatening ventricular arrhythmias not responsive to other therapy; selected patients with refractory supraventricular arrhythmias/tachyarrhythmias associated with WPW.

DOSE AND ROUTE OF ADMINISTRATION

Suggested Dose for Cardiac Arrest: Until results from additional studies become available, dosing recommendations for amiodarone in the setting of cardiac arrest will be largely empiric. One might consider IV loading of 150 to 500 mg over a period of 5 to 10 minutes—and repeating this dose 15 to 30 minutes later if needed. If successful, a maintenance infusion might be considered (Leak, 1986; Herre et al, 1989).

Dosing for Other Indications: See text.

COMMENTS

The treatment of choice for ventricular fibrillation is defibrillation. Although numerous factors may influence outcome (e.g., patient age, prearrest medical condition, precipitating cause), early recognition of cardiac arrest and prompt defibrillation are by far the most important determinants of survival. Practically speaking, *the likelihood of successful resuscitation with ultimate discharge from the hospital is exceedingly poor if the patient does not respond to countershock.*

Antiarrhythmic therapy (with lidocaine and/or bretylium) has been recommended for treatment of refractory ventricular fibrillation (ACLS Text, 1986). However, results from such treatment are generally disappointing and have not been shown to improve long-term prognosis. Clearly the need exists for new alternative treatment measures that are able to positively impact on survival when initial attempts at defibrillation are unsuccessful. Emergency use of amiodarone may offer a ray of hope in this regard *when the IV preparation of the drug becomes available for general use.*

Williams et al (1989) studied the use of IV amiodarone in a small, retrospective review of 14 patients who were victims of in-hospital cardiac arrest from ventricular tachycardia or ventricular fibrillation. Most of these patients had documented coronary artery disease and left ventricular dysfunction. Cardiac arrest was monitored in 13 of the patients, and resuscitative efforts were started promptly in all cases. Despite appropriate attempts at defibrillation and antiarrhythmic treatment with lidocaine, bretylium, and/or procainamide, refractory ventricular fibrillation persisted for *at least 30 minutes* in all patients (mean time = 75 minutes) before amiodarone was administered. Patients were then loaded with **IV amiodarone** (150 to 600 mg over 5 to 15 minutes). Repeat doses (up to a maximum total of 1,350 mg) were given to half of the patients.

Results of the study were eye-opening: *11 of the 14 patients were resuscitated, and 8 survived to leave the hospital.* In 4 of 11 patients, a single countershock after the loading dose of amiodarone restored normal sinus rhythm. In the remaining 7 survivors, several boluses of the drug were needed in addition to cardioversion to restore normal sinus rhythm.

Survivors were generally treated with an IV maintenance infusion of amiodarone (set at a rate of between 20 to 50 mg/hr). In addition, all patients required transient dopamine infusion to counteract hypotension (although this was primarily believed to be a consequence of the prolonged resuscitation rather than a direct adverse effect of IV amiodarone). Ventricular tachycardia recurred during hospitalization in only 3 of 11 survivors.

Despite the small size and retrospective nature of this study by Williams et al, it has important potential clinical implications. All study subjects were victims of prolonged cardiac arrest that had been refractory to *all other* standard treatment measures. Nevertheless, IV amiodarone successfully restored spontaneous circulation in 11 of 14 patients! Although it is clearly premature to routinely recommend early use of this drug for treatment of ventricular fibrillation that does not respond to initial attempts at countershock, the following approach may be reasonable:

---

1. Expedite recognition and treatment of ventricular fibrillation by standard measures:
   - Prompt initial defibrillation—with repeat countershock as per the recommended protocol
   - Early use of epinephrine
   - Lidocaine and/or bretylium for refractory ventricular fibrillation

2. Look for potentially treatable contributing causes:
   - Electrolyte disturbances, severe acidosis, hypoxemia, hypothermia, etc.

3. *Consider* alternative treatment measures relatively *early* in the process if the patient fails to respond:
   - Empiric trial of IV magnesium sulfate *and/or* **IV amiodarone** *and/or* IV β-blockers

4. Amiodarone may be especially useful for patients with cardiac arrest from *recurrent* ventricular tachycardia who are unable to maintain sinus rhythm with conventional antiarrhythmic therapy

---

Additional studies are needed to determine the true role (if any) of amiodarone in the treatment of refractory ventricular fibrillation/recurrent ventricular tachycardia.

> Discussion of the use of amiodarone outside of the setting of cardiac arrest extends beyond the scope of this book. As a result, we limit our comments to mention of several key points of interest about this drug (Med Letter, 1986; Skluth, Grauer, and Gums, 1989):
>
> - Amiodarone is a class III antiarrhythmic agent. As such, it prolongs the duration of the myocardial action potential and increases the refractory period without affecting the resting membrane potential of myocardial cells. The drug depresses sinus node function and prolongs the PR, QRS, and QT intervals.
>
> - Overall, amiodarone may be the most potent antiarrhythmic agent available for treatment of ventricular arrhythmias, supraventricular arrhythmias, and tachyarrhythmias associated with accessory pathway conduction (i.e., WPW).
>
> - The side-effect profile associated with long-term use of amiodarone is extensive and may result in adverse reactions affecting most major organ systems. Potential side effects include pulmonary fibrosis, liver function abnormalities, neurologic symptoms (ataxia, dizziness, tremor, neuropathy, mental status changes), photosensitivity, bluish gray skin discoloration, corneal microdeposits, and thyroid function abnormalities. In addition, amiodarone may produce adverse cardiac effects including exacerbation of heart failure

(from the drug's slight negative inotropic effect), proarrhythmia (including torsade de pointes), and marked bradycardia. Finally, amiodarone is associated with numerous drug interactions including warfarin, digoxin, and virtually all other antiarrhythmic agents. As a result of this extensive side effect profile, administration of long-term amiodarone therapy is probably best left to the specialist.

- The most unique feature of amiodarone is its tremendously long elimination half-life (of 20 to 100 days!). Antiarrhythmic effects after oral loading may not become apparent for days to *weeks* after initiation of oral therapy. Unfortunately, if any of the above cited adverse effects do occur, they are likely to persist for an extended period of time. Thus, long-term use of the drug is potentially problematic, and requires careful monitoring and regular follow-up.

- Dosing of amiodarone is highly variable, depending on individual patient characteristics and the arrhythmia being treated. Protocols for oral loading call for administration of between 600 to 1,600 mg daily for up to 4 to 8 weeks, followed by oral maintenance therapy of between 100 to 600 mg/day. In general, adverse effects are dose related and cumulative.

- Amiodarone may be given IV as an emergency treatment for life-threatening arrhythmias. An initial loading dose (of 3 to 5 mg/kg administered over a 5- to 10-minute period) may be followed by continuous infusion of the drug (at a rate of between 20 to 50 mg/hr). *IV amiodarone used in this manner may be highly effective in achieving initial control of life-threatening ventricular arrhythmias that do not respond to more conventional agents* (Herre et al, 1989).

In summary, the future may see amiodarone assume an increasingly important role in the emergency treatment of life-threatening ventricular arrhythmias and cardiac arrest:

- Empiric IV amiodarone (in a dose of 150 to 500 mg over 5 to 10 minutes) may be a reasonable option for the emergency care provider to consider when confronted with refractory ventricular fibrillation that fails to respond to standard treatment measures.

- For patients who are not in cardiac arrest, use of amiodarone (either IV or oral) generally falls within the realm of the specialist. In selected cases, the drug may be a life-saving measure in the management of malignant ventricular arrhythmias that have not responded to other treatment.

References

Abraham AS, Balkin J, Rosenmann D, Eylath U, Zion MM: Continuous intravenous infusion of magnesium sulfate after acute myocardial infarction, *Magnesium Trace Elem* 9:137–142, 1990.

American College of Cardiology/American Heart Association Task Force: Guidelines for the early management of patients with acute myocardial infarction, *Circulation* 82:664–707, 1990.

American Heart Association Subcommittee on Emergency Cardiac Care: Standards and guidelines for cardiopulmonary resuscitation (CPR) and emergency cardiac care (ECC), *JAMA* 255(suppl):2905–2992, 1986.

Armengol RE, Graff J, Baerman JM, Swiryn S: Lack of effectiveness of lidocaine for sustained, wide QRS complex tachycardia, *Ann Emerg Med* 18:254–257, 1989.

Barnett JC, Touchon RC: Short-term control of supraventricular tachycardia with verapamil infusion and calcium pretreatment, *Chest* 97:1106–1109, 1990.

Barton C, Callaham M: High-dose epinephrine improves the return of spontaneous circulation rates in human victims of cardiac arrest, *Ann Emerg Med* 20:722–725, 1991.

Belhassen B, Pelleg A: Acute management of paroxysmal supraventricular tachycardia: Verapamil, adenosine triphosphate or adenosine? *Am J Cardiol* 54:225–227, 1984.

Brown CG, Werman HA, Davis EA, Hamlin R, Hobson J, Ashton JR: The comparative effect of graded doses of epinephrine on regional cerebral blood flow in a swine model, *Ann Emerg Med* 15:1138–1144, 1986.

Brown CG, Werman HA, Davis EA, Hobson J, Hamlin RL: The effect of graded doses of epinephrine on regional myocardial blood flow during CPR in swine. *Circulation* 75:491–497, 1987.

Brown CG, Taylor RB, Werman HA, Luu T, Ashton J, Hamlin RL: Myocardial oxygen delivery/consumption during cardiopulmonary resuscitation: A comparison of epinephrine and phenylephrine, *Ann Emerg Med* 17:302–308, 1988.

Brown CG, Martin DR, Pepe PE, Stueven H, Cummins RO, Gonzales E, Jastrenski M, and the Multi Center High-Dose Epinephrine Group: A comparision of standard-dose and high-dose epinephrine in cardiac arrest outside the hospital, *N Eng J Med* 327:1051-1055, 1992.

Buxton AE, Marchlinski FE, Doherty JU, Flores B, Josephson ME: Hazards of intravenous verapamil for sustained ventricular tachycardia, *Am J Cardiol* 59:1107–1110, 1987.

Byerly WG, Hartmann A, Foster DE, Tannenbaum AK: Verapamil in the treatment of maternal paroxysmal supraventricular tachycardia, *Ann Emerg Med* 20:552–554, 1991.

Cairns CB, Niemann JT: Intravenous adenosine in the emergency department management of paroxysmal supraventricular tachycardia, *Ann Emerg Med* 20:717–721, 1991.

Callaham ML: High-dose epinephrine therapy and other advances in treating cardiac arrest, *West J Med* 152:697–703, 1990.

Callaham M, Barton CW, Kayser S: Potential complications of high-dose epinephrine therapy in patients resuscitated from cardiac arrest, *JAMA* 265:1117–1122, 1991.

Camm AJ, Garrat CJ: Adenosine and supraventricular tachycardia, *N Engl J Med* 325:1621–1629, 1991.

Cannon LA, Heiselman DE, Dougherty JM, Jones J: Magnesium levels in cardiac arrest victims: relationship between magnesium levels and successful resuscitation, *Ann Emerg Med* 16:1195–1199, 1987.

Chatterjee K: *Digitalis, catecholamines, and other positive inotropic agents.* In Parmley WW, Chaterjee K, editors: *Cardiology,* Philadelphia, 1990, Lippincott.

Coon GA, Clinton JE, Ruiz E: Use of atropine for brady-asystolic prehospital cardiac arrest, *Ann Emerg Med* 10:462–467, 1981.

Craddock L, Miller B, Clifton G, Krumbach B, Pluss W: Resuscitation from prolonged cardiac arrest with high-dose intravenous magnesium sulfate, *J Emerg Med* 9:469–476, 1991.

Crankin A, Goldroyd K, Chong E, Rae AP, Cobe SM: Value and limitations of adenosine in the diagnosis and treatment of narrow and broad complex tachycardias, *Br Heart J* 62:195–203, 1989.

Crespo SG, Schoffstall JM, Fuhs LR, Spivey WH: Comparison of two doses of endotracheal epinephrine in a cardiac arrest model, *Ann Emerg Med* 20:230–234, 1991.

Dasta JF: Assessing the phrase "renal dose" dopamine, *Crit Care Med* 19:843, 1991 (letter).

DiMarco JP, Sellers TD, Berne RM, West GA, Belardinelli L: Adenosine: Electrophysiologic effects and therapeutic use for terminating paroxysmal supraventricular tachycardia, *Circulation* 68:1254–1263, 1983.

DiMarco JP, Sellers TD, Lerman BB, Greenberg MI, Berne RM, Belardinelli L: Diagnostic and therapeutic use of adenosine in patients with supraventricular tachyarrhythmias, *J Am Coll Cardiol* 6:417–425, 1985.

DiMarco JP, Miles W, Akhtar M, Milstien S, Sharma AD, Platia E, McGovern B, Scheinman NM, Govier WC, and the Adenosine for PSVT Study Group: Adenosine for paroxysmal supraventricular tachycardia: Dose ranging and comparison with verapamil—assessment in placebo-controlled, multicenter trials, *Ann Int Med* 113:104–110, 1990.

Dolan DL: Intravenous calcium before verapamil to prevent hypotension, *Ann Emerg Med* 20:588–589, 1991 (editorial).

Garratt C, Linker N, Griffith M, Ward D, Camm J: Comparison of adenosine and verapamil for termination of paroxysmal junctional tachycardia, *Am J Cardiol* 64:1310–1316, 1989.

Gianopoulos JG: Cardiac disease in pregnancy, *Med Clin North Am* 73:639–651, 1989.

Goetting MG, Contreras E: Systemic atropine administration during cardiac arrest does not cause fixed and dilated pupils, *Ann Emerg Med* 20:55–57, 1991.

Gonzalez ER, Ornato JP, Garnett AR, Levine RL, Young DS, Racht EM: Dose-dependent vasopressor response to epinephrine during CPR in human beings, *Ann Emerg Med* 18:920–926, 1989.

Gonzalez ER, Ornato JP: The dose of epinephrine during cardiopulmonary resuscitation in humans: What should it be? *DICP: Ann Pharmacother* 25:773–777, 1991.

Grauer K, Cavallaro D, Gums J: New developments in cardiopulmonary resuscitation, *Am Fam Physician* 43:832–844, 1991.

Greenberg MI, Mayeda DV, Chrzanowski R, Brumwell D, Baskin SI, Roberts JR: Endotracheal administration of atropine sulfate, *Ann Emerg Med* 11:546–548, 1982.

Gums JG: Clinical significance of magnesium: a review, *Drug Intell Clin Pharm* 21:240–246, 1987.

Haft JI, Habbab MA: Treatment of atrial arrhythmias: Effectiveness of verapamil when preceded by calcium infusion, *Arch Intern Med* 146:1085–1089, 1986.

Herre JM, Sauve MJ, Malone P, Griffin JC, Helmy I, Langberg JJ, Goldberg H, Scheinman MM: Long-term results of amiodarone therapy in patients with recurrent sustained ventricular tachycardia or ventricular fibrillation, *J Am Coll Cardiol* 13:442–449, 1989.

Iseri LT, Chung P, Tobis J: Magnesium therapy for intractable ventricular tachyarrhythmias in normomagnesemic patients, *West J Med* 138:823–828, 1983.

Jameson SJ, Hargarten SW: Calcium pretreatment to prevent verapamil-induced hypotension in patients with SVT, *Ann Emerg Med* 21:84, 1992 (letter).

Jose AD, Taylor RR: Autonomic blockage by propranolol and atropine to study intrinsic myocardial function in man, *J Clin Invest* 48:2019–2031, 1969.

Kaiser SC, McLain PL: Atropine metabolism in man, *Clin Pharmacol Ther* 11:214–227, 1970.

Kastor JA: Multifocal atrial tachycardia, *N Engl J Med* 322:1713–1717, 1991.

Koehler RC, Michael JR, Guerci AD, Chjandra N, Schleien CL, Dean JM, Rogers MC, Weisfeldt ML, Traystman RJ, Beneficial effect of epinephrine infusion on cerebral and myocardial blood flows during CPR, *Ann Emerg Med* 14:744–749, 1985.

Koscove EM, Paradis NA: Successful resuscitation from cardiac arrest using high-dose epinephrine therapy, *JAMA* 259:3031–3034, 1988.

Kulick DL, Hong R, Ryzen E, Rude RK, Rubin JN, Elkayam U, Rahimtoola SH, Bhandari AK: Electrophysiologic effects of intravenous magnesium in patients with normal conduction systems and no clinical evidence of significant cardiac disease, *Am Heart J* 115:367–372, 1988.

Lang R, Klein HO, Weiss E, David D, Sareli P, Levy A, Guerrero J, Segni ED, Kaplinsky E: Superiority of Oral Verapamil Therapy to Digoxin in Treatment of Chronic Atrial Fibrillation. *Chest* 83:491–499, 1983.

Leak D: Intravenous amiodarone in the treatment of refractory life-threatening cardiac arrhythmias in the critically ill patient, *Am Heart J* 111:456–462, 1986.

Levine JH, Michael JR, Guarnieri T: Treatment of multifocal atrial tachycardia with verapamil, *N Engl J Med* 312:21–25, 1985.

Lin FC, Finley CD, Rahimtoola SH, Wu D: Idiopathic paroxysmal ventricular tachycardia with a QRS pattern of right bundle branch block and left axis deviation: A unique clinical entity with specific properties, *Am J Cardiol* 52:95–100, 1983.

Mader TJ: Adenosine: Adverse interactions, *Ann Emerg Med* 21:453, 1992 (letter).

Margolis B, DeSilva RA, Lown B: Episodic drug treatment in the management of paroxysmal arrhythmia, *Am J Cardiol* 45:621–626, 1980.

Mariani PJ: Pharmacotherapy of pregnancy-related SVT, *Ann Emerg Med* 21:229, 1992 (letter).

Martin D, Werman HA, Brown CG: Four case studies: High-dose epinephrine in cardiac arrest, *Ann Emerg Med* 19:322–326, 1990.

Mason JR, Marek JC, Loeb HS, Scanlon PJ: Intravenous propranolol in the treatment of repetitive ventricular tachyarrhythmias during resuscitation from sudden death, *Am Heart J* 110:161–165, 1985.

Massumi RA, Mason DT, Amsterdam EA, DeMaria A, Miller RR, Scheinman MM, Zelis R: Ventricular fibrillation and tachycardia after intravenous atropine for treatment of bradycardias, *N Engl J Med* 287:336–338, 1977.

McCabe JL, Adhar GC, Menegazzi JJ, Paris PM: Intravenous adenosine in the prehospital treatment of paroxysmal supraventricular tachycardia, *Ann Emerg Med* 21:358–361, 1992.

McGovern B, Garan H, Ruskin JN: Precipitation of cardiac arrest by verapamil in patients with Wolff-Parkinson-White syndrome, *Ann Intern Med* 104:791–794, 1986.

McGrath RB: In-house cardiopulmonary resuscitation: After a quarter of a century, *Ann Emerg Med* 16:1365–1368, 1987.

Medical Letter: Amiodarone, *Med Lett Drugs Ther* 28:49–50, 1986.

Medical Letter: Adenosine, *Med Lett Drugs Ther* 32:63, 1990.

Medical Letter: Drug Treatment of Cardiac Arrest, *Med Lett Drugs Ther* 34:30, 1992.

Meredith IT, Broughton A, Jennings GL, Esler MD: Evidence of a selective increase in cardiac sympathetic activity in patients with sustained ventricular arrhythmias, *N Engl J Med* 325:618–624, 1991.

Michael JR, Guerci AD, Koehler RC, Shi AY, Tsitlik J, Chandra N, Niedermeyer E, Rogers MC, Traystman RJ, Weisfeldt ML: Mechanisms by which epinephrine augments cerebral and myocardial perfusion during cardiopulmonary resuscitation in dogs, *Circulation* 69:822–835, 1984.

Miller JM, Josephson ME: *Ventricular arrhythmias.* In Parmley WW, Chatterjee K, editors: *Cardiology* Philadelphia, 1990, Lippincott.

Morisaki H, Takino Y, Ichikizaki K, Ochiai R: Sympathetic responses in out-of-hospital cardiac arrest, *J Emerg Med* 9:313–316, 1991.

Munoz A, Leenhardt A, Sassine A, Galley P, Puech P: Therapeutic use of adenosine for terminating spontaneous paroxysmal supraventricular tachycardia, *Eur Heart J* 5:735–738, 1984.

Myerburg RJ, Kessler KM, Zaman L, Conde CA, Castellanos A: Survivors of prehospital cardiac arrest, *JAMA* 247:1485–1490, 1982.

Niemann JT, Adomian GE, Garner D, Rosborough JP: Endocardial and transcutaneous cardiac pacing, calcium chloride, and epinephrine in postcountershock asystole and bradycardias, *Crit Care Med* 13:699–704, 1985.

Ornato JP: High-dose epinephrine during resuscitation: A word of caution, *JAMA* 265:1160–1161, 1991.

Paradis NA, Koscove EM: Epinephrine in cardiac arrest: A critical review, *Ann Emerg Med* 19:1288–1301, 1990.

Paradis NA, Martin GB, Rivers EP, Goetting MG, Appleton TJ, Feingold M, Nowak RM: Coronary perfusion pressure and the return of spontaneous circulation in human cardiopulmonary resuscitation, *JAMA* 263:1606–1113, 1990.

Paradis NA, Martin GB, Rosenberg J, Rivers EP, Goetting MG, Appleton TJ, Feingold M, Cryer PE, Wortsman J, Nowak RM: The effect of standard- and high-dose epinephrine on coronary perfusion pressure during prolonged cardipulmonary resuscitation, *JAMA* 265:1139–1144, 1991.

Perticone F, Adinolfi L, Bonaduce D: Efficacy of magnesium sulfate in the treatment of torsade de pointes, *Am Heart J* 112:847–849, 1986.

Podolsky SM, Varon J: Adenosine use during pregnancy, *Ann Emerg Med* 20:1027–1028, 1991.

Propp DA, Broderick K, Pesch D: Adenosine during pregnancy, *Ann Emerg Med* 21:453–454, 1992 (letter).

Rasmussen HS, Cintin C, Aurup P, Breum L, McNair P: The effect of intravenous magnesium therapy on serum and urine levels of potassium, calcium, and sodium in patients with ischemic heart disease, with and without acute myocardial infarction, *Arch Intern Med* 148:1801–1805, 1988.

Roden DM: Magnesium treatment of ventricular arrhythmias, *Am J Cardiol* 63:43G–46G, 1989.

Rose JS, Bhandari A, Rahimtoola SH, Wu D: Effective termination of reentrant supraventricular tachycardia by single dose oral combination therapy with pindolol and verapamil, *Am Heart J* 112:759–765, 1986.

Rossi AF, Burton DA: Adenosine in altering short- and long-term treatment of supraventricular tachycardia in infants, *Am J Cardiol* 64:685–686, 1989.

Roth A, Harrison E, Mitani G, Cohen J, Rahimtoola SH, Elkayam U: Efficacy and safety of medium- and high-dose diltiazem alone and in combination with digoxin for control of heart rate at rest and during exercise in patients with chronic atrial fibrillation, *Circulation* 73:316–324, 1986.

Schechter M, Hod H, Marks N, Behar S, Kaplinsky E, Rabinowitz B: Beneficial effect of magnesium sulfate in acute myocardial infarction, *Am J Cardiol* 66:271–274, 1990.

Scheinman MM, Thorburn D, Abbott JA: Use of atropine in patients with acute myocardial infarction and sinus bradycardia, *Circulation* 52:627–635, 1975.

Schoen MD, Parker RB, Hoon TJ, Hariman RJ, Ballman JL, Beekman KJ: Evaluation of the pharmacokinetics and electrocardiographic effects of intravenous verapamil with intravenous calcium chloride pretreatment in normal subjects, *Am J Cardiol* 67:300–304, 1991.

Semenkovich CF, Jaffee AS: Adverse effects due to morphine sulfate: Challenge to previous clinical doctrine, *Am J Med* 79:325–330, 1985.

Sharma AD, Klein GJ, Yee R: Intravenous adenosine triphosphate during wide QRS complex tachycardia: Safety, therapeutic efficacy, and diagnostic utility, *Am J Med* 88:337–343, 1990.

Singh BN, Nademanee K: Use of calcium antagonists for cardiac arrhythmias, *Am J Cardiol* 59:153B–162B, 1987.

Skluth H, Grauer K, Gums J: Ventricular arrhythmias: An assessment of newer therapeutic agents, *Postgrad Med* 85:137–153, 1989.

Steinberg JS, Katz RJ, Bren GB, Buff LA, Varghese PJ: Efficacy of oral diltiazem to control ventricular response in chronic atrial fibrillation at rest and during exercise, *J Am Coll Cardiol* 9:405–411, 1987.

Stewart RB, Bardy GH, Greene HL: Wide complex tachycardia: Misdiagnosis and outcome after emergent therapy, *Ann Intern Med* 104:766–771, 1986.

Steuven HA, Tonsfeldt DJ, Thompson BM, Whitcomb J, Kastenson E, Aprahamian C: Atropine in asystole: Human studies, *Ann Emerg Med* 13:815–817, 1984.

Stiell IG, Hebert PC, Weitzman BN, Wells GA, Raman S, Stark RM, Higginson LAJ, Ahuja J, Dickinson GE: High-dose epinephrine in adult cardiac arrest, *N Eng J Med* 327:1045-1050, 1992.

Thomas M, Woodgate D: Effect of atropine on bradycardia and hypotension in acute myocardial infarction, *Br Heart J* 28:409–413, 1966.

Till J, Shinebourne EA, Rigby ML, Clarke B, Ward DE, Rowland E: Efficacy and safety of adenosine in the treatment of supraventricular tachycardia in infants and children, *Br Heart J* 62:204–211, 1989.

Tobey RC, Birnbaum GA, Allegra JR, Horowitz MS, Plosay JJ: Successful resuscitation and neurologic recovery from refractory ventricular fibrillation after magnesium sulfate administration, *Ann Emerg Med* 21:92–96, 1992.

Tortolani AJ, Risucci DA, Powell SR, Dixon R: In-hospital cardiopulmonary resuscitation during asystole: Therapeutic factors associated with 24-hour survival, *Chest* 96:622–626, 1989.

Tzivoni D, Keren A: Suppression of ventricular arrhythmias by magnesium, *Am J Cardiol* 65:1397–1399, 1990.

Wellens HJJ: The wide QRS tachycardia, *Ann Med Intern* 104:879, 1986.

Wesley RC, Haines DE, Lerman BB, DiMarco JP, Crampton RS: Effect of magnesium sulfate on supraventricular tachycardia, *Am J Cardiol* 63:1129–1131, 1989.

Wesley RC, Resh W, Zimmerman D: Reconsiderations of the routine and preferential use of lidocaine in the emergent treatment of ventricular arrhythmias, *Crit Care Med* 19:1439–1444, 1991.

Whang R, Oei TO, Aikawa JK, Watanabe A, Vannatta J, Fryer A, Markanich M: Predictors of clinical hypomagnesemia, hypokalemia, hypophosphatemia, hyponatremia, and hypocalcemia, *Arch Intern Med* 144:1794–1796, 1984.

Whang R, Oei TO, Watanabe A: Frequency of hypomagnesemia in hospitalized patients receiving digitalis, *Arch Intern Med* 145:655–656, 1985.

Whang R, Ryder KW: Frequency of hypomagnesemia and hypermagnesemia: Requested vs routine, *JAMA* 263:3063–3064, 1990.

Williams ML, Woelfel A, Cascio WE, Simpson RJ, Gettes LS, Foster JR: Intravenous amiodarone during prolonged resuscitation from cardiac arrest, *Ann Int Med* 110:839–842, 1989.

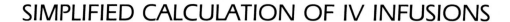

SIMPLIFIED CALCULATION OF IV INFUSIONS

The Rule of 250 ml

For the uninitiated, calculation of intravenous (IV) infusions may appear as a formidable task requiring a minimum of a Master's degree in mathematics to attain proficiency. In most cases, calculation of IV infusions is carried out by those assigned to the care of IV lines that have already been established—namely, by nurses and paramedics. Physicians often go no further than a request for the following:

"Please mix up a drip of drug X, *and run the infusion as fast as we need to*."

Practically speaking, the experienced nurse will usually have already anticipated the situation and be "ready and waiting" almost before the order is given. Occasionally, however, the team leader may find himself/herself working with code team members who are less familiar with the preparation of IV infusions. For this reason, *all* ACLS providers should at least be familiar with a method for formulating IV infusions of the most important drugs.

Another reason for learning how to prepare IV infusions is to successfully complete the ACLS Provider Course. Most ACLS Instructors will ask this information of the Code Leader during the MEGA CODE Station. Fortunately, the calculation of IV infusions for those drugs most commonly used in emergency cardiac care (and ACLS) *need not be difficult!* Application of a simplified and easily remembered rule greatly facilitates the process. The method we favor invokes the *"Rule of 250 ml,"* and works as follows:

Mix **1 unit** or *whatever* drug you are using in **250 ml** of D5W, and set the infusion to run at **15** to **30 drops/min.**

Application of this rule allows you to estimate an appropriate *initial* IV infusion rate for *most* of the essential drugs used in ACLS. Adjustments in dosing can then be made based on the patient's clinical response.

The KEY to the application of the **"Rule of 250 ml"** lies with determining the amount of drug contained in 1 "unit." Because the contents of a vial or ampule may vary from one hospital to the next (and are sometimes premixed in varying amounts by the pharmaceutical company), it is essential to become familiar with the drug formulary used in your institution. *Our calculations in this section assume the following:*

For the *antiarrhythmic agents,* **1 unit of drug** = 1 g of **lidocaine**
                                                              = 1 g of **procainamide**
                                                              = 1 g of **bretylium**

For the *catecholamines,* **1 unit of drug** = 1 mg (= 1 vial) of **isoproterenol**
                                                          = 1 mg (= 1 ampule) of **epinephrine** (in a 1:10,000 concentration for **SDE**)

For *dopamine,* **1 unit of drug** = 200 mg (= 1 ampule) of **dopamine**

Substitution into the **Rule of 250 ml** of the quantities listed above for "1 unit" of drug (for any of the three *antiarrhythmic agents*, two *catecholamines*, or *dopamine*) automatically results in an appropriately prepared initial IV infusion rate. For example:

For Preparing an IV Infusion for One of the *Antiarrhythmic Agents:*

Lidocaine—Mix **1 g** (i.e., 1 unit) of *lidocaine* in **250 ml** of D5W (or 2 g in 500 ml), and set the infusion to run at **30 drops/min** (= 2 mg/min).

Procainamide—Mix **1 g** (i.e., 1 unit) of *procainamide* in **250 ml** of D5W (or 2 g in 500 ml), and set the infusion to run at **30 drops/min** (= 2 mg/min).

Bretylium—Mix **1 g** (i.e., 1 unit) of *bretylium* in **250 ml** of D5W (or 2 g in 500 ml), and set the infusion to run at **15 drops/min** (= 1 mg/min).

The usual *initial* IV infusion rate for lidocaine and procainamide in the setting of cardiac arrest is 2 mg/min (= 30 drops/min). In contrast, it is more common to begin a bretylium infusion at 1 mg/min (= 15 drops/min).

As emphasized in Sections B and E of Chapter 12, many factors (e.g., age, body weight, hepatic function, and presence of heart failure) influence the rate of lidocaine clearance from the body. This may necessitate a lower rate of infusion for lidocaine (0.5 to 1 mg/min) after the acute stage.

For Preparing an IV Infusion for the *Catecholamines:*

Isoproterenol—Mix **1 mg** (i.e., 1 vial = 1 unit) of *isoproterenol* in **250 ml** of D5W, and set the infusion to run at **30 drops/min** (= 2 μg/min).

Standard Dose Epinephrine (SDE)—Mix **1 mg** (i.e., 1 ampule = 1 unit) of a *1:10,000 solution of epinephrine* in **250 ml** of D5W, and set the infusion to run at between **15 to 30 drops/min** (= 1 to 2 μg/min).

IV infusion of these catecholamines is initiated at a low rate (of 2 μg/min for isoproterenol, or 1 to 2 μg/min for epinephrine [when SDE is being used]). The rate of infusion may then be progressively increased as needed until the desired clinical effect is achieved.

In general, the rate of an isoproterenol infusion should not exceed 10 μg/min. In contrast, much higher doses of epinephrine (i.e., HDE) may be indicated for treatment of cardiac arrest (i.e., refractory ventricular fibrillation, asystole, or EMD) if SDE is ineffective (see the section on *Epinephrine* below).

For Preparing an IV Infusion for *Dopamine:*

Dopamine—Mix **200 mg** (i.e., 1 ampule = 1 unit) of *dopamine* in **250 ml** of D5W, and set the infusion to run at between **15** to **30 drops/min.**

Although the calculation of a dopamine infusion is somewhat complex, *the Rule of 250 ml may still be used to approximate an appropriate starting dose for IV infusion of this drug!* Setting the initial infusion rate at between 15 to 30 drops/min should deliver in the range of 2 to 5 μg/kg/min for most patients. The lower rate (i.e., 15 drops/min) may be preferable as a staring dose for patients who weigh less, and/or when preferential flow to the renal vascular bed is a high priority (i.e., dopaminergic effect of the drug). As for isoproterenol and

epinephrine, the rate of the dopamine infusion may then be progressively increased as needed depending on the patient's clinical response.

Being able to apply the Rule of 250 ml for the drugs we have listed should be more than sufficient for passing this aspect of the ACLS Provider Course. To do this, all one need remember is the Rule itself, and the quantity of drug contained in "1 unit" for each of the agents.

Derivation of the Rule of 250 ml takes the process one step further, and facilitates understanding the method of preparation.

Consider the following illustrative problems:

PROBLEM   **Make up a *lidocaine* infusion. How fast should the drip be set to infuse 2 mg of lidocaine per minute?**

ANSWER   Applying the Rule of 250 ml for any of the three *antiarrhythmic agents* (lidocaine, procainamide, or bretylium) suggests that **1 unit** of drug (i.e., 1 g) be mixed in **250 ml** (or 2 g in 500 ml) of D5W. The following calculation illustrates how doing so results in a concentration of 4 mg of lidocaine per ml:

$$\frac{\text{1 unit of drug}}{\text{250 ml}} = \frac{\text{1 g}}{\text{250 ml}} \left[\text{or } \frac{\text{2 g}}{\text{500 ml}} \right] = \frac{\text{4 g of drug}}{\text{1,000 ml}}$$

$$\frac{\text{4 g of drug}}{\text{1,000 ml}} = \frac{\text{4,000 mg}}{\text{1,000 ml}} = \frac{\text{4 mg}}{\text{ml}}$$

The problem posed above in this particular case is to determine how fast to set the infusion so as to deliver 2 mg of lidocaine per minute. Since we calculated the *concentration* of drug to be **4 mg/ml**, this means that in order to deliver 2 mg of lidocaine per minute, the drip would have to be set to infuse 0.5 ml/min. That is:

$$\frac{\text{4 mg}}{\text{ml}} \div 2 = \frac{\text{2 mg}}{\text{0.5 ml}}$$

The last piece of information required for determining the rate of the infusion is awareness of the *conversion factor* between *milliliters* and *drops* when a microdrip is used:

> **1 ml = 60 drops** for a **microdrip**

Thus, IV infusion with a microdrip set at a rate of **60 drops/min** will deliver the amount of drug contained in **1 ml** of fluid. It follows that:

• IV infusion at a rate of **30 drops/min** will deliver *half* this amount (i.e., the amount of drug contained in 1 ml ÷ 2) or:

> **30 drops/min** delivers **0.5 ml/min**

and

• IV infusion at a rate of **15 drops/min** will deliver *one-quarter* this amount (i.e., the amount of drug contained in 1 ml ÷ 4) or:

> **15 drops/min** delivers **0.25 ml/min**

In this particular case, setting the drip to infuse at a rate of 60 drops/min will deliver 4 mg of drug (since the concentration of lidocaine is 4 mg/ml). Thus, *the drip should be set to run in at a rate of* **30 drops/min** *to deliver half this amount (or 2 mg/min) of lidocaine.*

> For lidocaine then (at this same concentration), an IV infusion rate of:
> • **15** drops/min delivers **1 mg/min** of drug
> • **30** drops/min delivers **2 mg/min** of drug
> • **45** drops/min delivers **3 mg/min** of drug
> • **60** drops/min delivers **4 mg/min** of drug

We again emphasize that with the exception of HDE, the Rule of 250 ml works well for estimating an appropriate *initial* infusion rate for *each* of the six drugs we have listed (i.e., lidocaine, procainamide, bretylium, isoproterenol, SDE, and dopamine).

> Note that most manipulations in the above calculations involve *unit conversions* (e.g., 1 ml = 60 drops for a microdrip; 1,000 mg = 1 g; 1,000 μg = 1 mg, etc.) Thus, the *KEY* for determining the correct drug concentration and initial infusion rate is to *carefully maintain equivalent units of measure throughout each calculation!*

Application of the Rule of 250 ml for calculating an appropriate initial infusion rate for *isoproterenol* and *dopamine* is demonstrated in the next two illustrative problems.

PROBLEM   **Make up an *isoproterenol* infusion. How fast should the drip be set to achieve an initial infusion rate of 2 μg/min?**

ANSWER   Applying the Rule of 250 ml for the *catecholamines* (isoproterenol or epinephrine—when SDE is being used) suggests that **1 unit** of drug (i.e., 1 mg) be

mixed in **250 ml** of D5W. The following calculation illustrates how doing so results in a *concentration* of 4 μg/ml:

$$\boxed{\frac{1 \text{ unit of drug}}{250 \text{ ml}}} = \frac{1 \text{ mg}}{250 \text{ ml}} = \frac{4 \text{ mg}}{1,000 \text{ ml}} = \frac{4,000 \text{ μg of drug}}{1,000 \text{ ml}}$$

$$\frac{4,000 \text{ μg}}{1,000 \text{ ml}} = \frac{4 \text{ μg}}{\text{ml}} \left[\begin{array}{c} \text{which means that} \\ \text{there is} \end{array} = \frac{2 \text{ μg}}{0.5 \text{ ml}} \right]$$

Since the problem posed above is to determine the infusion rate needed to deliver 2 μg/min, the drip should again be set to infuse at a rate of **30 drops/min** (i.e., at 0.5 ml/min). Infusion at this rate will deliver 2 μg/min (since this is the amount of drug contained in each 0.5 ml of IV fluid).

PROBLEM   **Make up a *dopamine* infusion. How fast should the drip be set to achieve an initial infusion rate of 5 μg/kg/min for a patient who weighs 80 kg?**

ANSWER   Applying the Rule of 250 ml for *dopamine* suggests that **1 unit** of drug (i.e., 200 μg) be mixed in **250 ml** of D5W. The following calculation illustrates how doing so results in a concentration of 800 μg/ml:

$$\boxed{\frac{1 \text{ unit of drug}}{250 \text{ ml}}} = \frac{200 \text{ mg}}{250 \text{ ml}} = \frac{800 \text{ mg}}{1,000 \text{ ml}} = \frac{800,000 \text{ μg of drug}}{1,000 \text{ ml}}$$

$$\frac{800,000 \text{ μg}}{1,000 \text{ ml}} = \frac{800 \text{ μg}}{\text{ml}} \left[\begin{array}{c} \text{which means that} \\ \text{there is} \end{array} = \frac{400 \text{ μg}}{0.5 \text{ ml}} \right]$$

An initial infusion rate of 5 μg/kg/min entails delivery of **400 μg/min** of dopamine for a patient who weighs 80 kg (i.e., 5 × 80 = 400). Since 400 μg is the amount of drug contained in each 0.5 ml of IV fluid at the concentration calculated in this example, the drip should again be set to infuse at a rate of **30 drops/min.**

> As emphasized earlier in this section (and in Section B in the discussion of dopamine), the vasoactive effects of this drug depend on the rate of infusion. In the setting of cardiac arrest, IV infusion of the drug is most often begun at a rate of between 2 to 5 μg/kg/min (which comes out to about 15 to 30 drops/min for most patients). The rate of infusion is then progressively increased until the desired clinical effect is achieved. At higher infusion rates (i.e., ≥10 to 20 μg/kg/min), α-adrenergic (vasoconstrictor) effects predominate, and the actions of the drug become similar to those of norepinephrine. This usually occurs at infusion rates of *greater* than 60 drops/min.

EPINEPHRINE

As we acknowledged in the beginning of Section B of this chapter, the optimal dose of epinephrine for treatment of cardiac arrest remains unknown. For any given patient, dosing requirements will be influenced by a host of factors including the condition being treated (i.e. ventricular fibrillation, asystole, or EMD); the duration of the code until medication is administered; and patient specific variables such as age, body weight, the presence of underlying medical conditions, and the patient's response to other treatment measures.

The one point about epinephrine dosing that has become clear is that significantly higher doses than were used in the past may be needed by some patients to achieve and maintain adequate coronary perfusion pressure for as long as CPR is in progress.

Because the recommended *initial* infusion rate for SDE (of 1 to 2 μg/min) is *at least* 100-fold *less* than the initial rate commonly selected for IV infusion of HDE, it would appear preferable to use a different formulation for administration of these two dosing regimens. Incorporation of two modifications into the Rule of 250 ml allows it to be used in an alternative form for calculation of IV infusion with HDE:

1. Instead of the 1:10,000 dilution of drug that is used for preparing SDE infusions, consider using a **1:1,000 solution** of epinephrine. *This alteration increases the concentration of drug by a factor of 10, and thus facilitates IV infusion by minimizing the amount of fluid that needs to be administered for any given quantity of drug.* Whereas 10 ml of a 1:10,000 solution of epinephrine would have to be given to deliver 1 mg of drug, the same amount of epinephrine (1 mg) can be given in 1 ml of a 1:1,000 solution.

2. Use **50 mg** (instead of 1 mg) as the quantity of drug contained in **1 unit.** *This alteration increases the concentration of drug for an IV infusion of HDE by a factor of 50 compared to the concentration of drug for an IV infusion of SDE.*

Thus, preparation of IV infusion of *epinephrine* for treatment of cardiac arrest might proceed as follows:

For Preparation of **SDE** (**S**tandard-**D**ose **E**pinephrine): Mix **1 unit** of drug (i.e., 1 mg = 1 ml of a 1:10,000 solution) in **250 ml** of D5W, and set the infusion to run at **15 to 30 drops/min** (to achieve an *initial* infusion rate of 1 to 2 μg/min).

$$\boxed{\frac{1 \text{ unit of drug}}{250 \text{ ml}}} = \frac{1 \text{ mg}}{250 \text{ ml}} = \frac{4 \text{ mg}}{1,000 \text{ ml}} = \frac{4,000 \text{ μg of drug}}{1,000 \text{ ml}}$$

$$\frac{4,000 \text{ μg}}{1,000 \text{ ml}} = \frac{4 \text{ μg}}{\text{ml}} \left[\text{which means that there is} = \frac{2 \text{ μg}}{0.5 \text{ ml}} \right]$$

Infusion at a rate of **30 drops/min** (i.e., at 0.5 ml/min) will deliver 2 μg/min (since this is the amount of drug contained in each 0.5 ml of IV fluid at this concentration). Infusion at *half* this rate (i.e., at **15 drops/min,** or at 0.25 ml/min) will therefore deliver 1 μg/min. *Note that preparation of an IV infusion of SDE according to the Rule of 250 ml is virtually the same as preparation of an isoproterenol infusion.*

For Preparation of **HDE** (**H**igh-**D**ose **E**pinephrine): Mix **1 unit** of drug (i.e., **50 mg** = 50 ml of a **1:1,000** solution) in **250 ml** of D5W. The following calculation illustrates how doing so results in a *concentration* of 200 μg/ml:

$$\boxed{\frac{1 \text{ unit of drug}}{250 \text{ ml}}} = \frac{50 \text{ mg}}{250 \text{ ml}} = \frac{200 \text{ mg}}{1,000 \text{ ml}} = \frac{200,000 \text{ μg of drug}}{1,000 \text{ ml}}$$

$$\frac{200,000 \text{ μg}}{1,000 \text{ ml}} = \frac{200 \text{ μg}}{\text{ml}} \left[\text{which means that there is} = \frac{100 \text{ μg}}{0.5 \text{ ml}} \right]$$

Setting the *initial* infusion rate to run at **30 to 60 drops/min** will deliver 100 to 200 μg/min. *This rate can then be rapidly increased as needed until the desired clinical effect is achieved.*

IV Infusion of Other Drugs

The Rule of 250 ml is practical, as well as being easy to learn and remember. *It works.* It also encompasses what you will need to know about IV infusions to pass the ACLS Provider Course.

For those with a desire (or need) to know more, we conclude this section with two final concepts:

1. Calculation of IV infusion rates for three *other* drugs that do *not* follow the Rule (i.e., *dobutamine, nitroprusside,* and *nitroglycerin*).
2. Introduction of the **"Rule of 150 mg in 250 ml."**

Application of these concepts is again best demonstrated by the use of illustrative problems:

DOBUTAMINE

Dobutamine is a synthetic catecholamine with positive inotropic effects. It is most commonly used for treatment of patients with heart failure who maintain a normal (or near normal) blood pressure *(see Chapter 14 for further discussion on the clinical use of this drug).*

A dobutamine infusion is usually begun at a rate of 2.5 μg/kg/min. The rate of infusion may then be titrated upward as needed (with the usual range of infusion being between 2.5 to 10 μg/kg/min). *Calculation of a dobutamine infusion is best accomplished by application of the Rule of 150 mg in 250 ml (see below).*

NITROPRUSSIDE AND NITROGLYCERIN

Sodium nitroprusside and nitroglycerin are two potent vasodilating agents that share a number of indications in emergency cardiac care including treatment of hypertensive urgency/emergency and preload/afterload reduction (for treatment of patients in heart failure). Of the two, IV nitroprusside is the more potent arterial vasodilator (afterload reducer), whereas nitroglycerin exerts a relatively greater effect on the venous side (reducing preload). IV nitroglycerin also exerts a beneficial vasodilatory effect on the coronary arteries, making it an invaluable antiischemic agent *(see Section B in Chapter 12 and Chapter 14 for further discussion on the clinical use of these agents.)*

Although neither nitroprusside nor nitroglycerin follow the Rule of 250 ml (because the initial infusion rate is *not* 15 to 30 drops/min), preparation of an IV infusion for either agent may still be facilitated by using the same parameters as were suggested for preparation of an IV infusion of HDE. Therefore:

> To Prepare an IV Infusion of **IV Nitroprusside** or **Nitroglycerin**: Mix **1 unit** of drug **(= 50 mg)** in **250 ml** of D5W. As was the case for HDE, this results in a *concentration* of 200 μg/ml:

$$\boxed{\frac{1 \text{ unit of drug}}{250 \text{ ml}}} = \frac{50 \text{ mg}}{250 \text{ ml}} = \frac{200 \text{ mg}}{1,000 \text{ ml}} = \frac{200,000 \text{ μg of drug}}{1,000 \text{ ml}}$$

$$\frac{200,000 \text{ μg}}{1,000 \text{ ml}} = \frac{200 \text{ μg}}{\text{ml}}$$

IV infusion of *nitroprusside* and *nitroglycerin* is usually begun at a rate of **10 μg/min.** *The rate of infusion can then be carefully titrated upward as needed to obtain the desired clinical response.*

PROBLEM   **At what rate should the drip be set (for either *nitroprusside* or *nitroglycerin*) to achieve an initial IV infusion rate of 10 μg/min?**

ANSWER   At the concentration of drug derived above (i.e., 200 μg/ml), 1/20th of a ml would have to be infused each minute to deliver 10 μg of drug per minute (i.e., 200 ÷ 20 = 10 μg/min). Since **60 drops = 1 ml** with a microdrip, 1/20th of 1 ml will be 3 drops (i.e., 60 ÷ 20 = 3). Therefore *the drip should be set at* **3 drops/min** *to achieve an initial infusion rate of 10 μg/min.*

PROBLEM   **By how many drops per minute should a drip of either nitroprusside or nitroglycerin be increased to infuse an additional 10 μg each minute?**

ANSWER   Since we established above that a rate of 3 drops/min infuses 10 μg/min, *the drip would have to be increased by 3 drops each minute to infuse an additional 10 μg/min.* Thus:

- To infuse 20 μg/min, set the drip to infuse at a rate of 6 drops/min.
- To infuse 30 μg/min, set the drip to infuse at a rate of 9 drops/min.
- To infuse 40 μg/min, set the drip to infuse at a rate of 12 drops/min and so forth . . . .

PROBLEM   **What would be the *maximum* infusion rate recommended for nitroprusside for a patient who weighs 80 kg?**

ANSWER   The maximum recommended infusion rate for IV nitroprusside is 8 μg/kg/min. This comes out to 640 μg/min for an 80-kg patient (i.e., 80 × 8 = 640 μg/min).

At the concentration of drug derived above (i.e., 200 μg/ml), the maximum recommended infusion rate would therefore be 3.2 ml/min (640 ÷ 200). Because 60 drops = 1 ml with a microdrip, *the maximum recommended infusion rate of nitroprusside for a patient who weighs 80 kg is 192 drops/min (60 × 3.2).*

The Rule of 150 mg in 250 ml

When precision in the calculation of the rate of IV infusions is needed on a milligram per kilogram basis, the ***"Rule of 150 mg in 250 ml"*** becomes ideal. The Rule is especially helpful for determining the precise rate of infusion for drugs such as dopamine or dobutamine. Clinical application of the Rule involves two steps:

> 1. Mix **150 mg** of *whatever* drug you are using in **250 ml** of D5W. Doing so results in preparation of a drug concentration of 600 μg/ml (as illustrated by the calculation below):

$$\boxed{\frac{150 \text{ mg}}{250 \text{ ml}}} = \frac{600 \text{ mg}}{1,000 \text{ ml}} = \frac{600,000 \text{ μg of drug}}{1,000 \text{ ml}}$$

$$\frac{600,000 \text{ μg}}{1,000 \text{ ml}} = \frac{600 \text{ μg}}{\text{ml}} \left[\begin{array}{c} \text{which means that} \\ \text{there is} \end{array} = \frac{600 \text{ μg}}{60 \text{ drops}} = \frac{10 \text{ μg}}{\text{drop}} \right]$$

Because 1 ml = 60 drops with a microdrip, the resultant concentration of 600 μg/ml = 600 μg/60 drops = a concentration of **10 μg/drop** of IV fluid.

The second step in applying the Rule is to calculate the number of drops per minute at which to set the IV infusion. This is easily done by using the following formula:

> 2. IV infusion rate (in drops/min) $= \dfrac{\text{(Desired μ/kg/min)} \times \text{(Body weight in Kg)}}{10}$

PROBLEM   **Use the *Rule of 150 mg in 250 ml* to make up a *dopamine* infusion. How fast should the drip be set to achieve an initial infusion rate of 3 μg/kg/min for a patient who weighs 60 kg?**

ANSWER

> 1. Mix **150 mg** of *dopamine* in **250 ml** of D5W.

2. IV infusion rate (in drops/min) $= \dfrac{(\text{Desired } \mu g/kg/min) \times (\text{Body weight in Kg})}{10}$

IV infusion rate (in drops/min) $= \dfrac{(3\ \mu g/kg/min) \times (60\ kg)}{10}$

IV infusion rate $= 3 \times 60 \div 10 =$ **18 drops/min**

Thus with a mixture of 150 mg of dopamine in 250 ml of D5W, the infusion rate should be set at 18 drops/min to deliver 3 µg/kg/min for a patient who weighs 60 kg.

PROBLEM   Use the *Rule of 150 mg in 250 ml* to make up a *dobutamine* infusion. How fast should the drip be set to achieve an initial infusion rate of 2.5 µg/kg/min for a patient who weighs 80 kg? How fast will the drip be running at the upper limit of the usual therapeutic range (i.e., at 10 µg/kg/min)?

ANSWER

1. Mix **150 mg** of *dobutamine* in **250 ml** of D5W.

2. IV infusion rate (in drops/min) $= \dfrac{(\text{Desired } \mu g/kg/min) \times (\text{Body weight in Kg})}{10}$

Initial IV infusion rate (in drops/min) $= \dfrac{(2.5\ \mu g/kg/min) \times (80\ kg)}{10}$

Initial IV infusion rate $= 2.5 \times 80 \div 10 =$ **20 drops/min**

Upper limit infusion rate (in drops/min) $= \dfrac{(10\ \mu g/kg/min) \times (80\ kg)}{10}$

Upper limit infusion rate $= 10 \times 80 \div 10 =$ **80 drops/min**

Thus, with a mixture of 150 mg of dobutamine in 250 ml of D5W, the initial infusion rate should be set at 20 drops/min to deliver 2.5 µg/kg/min for a patient who weighs 60 kg. The rate of the infusion at the upper limit of the usual therapeutic range (i.e., at 10 µg/kg/min) will be 80 drops/min for this patient.

In summary, familiarity with the **Rule of 250 ml** facilitates recall of an easily applied method for calculating IV infusions for the drugs commonly used in ACLS (i.e., *lidocaine, procainamide, bretylium, isoproterenol, SDE,* and *dopamine*). Incorporation of two modifications (i.e., use of a 1:1,000 solution of epinephrine and use of 50 mg as the unit size) allows the Rule of 250 ml to be used in an alternative form for calculation of IV infusions with *HDE*.

For those with a desire (or need) to know more, additional modifications and application of the **Rule of 150 mg in 250 ml** allows calculation of IV infusion rates for *nitroprusside, nitroglycerin,* and *dobutamine* (at precise rates).

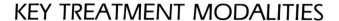

KEY TREATMENT MODALITIES

Precordial Thump

Technique: The precordial thump is a sharp, quick blow that is delivered with the fleshy part of the fist (hypothenar eminence) from a distance of 8 to 12 inches above the chest to the midportion of the sternum. *It should not be so forceful as to break any ribs.*

Indications: *Pulseless* rhythms in the absence of a defibrillator.

COMMENTS

The history of the precordial thump dates back to 1920 when Schott first used the procedure on a patient having Stokes-Adams attacks. Reports in the literature on the use of the thump had been limited since that time until the 1970s. During this period the group of Morgera et al (1979) were the most enthusiastic, reporting a success rate of almost 50% when the thump was administered to patients with sustained ventricular tachycardia that developed in a hospital setting.

> Less favorable results for the efficacy of the thump were obtained by Miller et al (1984), who reported on their experience with the use of this procedure in a prehospital setting. Among the 50 patients included in their study, a thump was administered for ventricular fibrillation in 23 cases and for ventricular tachycardia in 27 cases. None of those in ventricular fibrillation were converted out of this rhythm by the thump. In contrast, the maneuver was successful in converting 12% of the patients in ventricular tachycardia to a supraventricular rhythm with a pulse. However, in 44% of cases it had no effect, and in the remaining 44% of patients, administration of the thump resulted in *deterioration* of the rhythm (to ventricular fibrillation, pulseless idioventricular rhythm, or asystole). The results of this study make it clear that *the thump is NOT a benign procedure.* On the contrary, these authors found the thump to be detrimental more often than helpful, and advocated *against* its routine use in a prehospital setting.

Several practical issues are raised by these results:
1. What is the mechanism of the thump?
2. Why should the thump be effective for some patients, yet detrimental to others?
3. *When should emergency care providers administer this procedure in actual practice?*

> The thump appears to be most effective in terminating rhythms that are dependent on a reentrant pathway. Perhaps the best example of an arrhythmia with this mechanism is *sustained ventricular tachycardia.* Mechanical energy generated by the maneuver produces a low amplitude depolarization (of approximately 2 to 5 joules) that may be potent enough to interrupt a reentrant pathway arrhythmia *if it occurs at an opportune time during the cardiac cycle.* On the other hand, if the thump is delivered during the *vulnerable period,* it may precipitate ventricular fibrillation in much the same manner that the

"R-on-T" phenomenon does. The previous cited study by Miller et al suggests that this latter effect (i.e., precipitation of ventricular fibrillation) is significantly more likely to occur following a thump than is successful conversion to sinus rhythm.

Synchronized cardioversion is an extremely effective modality for treatment of sustained ventricular tachycardia. This is because the substrate for perpetuation of this tachyarrhythmia is most often a macro-reentry pathway. As a result, the arrhythmia commonly responds to cardioversion attempts at surprisingly low energy levels (of as little as 10 to 20 joules). In contrast, much higher energy levels are generally needed to convert a patient out of ventricular fibrillation, since electrical activity in this condition is totally chaotic.

> Practically speaking, it is exceedingly difficult to design a study to demonstrate how energy requirements for defibrillation change with time. Nevertheless, it is thought that extremely low energies (of as little as 5 to 10 joules) may be sufficient to terminate ventricular fibrillation if countershock can be applied at an early enough point in the process (Lown, 1980; Caldwell et al, 1985). Energy requirements for defibrillation appear to increase dramatically (almost *exponentially*) within seconds after the onset of cardiac arrest. Thus for the thump to have a realistic chance at being effective in terminating ventricular fibrillation, *it must be delivered as soon as possible after the onset of this rhythm.*
>
> On *rare* occasions, prompt delivery of a precordial thump has also been shown to convert patients out of asystole (Patros and Goren, 1983; Caldwell et al, 1985). The mechanism of the thump in this situation is unknown, although one might speculate that fine ventricular fibrillation could have been masquerading as asystole in some of these cases.

Our Suggestions for Use

In the past, recommendations for the thump were to employ the maneuver for ventricular tachycardia and fibrillation when the onset of these rhythms was monitored. However, concern for the potential of the procedure to *worsen* the arrhythmia (and precipitate ventricular fibrillation or asystole) led to deemphasis of the thump.

Practically speaking, we find it easiest to conceptualize indications for the use of the thump by thinking of the maneuver as a *"No-lose"* procedure:

> We tend to reserve the thump for patients presenting with *pulseless* rhythms, especially when a defibrillator is not available. If delivered within the early moments of a cardiac arrest, it may occasionally convert a patient out of pulseless ventricular tachycardia, ventricular fibrillation, or even asystole. If out in the field and without access to a defibrillator, there is really *nothing to lose* (and everything to gain) by attempting the maneuver. *The patient will die without it.* In the prehospital setting, it is important not to delay delivery of the thump because energy requirements for converting a patient out of ventricular fibrillation increase rapidly!
>
> On the other hand, if a patient develops ventricular tachy-

cardia or fibrillation and a defibrillator is readily available, use of this device is clearly preferable to administration of the thump. Should the defibrillator be "moments away" (as is usually the case when someone arrests in the intensive care unit or in an emergency department), the option of whether to thump should be at the discretion of the rescuer on the scene. The thump offers the advantage of *speed*, but it has the definite drawback of delivering its mechanical input at an unpredictable point in the cardiac cycle.

Finally, if the patient is in sustained ventricular tachycardia *with* a pulse, do *NOT* use the thump!!! Because of the substantial chance of converting this rhythm to a more malignant one, *there is simply too much to lose by administering a thump in this situation*. If the patient in sustained ventricular tachycardia remains hemodynamically stable, a trial of medical therapy may be reasonable. If the patient is (or becomes) hemodynamically unstable, delivery of an electrical impulse at a *predictable* point in the cardiac cycle (i.e., on the upstroke of the R wave) with *synchronized cardioversion* is much safer and offers a far greater chance for successful conversion to sinus rhythm than does the random delivery of electrical output provided by the thump.

Cough Version

Description: The patient is instructed to *"Cough hard, and keep coughing!"* as soon as the arrhythmia is noted (Schultz and Olivas, 1986).

Indications: At the onset of ventricular tachycardia, ventricular fibrillation, or asystole *before* consciousness is lost.

COMMENTS

As we will discuss in Chapter 10 (on *New Developments in CPR*), it is no longer thought that the principal mechanism for blood flow with CPR is the result of a "squeezing" of the heart between the sternum and vertebral column. Instead, increases in intrathoracic pressure and development of a pressure gradient between the intrathoracic and extrathoracic compartments are thought to play a much more important role. A large part of the impetus for advancing this theory resulted from observation in the cardiac catheterization laboratory that forceful and repetitive coughing (i.e., *"Cough CPR"*) could sustain consciousness for periods of *up to 90 seconds* in patients with pulseless ventricular tachycardia, ventricular fibrillation, or asystole! Intrathoracic pressures as high as 140 mm Hg are produced by such coughing, and are somehow able to generate adequate blood flow *despite* the presence of a nonperfusing rhythm.

It is still not known whether the mechanism of action for cough version is the result of improved coronary perfusion, stimulation of the autonomic nervous system, or conversion of mechanical energy from the cough into an electrical depolarization (since up to 25 joules of kinetic energy may be generated by a cough!). *What is known is that vigorous coughing occasionally converts malignant arrhythmias to normal sinus rhythm* (Caldwell et al, 1985; Schultz and Olivas, 1986).

Since the original description of cough CPR by Criley et al in 1976, instructing patients to cough at the onset of nonperfusing rhythms has become a standard practice in many cardiac catheterization laboratories. However, the technique is still largely ignored by all too many other emergency care providers who rarely seem to invoke coughing at the onset of a malignant arrhythmia.

Our Suggestions for Use

Don't forget about **cough version!!!!** Consider using this technique at the bedside or in the field for *any* patient who remains conscious in the face of a sustained malignant arrhythmia.

Clinically, the most commonly encountered situation in which cough version may be applied is for patients in ventricular tachycardia with a pulse. However, one should not forget the procedure is *also* indicated for pulseless ventricular tachycardia, ventricular fibrillation, and asystole. Practically speaking, because consciousness is so rapidly lost with these latter rhythms, it will usually be impossible for the rescuer to react in time to instruct the patient to begin coughing. Consequently, for individuals with repeated episodes of ventricular tachycardia, one might consider formulating a *prearranged signal* with the patient to indicate that immediate coughing (at 1- to 3-second intervals) must begin. If cough version is successful, it will either convert the rhythm or "buy time" (i.e., maintain perfusion) until definitive therapy can be administered.

Defibrillation

Indications: Ventricular fibrillation, *pulseless* ventricular tachycardia, and asystole (if the possibility exists that the rhythm may really be fine ventricular fibrillation).

Recommended Energy Levels for Adults:
Initial defibrillation attempt—200 joules
2ⁿᵈ defibrillation attempt—300 joules
3ʳᵈ defibrillation attempt—360 joules
Subsequent defibrillation attempts—360 joules (although it may be reasonable to drop back to 200 joules at a later point in the code)

KEY Concept: *The sooner a patient in ventricular fibrillation is defibrillated, the better the chance for survival.*

COMMENTS

Electrical defibrillation is by far the most important treatment modality for the patient in ventricular fibrillation. Convincing studies have shown that if emergency medical service personnel are allowed to do nothing other than defibrillate victims of cardiac arrest, lives will be saved.

The *KEY* determinant of survival for a patient who develops ventricular fibrillation is *time*. Practically speaking, if the patient does not have an underlying irreversible condition, the likelihood that an initial countershock attempt will successfully convert ventricular fibrillation to a rhythm with a pulse is *inversely proportional* to the time from patient collapse until delivery of the electrical discharge.

Energy requirements for electrical conversion of ventricular fibrillation increase dramatically *within* seconds (Winkle et al, 1990). As a result, realistic chances for survival drop off *exponentially* with time, and are markedly reduced when defibrillation is delayed for more than 3 minutes into the code (Hargarten et al, 1990). Prompt performance of CPR—*in and of itself*—will not prevent further deterioration of the rhythm (i.e., to asystole), although it may prolong the period of potential "viability" (i.e., responsiveness to defibrillation) for an additional 1 to 2 minutes (Enns et al, 1983; Eisenberg et al, 1990).

In contrast to the completely unexpected occurrence of out-of-hospital cardiac arrest, when ventricular fibrillation occurs in a setting in which trained medical personnel are able to anticipate this possibility (and are well equipped to handle the situation), defibrillation is almost uniformly successful. This concept is best illustrated by the experience accrued in carefully supervised, cardiac rehabilitation programs in which up to 100% of patients who develop ventricular fibrillation during monitored exercise activity can be resuscitated (Hossack and Hartwig, 1982). Clearly, *the sooner a patient in ventricular fibrillation can be defibrillated, the better the chance for survival.*

Despite the critical importance of prompt defibrillation, this procedure is not without risk. Thus, defibrillation of victims of out-of-hospital cardiac arrest by paramedics at the earliest opportunity will precipitate development of *refractory asystole* in up to one third of cases (Martin et al, 1986). Precipitation of asystole by defibrillation is especially likely to occur in patients who had been unresponsive for a significant period of time prior to arrival of EMS rescue personnel. Nevertheless, the chance for *meaningful* survival from cardiac arrest (i.e., survival with intact neurologic function) is still greatest when defibrillation is carried out *at the first possible moment* after arrival on the scene (Martin et al, 1986). Delay of defibrillation for intubation, establishment of IV access, and/or administration of drugs is not justified.

Theoretically, there is no limit to the number of times that a patient in ventricular fibrillation can be defibrillated. Clinically, the best opportunity for converting a patient out of ventricular fibrillation clearly lies with the first countershock attempt. The success rate drops off significantly with the second shock and continues to decrease with each subsequent countershock attempt. Practically speaking, the chance for meaningful survival for a victim of out-of-hospital cardiac arrest becomes extremely small if ventricular fibrillation fails to respond after five countershocks, and it is almost nil if ventricular fibrillation persists beyond nine countershocks (Hargarten et al, 1990).

Theoretic Concepts

The theory behind electrical defibrillation is simple: In an attempt to eliminate the chaotic asynchronous activity of ventricular fibrillation, a current is passed through the heart. If defibrillation is successful, the mass of individual cardiac cells will be depolarized. Ideally, they will then *repolarize* in a uniform manner with resumption of organized and coordinated contractile activity.

It appears that involvement of a "critical mass" of myocardium is required to *sustain* ventricular fibrillation. This explains why spontaneous resolution of ventricular fibrillation may occasionally be seen. The phenomenon is especially likely to occur in the neonate (because of their smaller heart size), and on rare occasions in previously healthy adults with otherwise normal hearts. In contrast, development of ventricular fibrillation in a diseased heart is much more likely to be a self-perpetuating process since the initial asynchrony of the fibrillating heart facilitates propagation of further asynchrony (Ewy, 1982).

In view of the above, it would seem that depolarization of the entire myocardium is *not* necessarily essential for successful defibrillation. Instead, it may be enough to depolarize just enough myocardium so that a critical mass of fibrillating cells no longer exists. This may explain why defibrillation at relatively low energy levels is sometimes effective in restoring sinus rhythm.

The strength (i.e., energy) of a defibrillation attempt is most often expressed in *joules* (or *watt-seconds*), where:

$$\text{Energy} = \text{Power} \times \text{Duration}$$
$$\text{(joules)} \quad \text{(watts)} \quad \text{(seconds)}$$

In the early days of defibrillation, it was of paramount importance to distinguish between the amount of electrical energy *stored* in a machine and the actual amount *delivered* with each countershock (i.e., "delivered" energy). Variability between these two parameters was sometimes so great that a defibrillator indicating 400 joules might deliver anywhere from 155 to 400 joules (Parmley et al, 1982)!

Defibrillator efficiency has markedly increased in recent years. Although a discrepancy may still occasionally exist between "stored" and "delivered" energy (due to internal resistance of the defibrillator), the difference is much less than in the past, and will rarely be of clinical significance.

It is important to emphasize that it is *current* passing through the chest (and *not* voltage!) that actually defibrillates.

Despite the fact that current defibrillates, convention still holds that calibration of defibrillators be designated in units of energy (i.e., joules or watt-seconds) rather than current. As might be expected, this practice is the source of some confusion.

The relationship between current, voltage, and resistance for any electrical circuit is as follows:

$$\text{Current (amperes)} = \frac{\text{Potential (volts)}}{\text{Resistance (ohms)}}$$

According to this formula, the amount of current that will flow through the circuit for any given voltage will depend on the electrical *resistance* (or *impedance*) of the circuit. Because of the inverse relationship in the formula, it can be seen that *less current will flow through the circuit if resistance increases.* Conversely, current flow will *increase* if resistance is reduced.

> This same relationship holds true in the clinical setting for electrical defibrillation. That is, the amount of current that will penetrate the chest wall to defibrillate the heart will vary *inversely* with the **transthoracic resistance (TTR)** to the passage of this current. If, for whatever reason TTR is increased, less current will penetrate the chest (and the efficacy of that defibrillation attempt will be correspondingly less). On the other hand, if TTR can be lowered, current flow will increase. Thus, *the best way to optimize current flow (and the efficacy of defibrillation) at any given voltage is to minimize TTR.*

As a result of the relationship between current and resistance, clinical factors that affect TTR will clearly play an important role in determining the amount of energy that penetrates the heart with each defibrillation attempt.

Factors known to affect TTR include:
1. The amount of energy selected for defibrillation
2. The time interval between successive shocks
3. The total number of shocks delivered
4. Size of the paddle electrodes
5. The interface used between the electrodes and the chest wall
6. Chest wall configuration
7. The pressure exerted on the electodes against the chest wall
8. The phase of ventilation of the patient at the time of defibrillation

---

The higher the energy selected for any given countershock attempt, the lower the TTR will tend to be. This raises the question of what the optimal energy for defibrillation should be? Much controversy centered around this point during the 1970s, and significant effort was directed at designing defibrillators capable of delivering high-energy countershocks (i.e., ≥400 joules with each countershock attempt). Although a *dose-weight* relationship (that lower defibrillation energies are adequate to defibrillate lower weight individuals) appears to exist in animals, infants, and small children, *body weight per se is probably not a major determinant of the amount of energy needed for defibrillation of adults!* (Kerber et al, 1981; Ewy, 1982).

> In animal studies, body weight often varies by a factor of 10. In contrast, body weight among adult human subjects will usually not vary by more than a factor of 2 (or at most 3). As a result, countershock attempts in the mid-energy range (i.e., using 200 to 300 joules) will often be effective for defibrillating adults of various body sizes.

Defibrillation is not benign. The greater the energy delivered with any given countershock attempt, the greater the

chance of producing additional injury to the conduction system. It would therefore seem preferable to try to limit the amount of energy used to the *lowest level possible* at which defibrillation will be successful. Unfortunately, it is extremely difficult clinically to predict the optimal amount of energy to use. Beginning at too low a level risks excessively delaying the process of defibrillation. Beginning too high may produce further damage to the conduction system (which would be deleterious if the patient is ever converted out of ventricular fibrillation).

> Recommendations for defibrillation from the 1986 Guidelines for ACLS reflected the American Heart Association's attempt at obtaining an optimal balance between these parameters. Preference for an initial defibrillation attempt at 200 joules was based largely on the work of Weaver et al (1982). In his study of subjects with out-of-hospital ventricular fibrillation, use of a lower energy (of 175 joules) for the initial attempt at defibrillation was found to be *equally effective* in converting patients out of ventricular fibrillation as was 320 joules, but resulted in less conduction system damage (in the form of AV block or asystole), as was evidenced by the postconversion rhythm.

The Effect of Specific Factors on TTR

The *number* of countershocks delivered to a patient in ventricular fibrillation exerts a *cumulative* effect on TTR. TTR is also affected by the time interval between successive shocks. Thus delivery of *multiple countershocks in rapid succession* is likely to significantly reduce TTR, and increase the amount of current flowing through the chest at any given energy level. This is the rationale for the recommendation to *minimize time* between countershock attempts.

> Practically speaking, the reduction in TTR that occurs between successful countershock attempts is relatively modest (Kerber et al, 1981). As a result, it has been common practice to progressively raise the energy level selected for successive countershock attempts (from 200- to 300- to 360 joules) so as to ensure that a significantly greater amount of current will pass through the chest with each defibrillation.

Clinically, another question that often arises relates to the amount of energy to use if ventricular fibrillation *recurs* (rather than persists) during the resuscitation effort. Although in the past, it had been recommended to reinitiate defibrillation "at the energy level that had previously resulted in successful defibrillation" (JAMA Suppl, 1986), *it may be equally reasonable to routinely drop back to an energy level of 200 joules if ventricular fibrillation recurs.*

> As indicated above, there is a *cumulative* (albeit modest) reduction in TTR with each successive countershock attempt. Thus, a tenth attempt at defibrillation with 200 joules should encounter a significantly lower TTR than the first few attempts at defibrillation—*and should therefore be associated with a significantly greater amount of current flow at any given energy level.* In addition, there are a host of other impossible-to-control-for patient-specific variables (such as metabolic condition and state of oxygenation) that may be affected by the resuscitation effort, and that may therefore affect fibrillation threshold and the amount of energy needed for successful defibrillation. As a result, in certain patients reducing the selected energy level

to 200 joules could be more than adequate for defibrillation at a later point in the code *despite the fact that 300 to 360 joules may have been essential early on.* In the event that this lower energy level is not successful, it can always be increased (to 300 to 360 joules) for subsequent defibrillation attempts.

Other factors that may affect TTR include *paddle size, paddle placement* and *pressure,* and the *interface* used. Up to a point, TTR will decrease with increasing electrode paddle size. Thus, a greater than 20% reduction may be noted when 12.5-cm diameter paddles are used to defibrillate adults instead of the standard 8-cm paddles (Ewy, 1982).

> Another reason for selecting optimal paddle size is that larger paddles are less likely to concentrate current and produce conduction system damage. In children, optimal paddle size is determined by choosing the largest electrode diameter that will allow good skin contact with the entire paddle surface.

The recommended position for paddle placement is to put one paddle under the right clavicle (just to the right of the sternum), while the other is placed lateral to the left nipple (in the anterior axillary line). Exerting firm downward pressure (of approximately 25 lb) on each paddle may further reduce TTR by as much as 25% (Kerber et al, 1980).

> Even the phase of respiration at the time of defibrillation may affect TTR. Thus, TTR appears to be lowest when countershock is performed during expiration because the distance between paddle electrodes and the heart is least at this moment. *Air (in the inflated lung) is not a good conductor of electricity.* Exerting firm downward pressure on the paddles helps lower TTR by ensuring forced expiration of the victim.

Chest wall configuration (especially chest *width*) may play an important role in determining TTR (Kerber et al, 1981). Clinically, this factor becomes particularly relevant when lower energy levels are selected for defibrillation of individuals with a large chest diameter, since TTR is likely to be greatest in such instances. Higher outputs (i.e., 300 to 360 joules) may be needed more often for defibrillation to be successful in these patients. It is important to emphasize, however, that *TTR is NOT simply a function of body weight, size, and chest wall configuration.*

> That TTR can *not* be predicted solely on the basis of physical appearance is evident from the finding of a more than *fivefold* variation in TTR values among an unselected population of adults (of various body sizes) who were found in cardiac arrest (Kerber et al, 1988). *Even elderly, emaciated patients can occasionally have surprisingly high TTR values despite their seemingly negligible body mass.*

The final factor to consider regarding TTR is the *paddle-skin interface.* The skin serves as a potent electrical resistor between electrode paddles and the heart. Defibrillation without the use of a suitable interface is likely to result in a significant burn of the skin surface, and a lack of penetration of the defibrillator current.

> A number of electrode gels are commercially available to optimize conductivity. Care must be taken to avoid excessive application of the gel to the paddles, since this may result in *bridging* of current when the patient is defibrillated. Excessive application of gel could also leave a slippery residue that might make it more difficult to perform CPR.

> In a pinch, saline-soaked gauze pads may be used as a substitute for conductive medium, although they are not as effective as clear electrode gel. *(Alcohol-soaked sponges should NEVER be used, since vaporized alcohol may ignite from the defibrillation shock.)*

Practically speaking, the problem of selecting a suitable conductive medium for defibrillation has been simplified by development of *disposable electrode pads.* Although conductivity with this product is not quite equal to that of some of the more efficient electrode gels, routine use of electrode pads eliminates the potential hazards of bridging and leftover electrode gel (i.e., leaving a slippery surface on the chest wall). It may also save time by eliminating a step (application of gel) in the defibrillation process.

Recent Developments: Potential Clinical Applications

Until recently, there was no practical way to clinically determine TTR (and adjust current delivery accordingly) at the scene of a cardiac arrest. The development of newer (current-based) defibrillators holds promise of being able to do so in the near future. Insight into potential clinical application of this exciting advance is provided from a study by Kerber et al (1988):

> TTR was measured in a series of more than 300 patients who were cardioverted or defibrillated for ventricular fibrillation, ventricular tachycardia, atrial fibrillation, or atrial flutter. Among the 100 patients in the study who were treated for ventricular fibrillation, a total of 323 unsynchronized countershocks were delivered. As alluded to previously, TTR values varied significantly among study subjects (from a high value of 150 ohms, to a low value of 28 ohms). When TTR was low (i.e., less than 70 ohms), defibrillation at an extremely low energy level (of 100 joules) successfully converted patients out of ventricular fibrillation 84% of the time! In contrast, when resistance to the passage of current was high (i.e., when TTR values exceeded 70 ohms), defibrillation with 100 joules was successful only 36% of the time. However, indiscriminate use of higher initial energy levels (of 200 joules or more) for all patients in the study would *not* have optimized the chance for successful conversion to sinus rhythm. Paradoxically, selection of higher initial energy levels actually *decreased* the chance for successful defibrillation in certain patients.

A number of important clinical implications are suggested by the results of this study:

1. A significant percentage of patients will respond to defibrillation at surprisingly low energy levels (i.e., at 100 joules). The chance of successfully defibrillating a patient at a low energy level is best when TTR is low (since a relatively greater amount of current will pass through the chest wall of such individuals at any given energy level).
2. TTR values may vary by *more* than a factor of *five* in adult human subjects. *Body size and habitus are not reliable predictors of TTR values.*
3. The amount of current that passes through the chest wall is directly influenced by TTR. Current flow at any given energy level may therefore also vary in

direct response to any of the factors that affect TTR. Thus implementation of a specified defibrillating protocol (such as the recommendation to administer 200- 300- and 360 joules for successive countershock attempts) will not standardize the amount of defibrillating current that a particular patient will receive.

4. *More energy is not necessarily better.* Although, in general, use of increasing energy levels enhances the likelihood of successful defibrillation, this relationship holds true *only up to a point.* Selection of higher energy levels beyond this point may paradoxically *decrease* the chance for successful defibrillation in a significant number of patients.

> Success rates for defibrillation in the study by Kerber et al continually improved as the amount of actual (i.e., measured) current flow increased from 21 to 41 amperes. The success rate for the initial countershock attempt was maximal (up to 93%!) when defibrillating current was found to be at the upper end of this range (i.e., between 38 and 41 amperes). However, with further increases in current, success rates for defibrillation dropped off. Success rates plummeted to 40% when measured current flow was in the highest range (i.e., more than 54 amperes).

5. In addition to reducing the chance for successful defibrillation, delivery of an excessively high defibrillating current may also be detrimental because it increases the likelihood of producing functional (conduction system) damage. Thus:

The amount of defibrillating current should *ideally* be limited to the *lowest possible value* that is still capable of successfully converting the patient out of ventricular fibrillation.

As we have already indicated, the clinical difficulty is in determining what the "lowest effective value" of current for successful defibrillation will be for any given patient at a particular moment in time during the resuscitation effort. Use of a defibrillator capable of *instantaneously* measuring TTR, and *automatically adjusting* the amount of energy selected to ensure delivery of a predesignated amount of current may provide the answer.

> Use of an *automatic* current-based (i.e., energy-adjusting) defibrillator should enable optimization of current flow delivery. Thus, for a patient who has an unexpectedly low TTR value, less energy will automatically be selected for the initial attempt at defibrillation than would probably be the case if a standard defibrillating protocol (beginning at 200 joules) was being followed. Conversely, a much higher initial energy level will be selected for defibrillation of a patient with an unexpectedly high TTR value. Moreover, knowing that TTR is unusually high in a particular patient justifies continued use of higher energy countershocks (of 360 joules or more) if ventricular fibrillation persists (or recurs).

Summary: Our Suggestions for Use of Defibrillation

At the present time, current-based defibrillators are not yet widely available for general use. As a result, determination of the energy level for defibrillation is still largely an *empiric* process. Keeping the following principles in mind may help in deciding how much energy to use:

---

1. Standardized (empiric) defibrillating protocols will select appropriate energy levels for defibrillation *most* of the time (Kerber et al, 1988). Their use has the decided advantage of facilitating the decision-making process.
2. Many factors affect TTR (and therefore affect the amount of current flowing through the chest wall at any given energy level). This is why energy requirements for successful defibrillation vary so greatly from one patient to the next *(and why surprisingly low energy levels will sometimes work).*
3. *Defibrillation is not benign.* Ideally, the lowest energy level likely to be successful should be selected. If this is not effective, a higher energy level can be used.
4. By far, the most important determinant of successful defibrillation is *time.* Although attention to factors affecting TTR may help to optimize current flow delivery, *they are clearly not a substitute for prompt defibrillation.*

Synchronized Cardioversion

Definition of Terms: The term *cardioversion* is often the source of much confusion. This is because the term is commonly interchanged (and mistakenly equated) with two other terms: *defibrillation* and *countershock.*

As discussed at the beginning of this section, **defibrillation** is the process of passing an electric current through the heart with the express intent of completely depolarizing all myocardial cells. The electrical discharge that is delivered with defibrillation is *unsynchronized,* which means that it occurs at an entirely *random* point in the cardiac cycle.

In contrast, use of the term **cardioversion** implies that the electrical discharge has been timed (i.e., *synchronized*) to occur at a designated point in the cardiac cycle. Doing so not only facilitates conversion of certain tachyarrhythmias to sinus rhythm, but it also minimizes the chance that the electrical impulse will exacerbate the arrhythmia (as may occur if the stimulus happens to be delivered during the vulnerable period).

> To avoid confusion about terminology, as well as to clarify the mode of delivery of the electrical impulse, we frequently refer to this procedure as *"synchronized cardioversion"* (rather than simply "cardioversion"). Although use of the

combined term in this manner may engender an element of redundancy, *it leaves no doubt as to how the operator is about to proceed* (which is really the *KEY* for ensuring a coordinated team effort in resuscitation).

Among emergency care providers, the third term— **countershock**—and its diminutive **"shock"** tend to be freely interchanged with the term *defibrillation*. We favor this usage, and unless otherwise specified, generally treat these three terms synonymously. We therefore separate them from the term *"cardioversion,"* and reserve our use of *defibrillation, countershock,* and *"shock"* for referring to delivery of an *unsynchronized* electrical impulse to a patient in ventricular fibrillation.

INDICATIONS/SUGGESTED ENERGY LEVELS FOR *EMERGENCY* USE OF SYNCHRONIZED CARDIOVERSION:

1. Treatment of **ventricular tachycardia** that is hemodynamically unstable, or that has not responded to antiarrhythmic therapy.

Most cases of ventricular tachycardia are surprisingly responsive to synchronized cardioversion with extremely low energy levels. Conversion of this tachyarrhythmia to sinus rhythm has been successful with as little as 1 joule, and up to 90% of cases respond to energy levels of *less* than 10 joules (Lown and DeSilva, 1982). Nevertheless, *we prefer to let the urgency of the situation serve as our guide for determining the amount of energy to use.* As a result, we favor use of relatively high initial energy levels (of 100 to 200 joules) for emergency cardioversion of an acutely decompensating patient. Lower initial energy levels (i.e., 50 joules) might be tried in a somewhat less urgent situation, as may be the case for a hemodynamically stable patient who has not responded to a trial of antiarrhythmic therapy.

2. Treatment of **supraventricular tachyarrhythmias** that have not responded to medical therapy, and/or that become hemodynamically unstable.

The supraventricular tachyarrhythmia that is most responsive to cardioversion is **atrial flutter.** Energy levels on the order of 25 to 50 joules are almost always successful in converting this arrhythmia to sinus rhythm. Although energy levels of less than 10 joules may also be effective, they are generally *not* recommended. This is because of the significant chance that cardioverting atrial flutter with extremely low energies will result in conversion of the rhythm to atrial fibrillation *instead* of sinus rhythm (Lown and DeSilva, 1982).

At the other end of the spectrum, **atrial fibrillation** is relatively resistant to synchronized cardioversion. As a result, higher initial energies are likely to be required, and *at least* 100 (if not 200) joules should probably be used for the first cardioversion attempt.

When cardioverting a patient with atrial fibrillation, it is important to pay particularly close attention to the monitor *immediately after* delivery of the electrical impulse. "Non-responsiveness" (i.e., failure to convert to normal sinus rhythm) should be differentiated from *transient* successful conversion in which sinus rhythm is *momentarily* restored, only to revert back to atrial fibrillation a few beats later. The former situation (i.e., "non-responsiveness") suggests that additional attempts at synchronized cardioversion (perhaps at higher energy levels) may be indicated. In contrast, momentary conversion to sinus rhythm with rapid reversion back to atrial fibrillation suggests that such additional attempts will also be unsuccessful at *maintaining* sinus rhythm (even if higher energy levels are used!). Electrical conversion to (and maintenance of) normal sinus rhythm may simply not be possible for such patients at that moment in time.

Practically speaking, cardioversion will not be required very often for treatment of **PSVT.** This is because most patients with this arrhythmia respond quite readily to pharmacologic treatment with verapamil or adenosine, and/or to application of vagal maneuvers. If cardioversion is needed, an initial energy of 75 to 100 joules is recommended. Higher energies can be tried if this is unsuccessful.

Cardioversion should *not* be used for treatment of *multifocal atrial tachycardia (MAT).* The key to management of this arrhythmia is diagnosis and treatment of the underlying cause (which is usually hypoxemia, often with accompanying metabolic abnormalities). Cardioversion of patients with MAT is unlikely to be successful at *maintaining* normal sinus rhythm, and it may be potentially dangerous.

Similarly, cardioversion should be avoided (if at all possible) for treatment of tachyarrhythmias in a patient with *digitalis toxicity.* This is because of the significant risk that this procedure may precipitate refractory ventricular arrhythmias in such patients. On the other hand, there appears to be virtually no increased risk of postconversion arrhythmias when cardioversion is performed on patients with therapeutic digoxin levels (Mann et al, 1985).

---

3. Treatment of **wide complex tachycardias of unknown etiology.**

Despite our most diligent efforts, it will *not* always be possible to determine (with certainty) the etiology of every cardiac arrhythmia. Acceptance of this clinical reality is particularly important when confronted with a wide complex tachyarrhythmia of unknown cause. Practically speaking, if the patient is (and/or becomes) hemodynamically unstable, the etiology of the arrhythmia no longer matters: *Synchronized cardioversion is IMMEDIATELY indicated.* On the other hand, if the patient remains hemodynamically stable, an initial trial of medical therapy may be preferable. If this is unsuccessful, synchronized cardioversion (on a somewhat less urgent basis) may then become indicated.

4. Treatment of **torsade de pointes.**

The most important aspect in the management of torsade de pointes is to identify and correct the underlying cause of the disorder. Administration of IV magnesium has become the medical treatment of choice. Overdrive pacing is the preferred treatment modality when withdrawal of the offending agent and medical therapy are ineffective. In spite of these measures, sustained episodes of the tachyarrhythmia may require immediate intervention. In such cases, synchronized cardioversion (with 50 to 200 joules) will usually be successful in *temporarily* converting the arrhythmia. Unfortunately, tachycardia episodes tend to recur (often repeatedly) until the underlying cause has been corrected.

COMMENTS

Synchronized cardioversion was born out of necessity. Following the successful use of closed-chest defibrillation in 1956, it became apparent that a therapeutic modality was needed for treatment of hemodynamically significant tachyarrhythmias that did not respond to pharmacologic therapy. Use of original defibrillating machines was unsafe for this purpose because the prolonged (150 to 250 millisecond) alternating current (AC) discharge they delivered was extremely likely to produce postconversion arrhythmias, asystole, or myocardial damage. Development of direct current (DC) capacitors (able to deliver the electrical impulse in as little as 4 to 30 milliseconds) and the ability to *synchronize* the discharge to the "nonvulnerable" period of the cardiac cycle made cardioversion a reality (Lown et al, 1962).

> The *vulnerable period* is the time during the cardiac cycle when the heart is most susceptible to developing ventricular fibrillation if stimulated by an electrical discharge. This period is approximately 30 milliseconds in duration. Temporally, it just precedes the apex of the T wave on the surface ECG. By synchronizing the electrical impulse to the height of the R wave (which by definition occurs *before* the T wave, and therefore before the vulnerable period), the risk of inducing a more malignant arrhythmia is minimized.

Cardioversion is most effective in the treatment of arrhythmias that depend on a *reentry* mechanism (i.e, atrial flutter, PSVT, and ventricular tachycardia). The process produces a single, brief electrical discharge that terminates the arrhythmia by interrupting the reentrant circuit.

Practical Considerations

Cardioversion may be used either electively or on an urgent (or emergent) basis. Discussion of purely elective cardioversion for patients with hemodynamically stable arrhythmias extends beyond the scope of this book.

Use of *emergent* (i.e., immediate) synchronized cardioversion is indicated for treatment of tachyarrhythmias in a patient who is acutely decompensating. Clinically, this situation most often occurs in patients with definite ventricular tachycardia, and/or a wide-complex tachycardia of uncertain etiology. The common denominator in such situations is that *time is at a premium*.

Consideration of the following ideas may help in preparing for the procedure:

> *Try to anticipate potential problems that might be encountered.* Occasionally cardioversion can precipitate malignant arrhythmias (including ventricular fibrillation) or asystole. As a result, it is essential to have a fully equipped crash cart nearby. Should the patient suddenly develop ventricular fibrillation, you'll need to turn off the synchronizer switch and immediately defibrillate (with 200 to 360 joules). If cardioversion results in asystole, atropine and/or immediate application of an external pacemaker are in order.

> Before cardioversion, a bed board should be placed under the patient in the event that CPR is needed. If the patient is awake and time permits, *sedation* (with 5 to 20 mg of IV diazepam, or other agent) is strongly advised to minimize discomfort (and hopefully induce amnesia for the event). If possible (i.e., if time permits), it may be preferable to call an anesthesiologist/nurse/anesthetist/respiratory therapist to the bedside to ensure the presence of qualified personnel to attend to the airway in the event that intubation is needed. Doing so *in advance* frees you to concentrate your efforts on directing resuscitation and managing any postconversion arrhythmias that occur.

> Last, be sure to continually monitor the patient throughout the procedure. Try to select an ECG monitoring lead that displays a tall R wave configuration if at all possible (since doing so may facilitate identification of both the QRS complex and synchronization spike).

emergency cardioversion may be performed as follows:

1. Apply conductive medium to the electrode paddles (or use disposable electrode pads), and place the paddles on the patient's chest in the same manner as for unsynchronized defibrillation.
2. Turn on the "synch" switch, and verify that the defibrillator is sensing the QRS complex.
3. Charge the defibrillator, making sure everyone is clear from the bed.
4. Simultaneously depress the buttons on each paddle. Unlike the case for defibrillation, *the buttons on each paddle must REMAIN depressed until the machine has discharged.*
5. Recheck the patient, the pulse, and the ECG monitor *immediately after* discharge to assess hemodynamic status and determine the postconversion rhythm.

> Two final caveats should be kept in mind. First, accept the clinical reality that, despite the best of intentions (and the

most diligent preparation), there may be times when the synchronized electrical impulse will simply not discharge. If a rapid attempt at troubleshooting does not resolve the problem, *do NOT persist in trying to cardiovert the patient.* Admittedly, an unsynchronized countershock is less optimal than synchronized cardioversion for treatment of ventricular tachycardia with a pulse. Nevertheless, *delivery of an unsynchronized discharge is far preferable to delivery of no discharge at all.* Practically speaking, unsynchronized countershock will work equally well much of the time *without* excessively increasing the risk of exacerbating the arrhythmia. Thus, if for whatever reason you find yourself *unable* to cardiovert a patient with a potentially life-threatening (i.e., hemodynamically unstable) tachyarrhythmia, we favor delivery of an unsynchronized countershock instead.

The other caveat worthy of mention relates to the difficulty that may occasionally be encountered when the rate of ventricular tachycardia is very rapid (i.e., well *over* 200 beats/min) and the QRS complex is especially wide. In this situation, the ECG tracing may take on the configuration of a sinusoid waveform, and it may become extremely difficult to differentiate between the QRS complex and the T wave. *If YOU find it difficult to distinguish between the QRS and the T wave, it is likely that the defibrillator will have the same difficulty.* Under such circumstances, delivery of an unsynchronized countershock may become preferable to synchronized cardioversion.

Cardiac Pacemakers

Technique: Application of **pacemaker therapy** may be accomplished by the use of *transvenous, transthoracic,* and/or *transcutaneous* pacing devices.

Indications: Generally accepted indications for *pacemaker therapy* include the following:

In the Setting of *Acute MI:*
- Mobitz II 2° AV block
- 3° AV block with *anterior* AMI
- New *bifascicular* bundle branch block
- New unifascicular bundle branch block *(controversial!)*
- Other hemodynamically significant bradyarrhythmias if they are resistant to medical therapy (i.e., severe sinus bradycardia; Mobitz I 2° AV block; 3° AV block with *inferior* AMI)

In the Setting of *Cardiac Arrest:*
- Mobitz II 2° AV block
- 3° AV block
- Slow idioventricular escape rhythm
- Asystole
- Refractory tachyarrhythmias, including torsade de pointes *(overdrive pacing)*
- Other hemodynamically significant bradyarrhythmias if they are resistant to medical therapy (i.e., severe sinus bradycardia; Mobitz I 2° AV block)

COMMENTS

The topic of cardiac pacing is a comprehensive one that extends well beyond the scope of this book. We therefore limit our comments in this section to those aspects of cardiac pacing that are pertinent to the emergency care provider in charge of an acutely unstable patient, and/or in the setting of cardiac arrest. Additional reference to indications for pacemaker therapy is made in Section D of Chapter 3 (under the discussion of the *Clinical Significance of the AV Blocks*), and in Section D of Chapter 12 on Acute Myocardial Infarction (under the discussion of *Autonomic Nervous System Dysfunction* and *Conduction System Disturbances*).

Practically speaking, the principal indication for emergency cardiac pacing can be summarized as follows:

Symptomatic and/or **hemodynamically significant** bradycardia

---

The cause of such bradycardia may be varied, and includes conditions such as marked sinus bradycardia, high-degree or complete AV block, slow idioventricular rhythm, asystole, and/or other conduction disturbances. Although a trial of medical therapy (i.e., use of drugs and/or fluid resuscitation) may be warranted, in most cases this treatment only serves as a *temporizing measure* until preparations for cardiac pacing can be made.

Clinically, the type of situation that is most likely to respond to medical therapy is a hemodynamically significant bradycardia that develops as the result of a sudden surge in parasympathetic tone. The setting in which this most commonly occurs is acute *inferior* infarction, especially during the first few hours after the onset of symptoms. Hypotension in this setting results not only from the bradycardia, but also from the inappropriate vasodilatation that so often accompanies the parasympathetic discharge. Repositioning (i.e., to the Trendelenburg position), infusion of IV fluid, a *tincture of time,* and/or small doses of IV atropine (if needed) will usually be effective in treating such patients.

In contrast, hemodynamically significant bradyarrhythmias that are not associated with excessive parasympathetic tone are much less likely to respond to medical therapy, and will usually require cardiac pacing for treatment. Practically speaking, except for patients who are seen during the early hours of acute inferior infarction, and those who develop bradycardia following a medical procedure or other stimulus likely to invoke a sudden surge in parasympathetic tone (e.g., as a result of vasovagal syncope, prolonged vomiting, or drug overdose), *most hemodynamically significant bradyarrhythmias that occur in the setting of cardiac arrest do not respond optimally to medical therapy.*

Pacemaker Options

Three types of cardiac pacemakers have been used in the emergency care setting: *transvenous* pacemakers, *transthoracic* pacemakers, and *transcutaneous* (external) pacemakers.

The most reliable pacemaking device (and the procedure of choice when time permits and an operator skilled in the technique is available) is the **transvenous pacemaker.** Insertion is accomplished through a major vein such as the brachial, subclavian, internal jugular, or femoral vein. The pacemaking wire is then advanced by means of a flow-directed, balloon-tipped catheter (with ECG monitoring), or under fluoroscopic guidance (if time allows and skilled personnel and equipment are on hand). In its final position, the pacemaker lies in the right ventricular apex.

Until recently, insertion of a **transthoracic pacemaker** was the procedure of choice for emergency pacing *when all else had failed* in the setting of cardiac arrest. Despite its invasive nature, the technique for insertion was simple: passage of a transthoracic needle through the skin at a point just to the left of the subxiphoid notch—with entry through the skin being accomplished at a 30° to 45° angle—and advancement of the needle while aiming for the sternal notch. After approximately three fourths of its length had been inserted, the inner trocar of the needle was withdrawn. Aspiration of blood with a syringe confirmed correct placement within the right ventricular cavity. The pacing wire was then introduced, and hookup made to the external energy source.

The principal advantage of this pacing technique was speed of insertion: Skilled operators could complete the procedure is *less* than 1 minute. Drawbacks included a high risk of complications (i.e., pneumothorax, hemothorax, hemopericardium), interference with external chest compression, and less than optimal reliability in performance. As a result, transthoracic pacing was usually reserved as a "last ditch effort" when all other treatment measures had failed. Arrival on the scene of the third type of pacemaking device has now virtually rendered the procedure obsolete.

The most exciting advance in pacemaker therapy has been development of the **transcutaneous (external) pacemaker.** First introduced by Zoll in 1952, this device fell out of favor when transvenous pacing became popular during the 1960s. Problems caused by the original external pacemaker were severe patient discomfort (from cutaneous sensory nerve and skeletal muscle stimulation) and significant stimulus artifact (from involuntary skeletal muscle contraction) that made interpretation of the surface ECG exceedingly difficult.

The device was modified and reintroduced in 1981. The improved model minimizes patient discomfort (from cutaneous sensory nerve stimulation and skeletal muscle contraction), and produces an easily interpretable ECG recording. Three additional features make this device extremely attractive as an emergency pacing procedure:

1. It is entirely noninvasive.
2. It is easily and rapidly applied.
3. It produces effective cardiac pacing in a majority of cases.

It should be emphasized that the external pacemaker is only a *temporizing* measure. Transvenous pacing is still the treatment of choice for patients who develop a severe conduction disorder that is likely to require a prolonged period of pacemaker support. However, when time is of the essence (as for a patient with asystole in cardiac arrest), and/or when transvenous pacing is not readily available, transcutaneous pacing may be a suitable (and much more rapidly instituted) alternative.

Moreover, in less critical situations when the need for transvenous pacing is uncertain (i.e., 3° AV block with an acceptable junctional response in the setting of an *inferior* AMI), ready availability of this *noninvasive* modality as *backup* in case the patient does decompensate may sometimes be preferable to routine prophylactic insertion of a transvenous pacemaker.

Practical Considerations

Despite improvements in technology that have been made, *pacemaker therapy is rarely a life-saving procedure in the setting of cardiac arrest.* Unfortunately, the overall prognosis for patients with bradyasystolic cardiac arrest is dismal *regardless* of whatever interventions are undertaken (Niemann et al, 1986; Syverud et al, 1986).

Most studies reported in the literature are retrospective in which pacemaker insertion was only attempted after all other resuscitative measures had been tried and failed. One could not reasonably expect any intervention to work under such circumstances.

Time appears to be a critical factor. Even when used in the prehospital setting with application of transcutaneous pacing within 15 minutes of the arrest—*and* with successful *electrical* capture—mechanical capture (i.e., development of an accompanying pulse) is rare, and long-term survival is not improved (Eitel et al, 1987).

The question remains as to whether emergency pacing could be lifesaving if it was applied sooner in the process—that is, within minutes of the onset of bradyasystolic arrest (and *before* the period of irreversibility has set in). Considering that up to 30% of cases of out-of-hospital cardiac arrest have a bradyarrhythmia as their cause, the potential impact of this issue is obvious. Perhaps resurgence of the noninvasive, rapidly instituted, transcutaneous pacemaker will enable EMS systems to improve these dismal statistics.

It should be emphasized that transcutaneous pacing is effective as treatment when meaningful (albeit slow) contractile activity is present (i.e., for treatment of hemodynamically significant bradycardia). However, pacing is usually not effective for treatment of asystole or EMD that occurs in the setting of cardiac arrest (Clinton et al, 1985; Zoll and Zoll, 1985). This is because the principal problem in these situations is *not* the lack of electrical activity, but rather the inability of the myocardium to generate effective contraction when appropriately stimulated.

Cardiac Pacing of Tachyarrhythmias

Cardiac pacing has also been used as a method for terminating supraventricular and ventricular tachyarrhythmias (Estes et al, 1989). In the case of torsade de pointes, magnesium sulfate has become the initial treatment of choice (see Section C in Chapter 16). However, if the rhythm persists despite medical therapy, *overdrive pacing* is indicated.

Although the use of pacing for termination of other tachyarrhythmias is most often attempted in the electrophysiologic laboratory, recent work by Grubbs et al (1992) suggests that emergency use of an *external pacemaker* to deliver an *asynchronous* burst (i.e., of 8 to 10 pulses at a current strength of 120 mA and a rate of 200 beats/min) may successfully terminate some cases of sustained, mono-morphic ventricular tachycardia.

Standard external pacemakers are usually constrained by an upper rate limit that prevents pacing at rates above 120 beats/min. However, use of an external tracking modification allows for connection to a standard atrial pacing box and acceleration of pacing to a much faster rate. Although it is important to appreciate that overdrive pacing is *not* benign (i.e., acceleration of the ventricular rate, and even precipitation of ventricular fibrillation may occur!), emergency use of this technique with an external pacemaker may provide a nonpharmacologic alternative for treating selected patients with sustained ventricular tachycardia that has not responded to medical therapy.

References

American Heart Association Subcommittee on Emergency Cardiac Care: Standards and guidelines for cardiopulmonary resuscitation (CPR) and emergency cardiac care (ECC), *JAMA* 255(suppl):2905-2992, 1986.

Caldwell G, Millar G, Quinn E, Vincent R, Chambearlain DA: Simple mechanical methods for cardioversion: Defense of the precordial thump and cough version, *Br Med J* 291:627-630, 1985.

Clinton JE, Zoll PM, Zoll R, Ruiz E: Emergency noninvasive external cardiac pacing, *J Emerg Med* 2:155-162, 1985.

Criley JM, Blaufuss AH, Kissel GL: Cough-induced cardiac compression: Self-administered form of cardiopulmonary resuscitation, *JAMA* 236:1246-1250, 1976.

Eisenberg MS, Horwood BT, Cummins RO, Reynolds-Haertle R, Hearne TR: Cardiac arrest and resuscitation: A tale of 29 cities, *Ann Emerg Med* 19:179-186, 1990.

Eitel DR, Guzzardi CJ, Stein SE, Drawbaugh RE, Hess DR, Walton SL: Noninvasive transcutaneous cardiac pacing in prehospital cardiac arrest, *Ann Emerg Med* 16:531-534, 1987.

Enns J, Tween WA, Donen N: Prehospital cardiac rhythm deterioration in a system providing only basic life support, *Ann Emerg Med* 12:478-481, 1983.

Estes NAM, Deering TF, Manolis AS, Salem D, Zoll PM: External cardiac programmed stimulation for noninvasive termination of sustained supraventricular and ventricular tachycardia, *Am J Cardiol* 63:177-183, 1989.

Ewy GA: *Defibrillation*. In Harwood AL, editor: *Cardiopulmonary resuscitation*, Baltimore, 1982 Williams & Wilkins.

Grubb BP, Tenesy-Armos P, Hahn H, Elliot L: The use of external, noninvasive pacing for the termination of ventricular tachycardia in the emergency department setting, *Ann Emerg Med* 21:174-176, 1992.

Hargarten KM, Stueven HA, Waite E, Olson DW, Mateer JR, Aufderheide TP, Darin JC: Prehospital experience with defibrillation of coarse ventricular fibrillation: A ten-year review, *Ann Emerg Med* 19:157-162, 1990.

Hossack KF, Hartwig R: Cardiac arrest associated with supervised cardiac rehabilitation, *J Cardiac Rehab* 2:402-408, 1982.

Kerber RE, Grayzel J, Hoyt R, Marcus M, Kennedy J: Transthoracic resistance in human defibrillation: Effect of body weight, chest size, serial same energy shocks, paddle size, and paddle contact pressure, *Med Instrum* 14:52-56, 1980.

Kerber RE, Grayzel J, Hoyt R, Marcus M, Kennedy J: Transthoracic resistance in human defibrillation: Influence of body weight, chest size, serial shocks, paddle size and paddle contact pressure, *Circulation* 63:676-682, 1981.

Kerber RE, Martins JB, Kienzle MG, Constantin L, Olshansky B, Hopson R, Charbonnier F: Energy, Current, and Success in Defibrillation and Cardioversion: Clinical Studies Using an Automated Impedance-Based Method of Energy Adjustment. *Circulation* 77:1038-1046, 1988.

Lown B, Amarasingham R, Neuman J: New method of terminating cardiac arrhythmias: Use of synchronized capacitor discharge, *JAMA* 182:548-555, 1962.

Lown B: *Cardiovascular collapse and sudden cardiac death*. In Braunwald E, editor: *Heart Disease*. Philadelphia, 1980, Saunders.

Lown B, DeSilva RA: *The technique of cardioversion*. In Hurst JW, editor: *The heart*. New York, 1982, McGraw-Hill.

Mann DL, Maisel AS, Atwood JE, Engler RL, Le Winter MM: Absence of cardioversion-induced ventricular arrhythmias in patients with therapeutic digoxin levels, *J Am Coll Cardiol* 5:882-888, 1985.

Martin TG, Hawkins NS, Weigel JA, Rider DE, Buckingham BD: Initial treatment of ventricular fibrillation: defibrillation or drug therapy? *Am J Emerg Med* 6:113-119, 1986.

Miller J, Tresch D, Harwitz L, Thompson BM, Aprahamian C, Darin JC: The precordial thump, *Ann Emerg Med* 13:791-794, 1984.

Morgera T, Baldi N, Chersevan D, Medugro G, Caerini F: Chest thump and ventricular tachycardia, *PACE* 2:69-75, 1979.

Niemann JT, Haynes KS, Garner D, Rennie CJ, Jagels G: Postcountershock pulseless rhythms: Response to CPR, artificial cardiac pacing, and adrenergic agonists, *Ann Emerg Med* 15:112-120, 1986.

Parmley WW, Hatcher CR, Ewy GA, Furman S, Redding J, Weisfledt ML: Task force V: Physical interventions and adjunctive therapy: Thirteenth Bethesda Conference on Emergency Cardiac Care, *Am J Cardiol* 50:409-420, 1982.

Patros RJ, Goren CC: The precordial thump: an adjunct to emergency medicine, *Heart Lung* 12:61-64, 1983.

Schultz DD, Olivas GS: The use of cough cardiopulmonary resuscitation in clinical practice, *Heart Lung* 15:273-280, 1986.

Syverud SA, Dalsey WC, Hedges JR: Transcutaneous and transvenous cardiac pacing for early bradyasystolic cardiac arrest, *Ann Emerg Med* 15:121-124, 1986.

Weaver WD, Cobb LA, Compass MK, Hallstrom AP: Ventricular defibrillation: A comparative trial using 175-J and 320-J shocks, *N Engl J Med* 307:1101-1106, 1982.

Winkle RA *et al*: Effect of duration of ventricular fibrillation in defibrillation efficacy on humans, *Circulation* 81:1477-1481, 1990.

Zoll PM, Zoll RH: Noninvasive temporary cardiac stimulation, *Crit Care Med* 13:925-926, 1985.

DRUGS THAT HAVE BEEN DEEMPHASIZED

Sodium Bicarbonate

How Dispensed: 44.6 mEq (7.5%) or 50 mEq (8.4%) per 50 ml ampule.

Indications: Extremely limited in the setting of cardiac arrest to severe metabolic acidosis that persists *beyond* the initial phase (i.e., beyond the first 5 to 15 minutes) of the resuscitation process—and/or cardiac arrest in a patient known to have a severe *preexisting* metabolic acidosis prior to the arrest—*if any sodium bicarbonate is indicated at all. . . .*

Precautions: Although sodium bicarbonate administration will correct the *arterial* blood pH value, treating arrest-induced acidosis in this manner can be counterproductive because it may lead to a paradoxic intracellular acidosis (as well as other adverse effects).

DOSE AND ROUTE OF ADMINISTRATION

IV Bolus: If the decision is made to administer sodium bicarbonate in the setting of cardiac arrest, an initial dose of 1 mEq/kg ($\approx$ 1 to 1.5 ampules) has been recommended). No more than half this amount should be given every 10 minutes. In the postresuscitation phase, sodium bicarbonate administration should be guided by ABG measurements.

COMMENTS

Despite the seemingly intuitive logic that administration of sodium bicarbonate to buffer acid should be beneficial in cardiopulmonary arrest, there is little objective data to back this up. During the early minutes of an arrest, the primary acid-base disturbance is respiratory acidosis. This results from hypoventilation. *If a victim of cardiopulmonary arrest can be adequately ventilated and perfused during this critical period, the need for sodium bicarbonate should be minimal.*

It appears that significant metabolic acidosis does *not* develop in cardiopulmonary arrest for at least some time (5 to 15 minutes?) after patient collapse (Sanders et al, 1984; Grundler et al, 1985; Callaham, 1990). Since the primary abnormality during these initial minutes is hyp**o**ventilation (i.e., *respiratory* acidosis), it would seem far more appropriate to correct this acidosis by improving ventilation (i.e., *hyp**er**ventilating the patient*) than by administering sodium bicarbonate.

> *Sodium bicarbonate therapy is NOT benign.* Adverse effects of excessive administration of this agent include extreme alkalosis, hyperosmolality, hypokalemia, sodium overload, shifting of the oxyhemoglobin dissociation curve leftward (with consequent impaired oxygen release to the tissues), and precipitation of convulsions, ischemia, and/or arrhythmias (Mizock,

1987). Moreover, unless adequate ventilation is achieved, carbon dioxide (CO_2) will tend to accumulate. Since CO_2 is freely diffusable across cellular and organ membranes, it readily enters the brain and heart where it may further depress function by producing a **paradoxic intracellular acidosis** (Grundler et al, 1985; Bersin et al, 1989). Administration of sodium bicarbonate only aggravates this process.

The manner in which a paradoxical intracellular acidosis may be produced by sodium bicarbonate therapy can best be explained by making use of the following equation:

$$H^+ + HCO_3^- \leftrightarrow H_2CO_3 \leftrightarrow H_2O + CO_2$$

According to this equation, acid (i.e., hydrogen ion = H^+) is neutralized by bicarbonate ion (= HCO_3^-) which is provided by administered sodium bicarbonate. This results in formation of a weak acid (carbonic acid = H_2CO_3), which subsequently breaks down into water (H_2O) and carbon dioxide (CO_2).

> The source of the problem in the above equation is the CO_2, because this gas is freely diffusable across cellular membranes. *Once inside the various body cells, CO_2 combines with H_2O to drive the above reversible equation back to the left.* That is, CO_2 and H_2O combine to form H_2CO_3, which then breaks down to produce HCO_3^- and H^+.
>
> Thus, the end result of trying to neutralize extracellular acidosis (i.e., an excess concentration of H^+ ions in the blood) by administration of IV sodium bicarbonate (i.e., HCO_3^-) will be to generate *additional* CO_2. This CO_2 readily diffuses into body cells (*including* the cells of the heart and brain). Excess CO_2 accumulates *within the cells*, and results in a reversal of the process whereby the above equation is now driven back to the left—ultimately leading to production of an excess concentration of *intracellular* H^+ ions. This results in a lowering of intracellular pH—and production of the *paradoxical intracellular acidosis* (Gazmuri et al, 1990; Kette et al, 1990).

In the setting of cardiac arrest, the old standby—**arterial blood gas (ABG) studies**—is *not* the dependable predictor of intracellular acid-base status that we used to think (Weil et al, 1986; Relman, 1986). Instead, it is the pH of mixed *venous* blood that most closely reflects the true pH within the cells (Nowak et al, 1987). Unfortunately, there is no *practical* way to rapidly determine the pH of mixed venous blood during a code.

> Studies have shown that a significant discrepancy (of up to several pH units) rapidly develops between arterial and mixed venous blood with the onset of cardiopulmonary arrest (Grundler et al, 1984; Weil et al, 1984 and 1985). As a result, severe venous hypercarbia and acidosis may simultaneously exist with arterial alkalosis. Fortunately, mixed venous aci-

dosis (and hence *intracellular* acidosis) can usually be corrected for the most part simply by hyperventilation. Elimination of excess CO_2 by hyperventilation helps to prevent the above cited equation from being driven back to the left.

In the past, one or more ampules of sodium bicarbonate were almost *reflexively* given at the onset of cardiopulmonary arrest, and repeated liberally thereafter until arterial blood pH values normalized. Although this practice often succeeded in correcting arterial pH (and made the emergency care provider feel better because ABG values "improved"), in the long run it exacerbated the situation by increasing the degree of intracellular acidosis (Bersin et al, 1989; Ayus and Krothapalli, 1989). We now appreciate that additional CO_2 generated as a result of IV-administered sodium bicarbonate readily diffuses into body cells and produces an intramyocardial and intracerebral acidosis. This effect ultimately leads to depression of both myocardial and cerebral function (Weisfeldt and Guerci, 1991).

> Surprisingly, ABGs obtained during cardiopulmonary resuscitation often demonstrate relatively normal PaO_2 readings. Such readings may well be misleading. Pulmonary blood flow is dramatically reduced in patients with cardiac arrest who are being resuscitated. High oxygen saturation values may result. It is important to realize that near "perfect" oxygen saturation in this situation is primarily a reflection of the prolonged time required for passage of blood through the pulmonary circuit. It indicates little about the much larger pool of stagnant, acidotic, hypercarbic, and hypoxic blood that resides in most body tissues.

Traditionally, the rationale for administering sodium bicarbonate to patients in cardiac arrest has been based on a number of assumptions: that such treatment would limit lactate production; that intracellular pH could be corrected in a predictable manner; and that survival would be improved. *None of these assumptions have proved to be true.* Instead, sodium bicarbonate administration has been shown to *impair* tissue oxygenation, an effect that leads to development of anaerobic metabolism and an *increase* in lactate production. Intracellular acidosis is exacerbated by bicarbonate therapy, and myocardial contractility is reduced (Bersin et al, 1989; Ayus and Krothapalli, 1989). Finally, as a result of the hypertonicity of sodium bicarbonate, aortic diastolic pressure is reduced and right atrial pressure increased—effects that lead to an overall reduction in coronary perfusion pressure (Kette et al, 1991). Most important, treatment with sodium bicarbonate has *never* been shown to improve survival (Mizock, 1987; Federiuk et al, 1991).

> A certain degree of metabolic acidosis may actually be beneficial in the setting of cardiac arrest. Oxygen delivery to the tissues is improved at a lower pH (as a result of a *rightward* shift in the oxyhemoglobin dissociation curve), and cellular adenosine triphosphate (ATP) energy stores are better preserved than in an alkalotic environment (Callaham, 1990).

Surprisingly, the amount of electrical energy required to defibrillate the heart does not appear to be significantly increased by acidosis. Therapeutic effects of catecholamines are admittedly blunted in an acidotic medium, but they are definitely *not* abolished. Utilization of larger amounts of catecholamines (i.e., high-dose epinephrine) should easily overcome any blunting in their effect (Callaham, 1990). Thus beyond assuring adequate ventilation, there seems to be little (or no) justification for rapid correction of arrest-induced metabolic acidosis—especially if arterial pH is 7.15 to 7.2 or higher. Even when arterial pH is lower than this, *trying to correct intraarterial pH with bicarbonate therapy may be harmful.*

In summary, with the usual scenario that occurs during cardiopulmonary arrest, the acidosis that develops appears to be primarily *respiratory* in nature during the early minutes after patient collapse. *Appropriate initial therapy should therefore be aimed at optimizing ventilation.* Sodium bicarbonate administration is probably *not* indicated for *at least* the first 5 to 10 minutes of the resuscitation effort—*if it is ever indicated at all* .... The only possible exception to this generality is for a patient who is known to have a severe *preexisting* metabolic acidosis (such as a patient with diabetic ketoacidosis)—and even then the value of bicarbonate therapy remains uncertain.*

Standard ABG studies in cardiac arrest cannot be relied upon because they do not accurately reflect the true state of *intracellular* homeostasis. Even if mixed venous blood gas studies were routinely available to emergency care providers, one would still be faced with the dilemma of knowing that IV sodium bicarbonate administration may paradoxically *exacerbate* the degree of intracellular acidosis, and ultimately result in depression of cerebral and myocardial function.

*Chronic dialysis patients may make up a special exception to the general rule of minimizing /avoiding the use of sodium bicarbonate during cardiopulmonary resuscitation—especially if it is known that several days have passed since their last dialysis treatment. Because such individuals are particularly likely to be acidotic and/or hyperkalemic before cardiac arrest, administration of sodium bicarbonate may produce a beneficial response (Evans, 1992).

Bretylium Tosylate

How Dispensed: 500 mg per 10 ml ampule
Indications: Refractory ventricular fibrillation (not responding to lidocaine); potentially life-threatening ventricular arrhythmias including ventricular tachycardia (as a third-line agent after lidocaine and procainamide).

DOSE AND ROUTE OF ADMINISTRATION

IV Bolus: Initially, administer about 5 mg/kg (≈ 1 ampule). Defibrillate. If patient is still in ventricular fibrillation, give a second dose of 10 mg/kg (1 to 2 ampules). This may be repeated every 15 to 30 minutes up to a total loading dose of 30 mg/kg.

IV Maintenance Infusion: Mix 1 g in 250 ml D5W, and begin the infusion at 15 to 30 drops/min (1 to 2 mg/min).

IV Loading Infusion for VT: Dilute 500 mg in 50 ml of D5W, and infuse over 10 minutes. This may be followed with an IV infusion at 1 to 2 mg/min.

COMMENTS

Bretylium is a quaternary ammonium compound that was initially used in the 1950s as an antihypertensive agent. The drug has a complex mechanism of action including *adrenergic stimulation* that results in an initial release of norepinephrine, followed several minutes later by *adrenergic blockade* (in which uptake of norepinephrine and epinephrine into postganglionic adrenergic nerve endings is prevented). This latter effect becomes the predominant one and accounts for the fact that following an initial increase in blood pressure, hypotension commonly occurs.

> Bretylium-induced hypotension has a particularly strong orthostatic component and is a major factor limiting use of this drug for ventricular tachycardia. Another result of bretylium-induced adrenergic blockade is that hypersensitivity to infused catecholamines (such as epinephrine, norepinephrine, or dopamine) may develop, heightening the response to these agents.

Bretylium is most effective in the treatment of *refractory ventricular fibrillation*. The drug exerts a potent *antifibrillatory* effect that facilitates subsequent electrical conversion.

> Practically speaking, dosing of bretylium for treatment of refractory ventricular fibrillation is somewhat empiric. Initially an IV bolus of about 5 mg/kg (or about 1 ampule) may be given. *Chemical conversion of the rhythm* (i.e., spontaneous conversion of ventricular fibrillation by the drug itself) is rare. It is therefore essential to continue CPR for at least 1 to 2 minutes *after* administering bretylium to allow adequate time for the drug to reach the central circulation *before* defibrillating. If there is no response, a second dose of 10 mg/kg (1 to 2 ampules) of drug may be given, circulated, and followed again by defibrillation.

The onset of action of bretylium following bolus injection is variable. Although the drug most often begins to exert its antifibrillatory effect within 2 minutes of administration, delays of as much as up to 10 to 15 minutes (or longer) have been reported (Dhurandhar et al, 1980; Haynes et al, 1981). *This suggests that resuscitation efforts should not be abandoned after giving bretylium until adequate time has passed to ensure that the drug has had a chance to act.* Following the second dose of bretylium, additional 10 mg/kg boluses of the drug may be administered at 15- to 30-minute intervals until the maximum dose (30 mg/kg) has been given.

> Because the duration of action of a bretylium bolus is between 2 to 6 hours, some protection against immediate recurrence of ventricular fibrillation is provided by this form of administration. Most emergency care providers also tend to initiate a prophylactic maintenance infusion (of *either* bretylium or lidocaine) as soon as the patient is converted to a normal rhythm in the hope of providing additional protection.

Recent years have seen a deemphasis in the use of bretylium as treatment of refractory ventricular fibrillation. Lidocaine is preferred as *initial* antifibrillatory treatment because it is equally effective as bretylium, and emergency care providers are much more familiar with its use. Lidocaine may also be a safer agent to use in this setting.

> At least theoretically, administration of bretylium could be counterproductive in the arrested heart because the vasodilatation it produces (as a result of sympathetic blockade) may adversely affect aortic diastolic pressure and coronary blood flow (Euler et al, 1986). If conversion to a spontaneously perfusing rhythm occurs, after effects of the bretylium bolus may result in residual hypotension.
>
> Despite potential adverse effects of bretylium-induced adrenergic blockade, this drug may still have a role in the treatment of selected patients with refractory ventricular fibrillation who fail to respond lidocaine. In this situation, the addition of one or more boluses of bretylium may act in a *synergistic* manner to enhance the antifibrillatory effect of lidocaine (Hanyok et al, 1988).

The use of bretylium for treatment of ventricular tachycardia has been deemphasized to an even greater degree. Currently, the drug is viewed as no more than a *third-line* agent for this indication, and probably should not be used unless optimal doses of procainamide and lidocaine have been tried and failed.

> When used to treat *ventricular tachycardia*, bretylium should be given as a *slow* IV loading infusion to minimize the risk of developing hypotension, and nausea and vomiting (in the awake patient) that may occur if the drug is administered too rapidly. One can dilute 500 mg in 50 ml of D5W, and set up an infusion to run in over a 10-minute period. If successful, IV loading may be followed by a maintenance infusion of the drug at 1 to 2 mg/min. Slower loading (i.e., over 30 minutes) and lowering the rate of the maintenance infusion to 0.5 mg/min may help to reduce the incidence of adverse effects from the drug.

It is important to emphasize that bretylium is *not* a first-line agent for treatment of PVCs. In fact, ventricular ectopy may actually *worsen* when bretylium is first administered because of the initial adrenergic stimulation (and release of norepinephrine) it produces (Castle, 1984; Lucchesi, 1984). As a result, lidocaine and procainamide are preferred for initial treatment of PVCs. *Only if malignant ventricular arrhythmias persist despite optimal administration of these two antiarrhythmic agents would a trial of bretylium seem warranted.*

In summary, bretylium is an effective antifibrillatory agent that may be indicated for the treatment of ventricular fibrillation that has not responded to repeated attempts at defibrillation, epinephrine, and lidocaine. In this situation, the addition of one or more boluses of bretylium could produce a synergistic antifibrillatory effect (with already administered lidocaine). If the decision is made to use bretylium in this setting, one should be sure to allow adequate time for the drug to act (i.e., up to 10 to 15 minutes) *before* concluding that the rhythm is truly refractory.

Use of bretylium for treatment of PVCs or ventricular tachycardia has been deemphasized.

In emergency cardiac care, calcium *chloride* is the most commonly administered form of this cation. It is important to realize that other calcium preparations are available, and that the amount of *elemental calcium* (i.e., the potency) of each preparation may vary significantly. For example, three times as much elemental calcium is contained in one 10-ml ampule of calcium chloride as in one 10-ml ampule of calcium gluconate (i.e., 270 mg compared to 90 mg). Thus, compared to calcium chloride, larger amounts of calcium gluconate are needed to obtain the same therapeutic effect. *Awareness of the particular preparation being administered is therefore essential.*

Calcium Chloride

How Dispensed: The 10% solution of calcium chloride contains 1,000 mg (13.6 mEq) of calcium per 10-ml syringe.

Indications: Limited in the acute care setting to *four* clinical situations: (1) hypocalcemia; (2) hyperkalemia; (3) asystole/marked bradycardia that occurs following administration of IV verapamil; and (4) as pretreatment before the use of IV verapamil.

Precautions: Calcium administration is contraindicated in the setting of digitalis toxicity. Caution is urged in patients with significant renal impairment.

DOSE AND ROUTE OF ADMINISTRATION

IV Dose/Calcium Pretreatment: Administer 500 to 1,000 (5 to 10 ml) of a 10% solution of calcium chloride over a 5- to 10-minute period.

Too rapid IV infusion of calcium may produce a generalized sensation of heat in the patient. This usually resolves if the rate of the infusion is slowed or temporarily stopped.

Excessive administration of calcium could potentially produce adverse effects (i.e., marked bradycardia or other arrhythmias). As a result, we share the concern urged by Jameson and Hargarten (1992), and favor use of the lower dose of calcium chloride (i.e., *no more* than half an ampule = ≤500 mg) for initial administration.

If the indication for replacement is less urgent (i.e., less severe hypocalcemia in a hemodynamically stable patient), calcium chloride may be added to the patient's IV solution and more gradually infused over a period of several hours.

COMMENTS

In the past, calcium chloride had been routinely recommended for treatment of asystole and EMD. No longer. Clinical data in support of these indications in the setting of cardiac arrest are lacking.

Previous reports on the use of calcium chloride in the setting of cardiac arrest were largely anecdotal, and included surgical patients (who were likely to be hypocalcemic from multiple blood transfusions) and patients with pulseless intraventricular conduction defects that were the result of hyperkalemia (Harrison and Amey, 1984; Stueven, 1984). Both of these conditions should have been *expected* to respond to calcium administration. If anything, experience with the use of calcium chloride for patients with prehospital cardiovascular collapse and asystole suggests that the drug is associated with an *unfavorable* outcome in a significant percentage of cases (Stueven et al, 1983; Stueven, 1984).

There are a number of reasons why administration of calcium may be deleterious in this setting. The drug was initially recommended out of a belief that "the inotropic state of the heart depended on calcium" (Redding et al, 1983). However, calcium *increases* ventricular excitability and *suppresses* sinus impulse formation. Given too rapidly or in an excessive amount, it may produce marked bradycardia or even asystole.

Studies have shown that routine administration of a 500-mg IV bolus of the drug (as had been previously recommended for cardiac arrest) results in dangerously high elevations of the serum calcium level (to a mean value of 15 mg/100 ml). Levels remain elevated for an average of 15 minutes after the drug is given (Dembo, 1981). Moreover, emergency administration of calcium to patients in cardiac arrest may induce spasm of the cerebral microvasculature and lead to cerebral hypoperfusion (White et al, 1983; Stempien et al, 1986). Current work on cerebrovascular preservation after cardiac arrest has focused on the use of calcium antagonists, and if anything suggests that administration of these agents may improve cerebral blood flow and enhance neurologic recovery. If calcium antagonists act to enhance cerebral blood flow (and help to "save" the brain), calcium chloride might well be expected to do the opposite.

In summary, the use of calcium chloride is now *contraindicated* for the treatment of asystole and EMD. Use of this agent in the emergency care setting is essentially limited to the following *four* special situations:

1. Hypocalcemia
2. Hyperkalemia (which responds acutely to administration of glucose/insulin and/or calcium infusion)
3. Asystole (or marked bradycardia) that occurs immediately following the use of a calcium antagonist (such as may be seen when IV verapamil is used to treat PSVT)
4. As pretreatment of patients with supraventricular tachyarrhythmias prior to administration of IV verapamil *(see Section B of Chapter 2 for additional information regarding the use of verapamil/calcium pretreatment of SVT).*

Isoproterenol

How Dispensed: 1-mg vials

Indications: As a *stopgap measure* (until pacemaker therapy can be initiated) for chronotropic support of hemodynamically significant bradyarrhythmias that have not responded to atropine.

DOSE AND ROUTE OF ADMINISTRATION

IV Infusion: Mix 1 mg in 250 ml D5W, and begin drip at 30 drops/min (2 µg/min). Titrate infusion to clinical effect. Rate of infusion should not exceed 10 µg/min.

COMMENTS

Isoproterenol is a pure β-adrenergic receptor stimulating agent which exerts an equipotent effect on β-1 and β-2 receptors. The former action results in enhanced myocardial contractility and an increase in heart rate (i.e., positive inotropic and chronotropic effects), whereas the β-2 adrenergic stimulating effect results in vasodilatation and a reduction in systemic vascular resistance.

Although in the past isoproterenol was recommended as the vasopressor of choice in the setting of cardiac arrest, the drug has been greatly deemphasized in recent years. Currently, the *only* indication for its use is as a *stopgap measure* (i.e., until pacemaker therapy can be initiated) for the treatment of hemodynamically significant bradyarrhythmias that have not responded to atropine. In this setting, *low-dose* infusion of the drug may provide effective *chronotropic* support. However, when used in higher doses

(i.e., >5-10 µg/min), adverse effects are much more likely to occur.

There are many reasons why isoproterenol has been deemphasized. Adverse effects of the drug include excessive acceleration of heart rate, arrhythmogenicity, increased myocardial oxygen consumption, hypotension, and decreased myocardial and vital organ perfusion.

The excessive tachycardia so commonly seen in association with isoproterenol infusion may be deleterious in several ways. Because of disproportionate shortening of the period of diastole, left ventricular filling time is curtailed. Tachycardia also increases myocardial oxygen consumption and predisposes the patient to myocardial ischemia and cardiac arrhythmias.

Hypotension is likely to result from the reduction in systemic vascular resistance. The effect is likely to further reduce aortic diastolic pressure and coronary perfusion. As a result, isoproterenol is now *contraindicated* as a treatment measure in the arrested heart (i.e., for ventricular fibrillation, asystole, or EMD). In the patient with a spontaneous circulation, the vasodilatory effect of isoproterenol tends to redistribute blood flow to *nonvital* organs (i.e., skin and skeletal muscle). This further compromises oxygen delivery to the heart, brain, and kidneys. Thus, when confronted with a patient in cardiac arrest or in a hemodynamically significant bradyarrhythmia, the use of a pressor agent with α-adrenergic (vasoconstrictor) activity (i.e., epinephrine or dopamine) appears to be far preferable to the use of isoproterenol.

References

American Heart Association Subcommittee on Emergency Cardiac Care: Standards and guidelines for cardiopulmonary resuscitation (CPR) and emergency cardiac care (ECC), *JAMA* 255(suppl):2905-2992, 1986.

Ayus JC, Krothapalli RK: Effect of bicarbonate administration on cardiac function, *Am J Med* 87:5-6, 1989.

Bersin RM, Chatterjee K, Arieff AI: Metabolic and hemodynamic consequences of sodium bicarbonate administration in patients with heart disease, *Am J Med* 87:7-14, 1989.

Callaham ML: High-dose epinephrine therapy and other advances in treating cardiac arrest, *West J Med* 152:697-703, 1990.

Castle L: Therapy of ventricular tachycardia, *Am J Cardiol* 54:26A-33A, 1984.

Dembo DH: Calcium in advanced life support, *Crit Care Med* 9:358-359, 1981.

Dhurandhar RW, Pickron J, Goldman AM: Bretylium tosylate in the management of recurrent ventricular fibrillation complicating acute myocardial infarction, *Heart Lung* 9:265-270, 1980.

Euler DE, Zeman TW, Wallock ME, Scanlon PJ: Deleterious effects of bretylium in hemodynamic recovery from ventricular fibrillation, *Am Heart J* 112:25-31, 1986.

Evans DH: Presumptive use of bicarbonate in cardiopulmonary resuscitation, *JAMA* 267:807, 1992 (letter).

Federiuk CS, Saners AB, Kern KB, Nelson, Ewy GA: The effect of bicarbonate on resuscitation from cardiac arrest, *Ann Emerg Med* 20:1173-1177, 1991.

Gazmuri RJ, Van Planta M, Weil MH, Rackow EC: Cardiac effects of carbon dioxide-consuming and carbon dioxide-generating buffers during cardiopulmonary resuscitation, *J Am Coll Cardiol* 15:482-490, 1990.

Grundler W, Weil MH, Yamaguchi M, Michaels S: The paradox of venous acidosis and arterial alkalosis during CPR, *Chest* 86:262, 1984 (abstract).

Grundler W, Weil MH, Rackow E, Falk JL, Bisera J, Miller JM, Michaels S: Selective acidosis in venous blood during human cardiopulmonary resuscitation: A preliminary report, *Crit Care Med* 13:886-887, 1985.

Hanyok JJ, Chow MSS, Kluger J, Fieldman A: Antifibrillatory effects of high dose bretylium and a lidocaine-bretylium combination during cardiopulmonary resuscitation, *Crit Care Med* 16:691-694, 1988.

Haynes RE, Chinn TL, Copass MK, Cobb LA: Comparison of bretylium tosylate and lidocaine in management of out-of-hospital ventricular fibrillation: A randomized clinical trial, *Am J Cardiol* 48:353-356, 1981.

Jameson SJ, Hargarten SW: Calcium pretreatment to prevent verapamil-induced hypotension in patients with SVT, *Ann Emerg Med* 21:68, 1992 (letter).

Kette F, Weil MH, Von Planta M, Gazmuri R, Rackow EC: Buffer agents do not reverse intramyocardial acidosis during cardiac resuscitation, *Circulation* 81:1660-1666, 1990.

Kette F, Weil MH, Gazmuri RJ: Buffer solutions may compromise cardiac resuscitation by reducing coronary perfusion pressure, *JAMA* 266:2121-2126, 1991.

Lucchesi BR: Rationale of therapy in the patient with acute myocardial infarction and life-threatening arrhythmias: A focus on bretylium, *Am J Cardiol* 54:14A-19A, 1984.

Mizock BA: Controversies in lactic acidosis: Implications in critically ill patients, *JAMA* 258:497-501, 1987.

Morris LR, Murphy MB, Kitabchi AE: Bicarbonate therapy in severe diabetic ketoacidosis, *Ann Int Med* 105:834-840, 1986.

Narins RG, Cohen JJ: Bicarbonate therapy for organic acidosis: The case for its continued use, *Ann Int Med* 106:615-618, 1987.

Nowak RM, Martin GB, Garden DL, Tomlanovich MC: Selective venous hypercarbia during human CPR: Implications regarding blood flow, *Ann Emerg Med* 16:527-530, 1987.

Redding JS, Haynes RR, Thomas JD: Drug therapy in resuscitaiton from electromechanical dissociation, *Crit Care Med* 11:681-684, 1983.

Relman AS: "Blood gases": Arterial or venous? *N Engl J Med* 315:187-188, 1986.

Sanders AB, Ewy GA, Taft TY: Resuscitation and arterial blood gas abnormalities during prolonged cardiopulmonary resuscitation, *Ann Emerg Med* 13:676-679, 1984.

Stacpoole P: Lactic acidosis: The case against bicarbonate therapy, *Ann Int Med* 105:276-279, 1986.

Stueven H, Thompson BM, Aprahamian C, Darin JC: Use of calcium in prehospital cardiac arrest, *Ann Emerg Med* 12:136-139, 1983.

Stueven HA: Calcium chloride: Reassessment of use in asystole, *Ann Emerg Med* 13:820-822, 1984.

Weil MH, Grundler W, Rackow EC, Bisera J, Miller JM, Michaels S: Blood gas measurements in human patients during CPR, *Chest* 86:282, 1984 (abstract).

Weil MH, Grundler W, Yamaguchi M, Michaels S, Rackow EC: Arterial blood gases fail to reflect acid-base status during cardiopulmonary resuscitation: A preliminary report, *Crit Care Med* 13:884-885, 1985.

Weil MH, Rackow EC, Trevino R, Grundler W, Falk JL, Griffel MI: Difference in acid-base stage between venous and arterial blood during cardiopulmonary resuscitation, *N Engl J Med* 315:153-156, 1986.

Weisfeldt ML, Guerci AD: Sodium bicarbonate in CPR, *JAMA* 266:2129-2130, 1991.

White BC, Winegar CD, Wilson RF, Hochner PJ, Prombley JH: Possible role of calcium blockers in cerebral resuscitation: A review of the literature and synthesis for future studies, *Crit Care Med* 11:202-207, 1983.

CHAPTER 3

BASIC ARRHYTHMIA INTERPRETATION

BASIC PRINCIPLES AND SYSTEMATIC APPROACH

In order to effectively manage a cardiac arrest, one has to be able to rapidly and accurately diagnose cardiac arrhythmias. The goal of this chapter is to present a readily mastered approach to aid in rapid recognition and interpretation. We will then run through the gamut of arrhythmias that are likely to be encountered during a cardiac arrest and show how the method may be applied. Discussion of more subtle arrhythmias is deferred until Chapters 15 and 16.

Heart Rate

Before tackling the intricacies of rhythm analysis, it is important to feel comfortable calculating heart rate. Many methods exist for doing this. Perhaps the easiest to master is simply to *take 300 and divide it by the number of large boxes in the R-R interval*. Explanation of this method is as follows. The dimensions of small and large boxes on ECG grid paper are 1 mm and 5 mm, respectively. Since the usual speed of recording is 25 mm/sec, the amount of time needed to travel the distance represented by each small box (1 mm) is $\frac{1}{25}$th (0.04) of a second *(Fig. 3A-1)*. By the same reasoning, the amount of time needed to travel the distance represented by each large box (5 mm) is 5 × 0.4 = 0.20 seconds.

If a QRS complex were to occur every large box (every 0.20 sec) as shown in Figure 3A-1, then 5 QRS complexes would occur in 1 second (5 × 0.20 = 1 sec). Since there are 60 seconds in a minute, the heart rate would be 300 beats/min (5 beats/sec × 60 sec = 300 beats/min). *Thus, if a QRS complex occurs every large box, the heart rate will be 300 beats/min.* If the rate were only half as fast (if a QRS complex occurred every 2 large boxes), it would be 150 beats/min (300 ÷ 2 = 150 beats/min). A heart rate one third as fast (a QRS occurring every 3 large boxes) reflects a rate of 100 beats/min (300 ÷ 3); a QRS complex every 4 large boxes, a rate of 75 beats/min (300 ÷ 4); and so forth *(Fig. 3A-2)*.

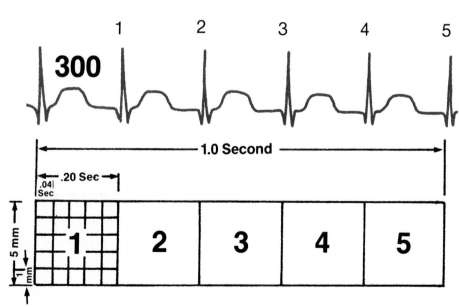

Figure 3A-1.   Dimensions of small and large boxes on standard ECG grid paper.

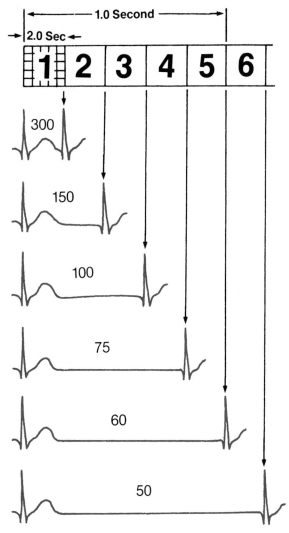

Figure 3A-2. Simplified method for rapid estimation of heart rate when the rhythm is regular. *Divide 300 by the number of large boxes in the R-R interval.* Applying this method, it can be seen that if a QRS complex occurred every 6 large boxes, the heart rate would be 50 beats/min (300 ÷ 6 = 50).

Before calculating the heart rate of any arrhythmia, it is important to determine if the rhythm is *regular*. Although this can usually be done quite readily by inspection, subtle variations in regularity may sometimes be missed by this method. When in doubt, regularity of the rhythm may be confirmed by measuring each R-R interval with a pair of **calipers*** (or by marking down the R-R interval on a sheet of paper and checking to see if each beat is on time).

*There appears to be an imagined "aura" surrounding the use of calipers, with the expectation (assumption) by many that *he or she who uses calipers must be an expert in arrhythmia interpretation.* As a result, our suggestion to use **calipers** may initially seem quite intimidating (if not downright overwhelming) to the beginning or less experienced interpreter. *This need not be the case!* With a minimum of practice, the use of calipers soon becomes a natural part of rhythm interpretation. The benefits of such use are immediately clear, as rates are much more rapidly calculated and seemingly subtle relationships between atrial and ventricular activity become ever so obvious. Resistance on the part of some experienced clinicians to use calipers is not borne out of increased knowledge, but instead arises from their failure to accept this fact.

When the rhythm is regular, the easiest way to determine the R-R interval is to select a QRS complex that begins on a *heavy* line and to count over to where the next QRS complex occurs.

PROBLEM   **Apply the method for calculating heart rate shown in Figure 3A-2 to the examples shown in *Figures 3A-3* through *3A-6.***

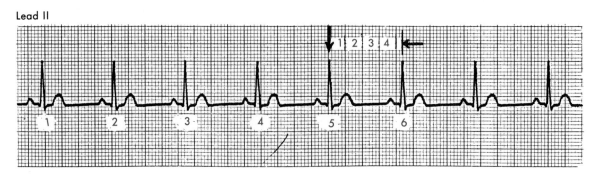

Figure 3A-3

Lead II

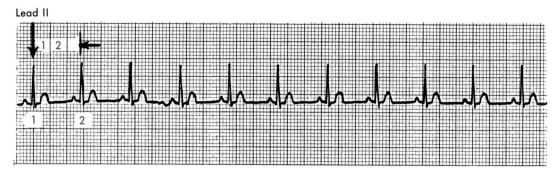

Figure 3A-4

Lead II

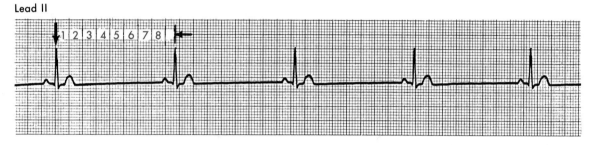

Figure 3A-5

Lead II

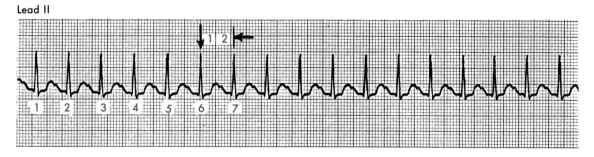

Figure 3A-6

ANSWER TO FIGURE 3A-3   The rhythm is regular. The upstroke of the R wave of beat #5 occurs on a heavy line. The R wave of beat #6 is a little over four large boxes away. Thus the R-R interval is between four and five large boxes, and slightly closer to the former. If it were exactly four large boxes, the rate would be 75 beats/min (300 ÷ 4). If it were five large boxes, the rate would be 60 beats/min (300 ÷ 5). The rate is about 70 beats/min.

ANSWER TO FIGURE 3A-4   Again the rhythm is regular. Using beat #1 (which falls on a heavy line) as a starting point and counting over, the R-R interval is just *less* than three large boxes. If it were exactly three large boxes, then the rate would be 100 beats/min. Since the rate is a little faster than this, we estimate it to be about 105 beats/min.

ANSWER TO FIGURE 3A-5   The rhythm is *slow* but regular. The R-R interval is between eight and nine large boxes. If it were eight boxes, the heart rate would be 38 beats/min (300 ÷ 8). If it were 10 boxes, the rate would be 30 beats/min (300 ÷ 10). The heart rate is therefore about 35 beats/min.

ANSWER TO FIGURE 3A-6   The rhythm is *rapid* but regular. Using beat #6 as a starting point and counting over, the R-R interval is just over two large boxes. Thus the rate is just under 150 beats/min, or about 140 beats/min.

When the heart rate is extremely rapid (between 150 and 300 beats/min), accurate estimation becomes difficult since minor discrepancies in how one measures the R-R interval may exert a disproportionately large effect on the calculated rate. Not accounting for the thickness of one's calipers (or even of the QRS complex itself) may throw the estimate off by as much as 20 to 30 beats/min!

Lead II

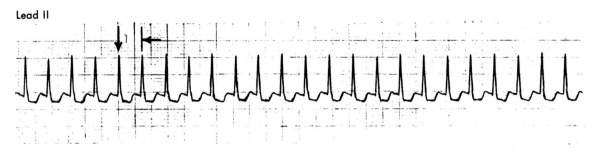

Figure 3A-7.　　Is the heart rate above or below 200 beats/min?

PROBLEM　　**Calculate the heart rate of the rhythm shown in *Figure 3A-7. Is the rate above or below 200 beats/min?***

ANSWER TO FIGURE 3A-7　　The rhythm is extremely rapid but regular. Because the R-R interval is between one and two large boxes, the heart rate must be between 150 and 300 beats/min. However, it is difficult to tell by the method just presented whether the rate is above or below 200 beats/min.

Figure 3A-7A illustrates a useful way of overcoming this difficulty. When the rate is fast and regular, *measure the R-R interval of **every other beat.*** Dividing 300 by this number will yield *one half* the actual rate. Simply double this number to determine the actual rate.

If one picks a QRS complex that falls on a heavy line in Figure 3A-7A (beat #5 will do), it can be seen that the R-R interval of every other beat is just *under* three large boxes. Thus, *half the rate* must be a little more than 100 beats/min (≈105 beats/min). The actual rate in Figure 3A-7A is therefore about 210 beats/min.

> As stated above, the R-R interval of the rhythm in Figure 3A-7A is between one and two large boxes. If it were exactly one large box (five small boxes), the heart rate would be 300 beats/min. If it were exactly two large boxes (10 small boxes), the rate would be 150 beats/min. One might reason that if an R-R interval of five small boxes reflects a heart rate of 300 beats/min and one of 10 small boxes reflects a rate of 150 beats/min, each small box should represent an increment of 30 beats/min. By this line of reasoning, an R-R interval of 1½ large boxes (7½ small boxes) might be expected to represent a heart rate midway between 300 and 150 beats/min, or 225 beats/min.

Unfortunately, calculation of heart rate is not quite so simple! The incremental change in heart rate for each small box is *not* equal. This concept is illustrated in *Figure 3A-8*.

Note in Figure 3A-8 that there is a 50 beat/min decrement in heart rate (from 300 to 250 beats/min) when the R-R interval lengthens from five to six small boxes, but only a 17 beat/min decrement (from 167 to 150 beats/min) when it lengthens from nine to ten small boxes. Decrements become nearly equal once the heart rate drops below 100 beats/min.

PROBLEM　　**Return to *Figure 3A-6* and determine the number of small boxes in the R-R interval. Refer to *Figure 3A-8* to determine the heart rate.**

ANSWER　　The upstroke of the R wave of the sixth QRS complex in Figure 3A-6 occurs precisely on a heavy line. Counting over, the R-R interval is 11 small boxes in duration. Therefore, according to Figure 3A-8, the heart rate should be 136 beats/min.

> Practically speaking, dividing 300 by the number of large boxes in the R-R interval will *almost always* yield accurate enough heart rate estimation for our purposes. For those with an interest in more precise heart rate determination, particularly in the presence of rapid heart rates, referral to Figure 3A-8 may be helpful.

RHYTHM DETERMINATION

The key to dysrhythmia interpretation is to apply a *systematic* approach. In addition to estimating heart rate, four basic points should be considered for every arrhythmia that is analyzed. We incorporate these points into the *four basic questions (Table 3A-1).*

Lead II

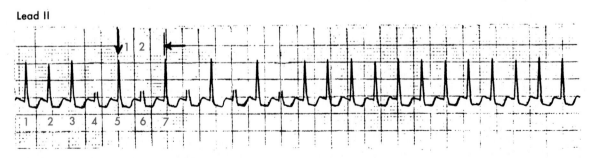

Figure 3A-7A.　　The ***every-other-beat method*** for estimating heart rate when the rhythm is fast and regular.

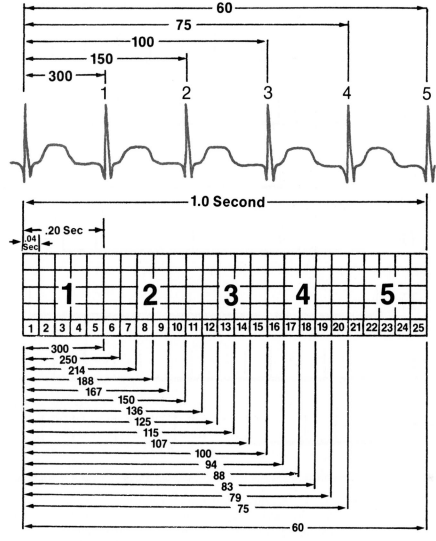

Figure 3A-8.   Graph for more accurate calculation of heart rate. Note that the incremental change in heart rate for each small box is *not* equal!

Table 3A-1

Approach to Rhythm Analysis
A. Heart Rate Estimation
B. Rhythm Analysis: The Four Questions
1. *Is the rhythm regular?*
2. *Are there P waves?*
3. *Is the QRS wide or narrow?*
4. *Is there a relationship between P waves and the QRS complex?*

1) IS THE RHYTHM REGULAR?

We have already alluded to the importance of regularity in rhythm interpretation. Determination of the degree of regularity (or lack thereof) usually provides the first clue to the etiology of an arrhythmia. In most instances, assessment of regularity will be obvious from inspection. *Figure 3A-9* schematically demonstrates how rhythms may be *precisely* regular, *almost* regular (with slight beat-to-beat variation), regular with the exception of an occasional early *(premature)* or late-occurring *("escape")* beat, *irregularly irregular*, or irregular in a certain pattern (i.e., with a "regular irregularity," or *group beating*).

Try your hand at using calipers to verify the relationships given in the legend of Figure 3A-9. Admittedly, the subtle beat-to-beat variability of pattern B is often of little clinical significance. Note that with patterns C and D, the interval *after* the early **(X)** or late **(Y)** complex also differs from the usual rate before the underlying regular pattern resumes. The irregular irregularity (i.e., continual variation) of the rhythm in pattern E is obvious from inspection. However, slight (but definite) irregularity of the rhythm is much more difficult to

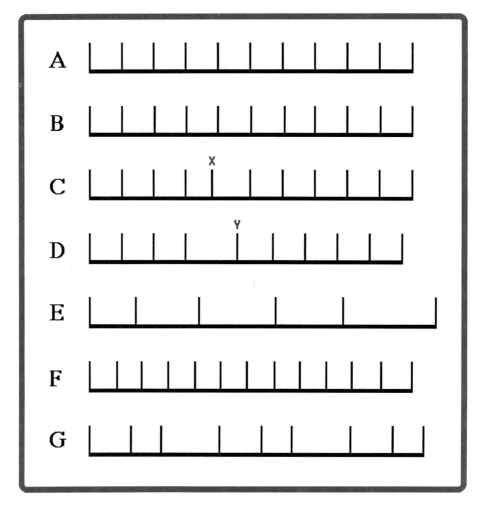

Figure 3A-9.   Schematic demonstration of the different patterns of rhythm regularity. **A,** Precisely regular rhythm. **B,** Almost regular rhythm (with slight beat-to-beat variation). **C,** Regular rhythm except for an early-occurring beat (*premature* beat **X**). **D,** Regular rhythm except for a late-occurring beat (*"escape"* beat **Y**). **E,** Irregularly irregular slower rhythm. **F,** Irregularly irregular rapid rhythm. **G,** Regularly irregular rhythm *(group beating)*.

recognize visually (i.e., without use of calipers) when the rate is rapid (pattern F). Finally, despite its irregularity, a definite pattern (of three grouped beats) is present in G. *As we progress through this chapter, clinical implications of each of these patterns will soon become clear.*

2) ARE THERE P WAVES?

Detection of *P waves* is the cornerstone of rhythm analysis. By definition, the P wave should *always* be upright in standard lead II with normal sinus rhythm. This is because orientation of the electrical impulse as it travels from the sinoatrial (SA) node to the atrioventricular (AV) node is virtually parallel to lead II *(Fig. 3A-10).* Under normal circumstances, **if the P wave is not upright in lead II, normal sinus rhythm cannot be present!**

The *only* exceptions to the general rule that the P wave in lead II is always upright with normal sinus rhythm is if there is lead misplacement or dextrocardia.

QUESTION   **Which exception to this rule would you expect to be more common—lead misplacement or dextrocardia?**

ANSWER   Lead misplacement probably accounts for 99% of the exceptions to this rule (in which there is P wave negativity in lead II despite sinus rhythm). Lead misplacement is especially likely to occur under the stressful situation of running a cardiac arrest.

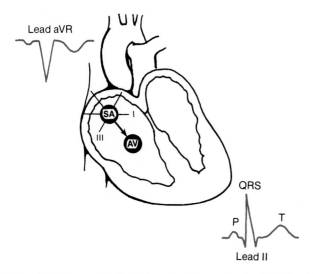

Figure 3A-10. By definition, the P wave in lead II should *always* be upright with normal sinus rhythm. (The *only* exceptions to this rule are if there is dextrocardia or lead misplacement.)

> *If QRS duration is **greater** than **half** a large box, the QRS complex is wide.*

A caveat to keep in mind when assessing QRS duration is that occasionally a portion of the QRS complex may be *iso-electric* (lie on the baseline). When this happens one may get the false impression that in a particular lead the QRS complex is shorter than it really is. To avoid this pitfall, whenever possible one should try to survey the ECG in more than one lead.

When the QRS complex is *narrow* (≤0.10 second), the electrical impulse almost always has a *supraventricular* origin. That is, the impulse originates from the SA node, the AV node, or from elsewhere in the atria (i.e., from anywhere *above* the dotted line in *Fig. 3A-11*). Rarely it may arise from a site low down in the conduction system (below

> Thus, *practically speaking, if the P wave is not upright in lead II, you don't have sinus rhythm!* Recognition of P wave negativity in lead II (and/or the absence of a distinct, upright P wave in this lead) is therefore a strong clue that some other rhythm (e.g., junctional rhythm, atrial flutter, or ventricular tachycardia) is present.

3) IS THE QRS COMPLEX WIDE OR NARROW?

Width of the QRS complex is a most helpful determinant of the site of origin of the electrical impulse. The usual upper limit of normal for duration of the QRS complex in adults is 0.10 second. A QRS duration of 0.11 second is "borderline," whereas one of 0.12 second or greater is definitely prolonged.

Previously we have indicated that each large box on ECG grid paper corresponds to 0.20 second in time. *One half* of a large box therefore corresponds to 0.10 second in time. This makes it easy to tell at a glance if the QRS complex is prolonged:

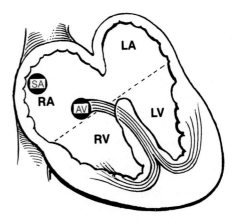

Figure 3A-11. In general, when the QRS complex is narrow, the electrical impulse will be of *supraventricular* origin (i.e., originate from *above* the *dotted line*). A widened QRS complex is likely to have a ventricular site of origin (i.e., originate from *below* the *dotted line*) unless something has happened to alter ventricular conduction.

the dotted line) such as the bundle of His or one of the bundle branches.

On the other hand, when the QRS complex is *widened* (≥0.12 second), the site of origin may not be so certain. Although widening of the QRS complex suggests a ventricular site of origin, the impulse could still be supraventricular if something has happened to alter ventricular conduction.

The Pathway of Normal Conduction

With normal sinus rhythm, the electrical impulse originates in the SA node, the principal pacemaker of the heart. From there it spreads through the right and left atria on its way to the AV node. The impulse then enters the ventricular conduction system, from which it will be carried to all parts of the ventricles (Fig. 3A-11).

When the ventricular conduction system is functioning normally, the time required for conduction of the electrical impulse from the SA node throughout the ventricular myocardium is short. Such conduction results in a narrow QRS complex. Should the impulse originate from another supraventricular site instead of the SA node (from either the right or left atria or from the AV node), it will still pass through the ventricular conduction system en route to activating the ventricles. Therefore, under normal circumstances the QRS complex will be narrow and of similar morphology for normal sinus beats, AV nodal beats, and beats originating from elsewhere in the atria–since the same conduction pathway through the ventricles will have been used.

Should there be a defect in ventricular conduction (as in *bundle branch block*) or should ventricular conduction be abnormal *(aberrant)* due to incomplete recovery of a portion of the conduction system following a premature beat, both the path and the time for the electrical impulse to travel through the ventricles will be altered. In such cases, the QRS complex may change in morphology and become *widened* despite a supraventricular origin.

4) *IS THERE A RELATIONSHIP BETWEEN P WAVES AND THE QRS COMPLEX?*

Determination of the relationship between P waves and QRS complexes is critical to rhythm analysis. In analyzing any given rhythm strip, it is probably easiest to first identify QRS complexes. One can then look to see if P waves precede each QRS. If they do, are P waves related *("married")* to their respective QRS complex?

With **normal sinus rhythm**, every QRS complex is preceded by a normal appearing P wave (i.e., a P wave that is upright in lead II) with a *constant* PR interval. That is, each atrial impulse is conducted to the ventricles. If AV conduction is normal, the PR interval will be ≤0.20 second (or *not greater* than a large box in duration). With **1° AV block,** each atrial impulse is still conducted to the ventricles with a constant PR interval, but the time required for AV conduction is prolonged (to ≥0.21 second). With more advanced degrees of AV block, conduction of

one or more atrial impulses to the ventricles is prevented *("blocked")*, and the relationship between P waves and QRS complexes is altered.

It doesn't matter in which order the Four Questions are asked. In fact it will often be advantageous to alter the order. What *is* important, however, is to *always* ask yourself *each* of these questions when analyzing *any* arrhythmia. Even when the answer is obvious, mentally checking off these four points as a matter of routine will prove invaluable for organizing one's approach to dysrhythmia interpretation. Especially when confronted with more difficult arrhythmias, adherence to this systematic technique will be extremely helpful in narrowing the list of diagnostic possibilities.

PROBLEM   **Return to *Figures 3A-3* and *3A-4*. Analyze these rhythms by the Four-Question approach shown in Table 3A-1.**

ANSWER TO FIGURE 3A-3   The rhythm is regular and the heart rate is 70 beats/min. The QRS complex is of normal duration (≤0.10 second, or clearly *not greater* than one half of a large box in duration). Each QRS is preceded by a P wave with a constant, normal (≤0.20 second) PR interval. This is *normal sinus rhythm.*

Normal Sinus Rhythm

By convention, we define normal sinus rhythm in an adult to have a rate between 60 and 100 beats/min. Sinus conduction with a faster ventricular rate is termed sinus *tachycardia*, whereas a slower rate is sinus *bradycardia*. Neither sinus bradycardia nor sinus tachycardia necessarily represent a disease state, and both are commonly found among normal individuals.

The limits for sinus bradycardia and sinus tachycardia are very different in the pediatric age group (as we will see in Section D of Chapter 17). Thus a heart rate of 75 beats/min constitutes sinus bradycardia for an infant, whereas one of 130 beats/min is perfectly normal for this age group. For the purpose of this introductory chapter on arrhythmia interpretation, unless we specifically state otherwise, you can safely assume that all rhythms shown are from adult patients.

ANSWER TO FIGURE 3A-4   The rhythm is regular and the heart rate is 105 beats/min. The QRS complex is narrow, and each beat is preceded by a normal, upright P wave with a constant PR interval. This is *sinus tachycardia.*

PROBLEM   **What about the rhythm shown in *Figure 3A-12*? In what way does this arrhythmia differ from those we have examined up to now?**

Lead II

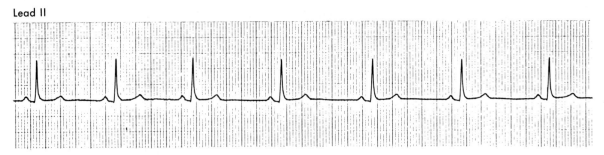

Figure 3A-12

ANSWER TO FIGURE 3A-12   Although at first glance this rhythm may appear to be regular, measurement with calipers reveals a slight (but definite) irregularity. The R-R interval is between five and six large boxes, putting the rate between 50 and 60 beats/min. Each QRS complex is preceded by a normal-appearing, upright P wave, and the PR interval is normal. This is *sinus brady-cardia* and *arrhythmia*.

Sinus Arrhythmia

Sinus arrhythmia is an extremely common normal finding among children and young adults, in whom heart rate often varies with respiration. Although sinus arrhythmia may also occur normally in the elderly, it is usually not related to respiration in this age group and sometimes is the precursor of *sick sinus syndrome*.

The rate of even "normal sinus rhythm" may often vary slightly from beat to beat (as in pattern B of Fig. 3A-9). To diagnose sinus *arrhythmia* (and to distinguish it from the slight normal variation in rate that may occur with normal sinus rhythm), there should be a difference of *at least* 0.08 second between the shortest and longest R-R intervals.

Despite the existence of this criterion, the presence of sinus arrhythmia is frequently overlooked (and/or not noted) in practice because subtle differences in heart rate are easy to miss unless one meticulously measures each R-R interval on every tracing. *Clinically, sinus arrhythmia is usually of little significance.* More marked variations in the R-R interval (>0.20 second), however, should probably at least be noted.

PROBLEM   **Examine the rhythm shown in *Figure 3A-13*. From where in the conduction system would you expect this rhythm to arise?**

ANSWER TO FIGURE 3A-13   The rhythm is regular, and the R-R interval is between five and six large boxes. Thus, the heart rate is about 55 beats/min. The QRS complex is of normal duration, but there are no P waves! This is *AV nodal* (or *junctional*) *rhythm.*

Junctional (AV Nodal) Rhythm

We have already indicated that the SA node is the principal pacemaker of the heart, and that with normal sinus rhythm it usually fires at a rate of between 60 and 100 beats/min. Should something happen to the SA node's pacesetting ability, other areas of the heart with inherent automaticity may take over the pacemaking function. With an inherent rate of 40 to 60 beats/min, the AV node is usually next in line. Should the AV nodal pacemaker also fail, a ventricular pacemaker at a rate of between 30 and 40 beats/min may take over. In the event that no other area of the heart takes over the pacesetting function, asystole will result.

The **usual range** of heart rates in adults for various rhythms is:

NSR (Normal sinus rhythm)—60 to 100 beats/min

AV nodal (junctional) escape rhythm—40 to 60 beats/min

Idioventricular escape rhythm—30 to 40 beats/min

Lead II

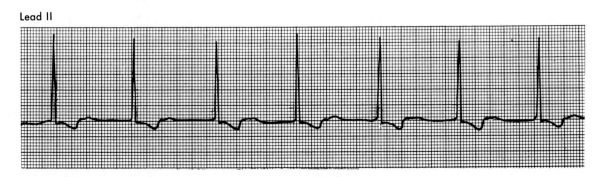

Figure 3A-13

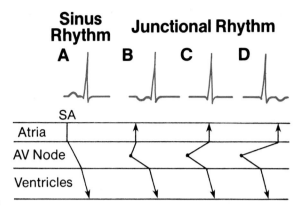

Sinus Rhythm   Junctional Rhythm

Figure 3A-14.   With junctional rhythm, the P wave in lead II will be inverted and precede, occur simultaneously, or follow the QRS complex (Panels **B, C,** and **D,** respectively)

An additional point to be made about junctional rhythms deals with the atrial activity that one is likely to see with this rhythm. In Figure 3A-10, we emphasized how with normal sinus rhythm the P wave should always be upright in lead II. This is because orientation of the electrical impulse as it travels from its origin in the SA node toward the AV node is virtually parallel to lead II.

PROBLEM   **What would you expect P waves to look like in lead II if the electrical impulse originated from the AV node instead of the SA node?**

ANSWER   With junctional rhythm, P waves tend to be inverted in lead II and either occur before or after the QRS complex, or are hidden within it. This concept is illustrated in the *laddergram** shown in *Figure 3A-14.* Panel A of the laddergram represents the sequence of events that occurs with normal sinus rhythm. The impulse originates from the SA node and then travels through the atria, AV node, and ventricles. In contrast, with *junctional rhythm* (panels B, C, and D), the electrical impulse originates from the AV node. P waves now travel backward *(retrograde)* from the AV node to depolarize the atria. Consequently, atrial activity (P waves) are *negative* (inverted) in lead II. If retrograde conduction is extremely rapid, inverted P waves will *precede* the QRS complex (Fig. 3A-14, panel **B**). If retrograde conduction is slow, the atria will not be depolarized until *after* the ventricles, and retrograde P waves will *follow* the QRS complex (Fig. 3A-14, panel **D**). However, if the speed of retrograde conduction is about equal to the speed of forward *(antegrade)* conduction through the ventricles, the inverted P waves will occur *simultaneously*

---

*A **laddergram** is an extremely useful teaching tool for helping to understand the mechanism of various cardiac arrhythmias. We emphasize that learning how to construct laddergrams is far from an easy task, and extends well beyond the core content of this chapter. *You will NOT need to draw laddergrams to successfully complete the ACLS course.* Despite the difficulty in learning to construct laddergrams, learning how to read them is relatively easy. For this reason, and because they provide a wealth of information, we introduce laddergrams here and periodically illustrate concepts with this technique.

with the QRS complex and be hidden within it (Fig. 3A-14, panel **C**).

PROBLEM   **Examine *Figure 3A-15.* Note that P waves are absent. Is this likely to be a junctional rhythm?**

ANSWER TO FIGURE 3A-15   The rhythm is regular at a rate of 130 beats/min (the R-R interval is between two and three boxes, and is closer to the former). The QRS complex is *wide* ($\geq$0.12 second), and no P waves are evident. Although this could be a junctional tachycardia (with the wide QRS complex being due to either preexisting bundle branch block or aberrant conduction), *ventricular tachycardia* must be assumed until proven otherwise!

Regular Wide QRS Complex Tachycardias

An extremely common and critically important problem in managing cardiac arrest is determining the cause of regular wide QRS complex tachycardias. *Five* entities should always come to mind:

1. Ventricular tachycardia
2. VENTRICULAR TACHYCARDIA
3. **VENTRICULAR TACHYCARDIA**
4. Supraventricular tachycardia (SVT) with preexisting bundle branch block
5. SVT with aberrant conduction

The onus of proof must always be to show that a wide QRS complex tachycardia is not ventricular tachycardia, rather than the other way around. Although the QRS complex in the above example does not appear to be particularly bizarre, it *is* wide and evidence of atrial activity is lacking. QRS morphology with junctional rhythms is similar (if not identical) to QRS morphology with normal sinus rhythm. Usually the QRS is narrow. Statistically, the overwhelming majority of wide QRS complex tachycardias are ventricular in origin. Therefore, unless previous rhythm strips demonstrate sinus conduction with identical QRS morphology, or there is unequivocal evidence in favor of aberrancy, one has to assume that the rhythm in Figure 3A-15 is ventricular tachycardia.

PROBLEM   **From where in the conduction system do you suppose the three dysrhythmias shown in *Figures 3A-16* through *3A-18* come from?**

ANSWER TO FIGURE 3A-16   The rhythm is regular, and the R-R interval is a little over six large boxes. The rate is therefore just under 50 beats/min. No P waves are seen, and the QRS complex is wide. Although a junctional rhythm with a preexisting bundle branch block cannot absolutely be ruled out, one must again assume a ventricular etiology. This rhythm is known as an *accelerated idioventricular rhythm (AIVR).*

Accelerated Idioventricular Rhythm

Accelerated idioventricular rhythm (AIVR) is an *escape rhythm* that usually arises when the sinus pacemaker fails. The

Lead II

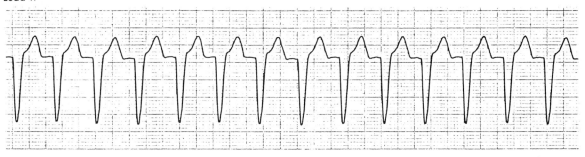

Figure 3A-15

Lead II

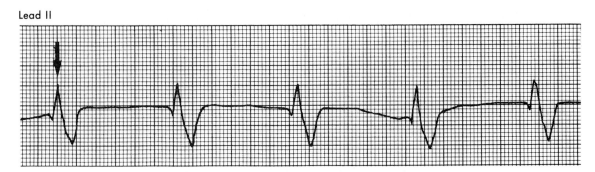

Figure 3A-16

Lead II

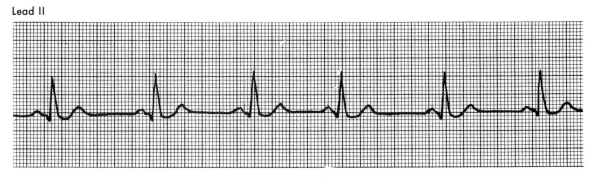

Figure 3A-17

Lead II

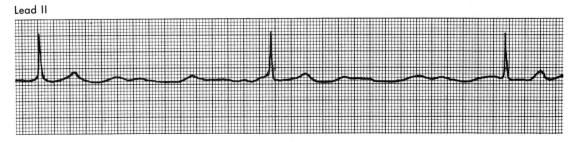

Figure 3A-18

ventricular rate in adults is between 50 and 110 beats/min. The rhythm is termed *accelerated* because it is faster than the usual idioventricular rate of 30 to 40 beats/min.

In general, AIVR is a *benign* rhythm that only rarely degenerates to rapid ventricular tachycardia. It is commonly seen in the setting of acute myocardial infarction. Frequently the patient is entirely asymptomatic and does not need to be treated. However, if the rhythm is accompanied by hypotension, measures should be taken to speed up the rate.

At times it is hard to be sure from one monitoring lead alone where the QRS complex ends and the ST segment begins. This is the case in Figure 3A-16. Regardless of whether the deep negative deflection represents an S wave or the ST segment, however, it is clear that the QRS complex is widened.

ANSWER TO FIGURE 3A-17
The R-R interval is slightly irregular and averages between five and six boxes. Thus, the rate is between 50 and 60 beats/min. Close inspection of the QRS complex reveals it to be wide; it is at least three small boxes in duration (0.12 second). Yet unlike the rhythm in Figure 3A-16, each QRS complex *is* preceded by a normal-appearing P wave with a constant PR interval. Clearly a sinus mechanism is operative here. *Sinus bradycardia* is present (since the rate is under 60 beats/min), and there is *sinus arrhythmia* (because the R-R interval varies). QRS prolongation is explained by the existence of a preexisting intraventricular conduction delay (bundle branch block).

ANSWER TO FIGURE 3A-18
This is an excellent example of how our method for calculating heart rate works even when the rhythm is exceedingly low. The R-R interval is almost 15 boxes in duration. Dividing 300 by 15, we estimate the heart rate to be about 20 beats/min.

Although one might be tempted to call many of the small undulations in the baseline of this tracing P waves, *no definite atrial activity is present!* The undulations seen here are commonly noted in tracings obtained while cardiopulmonary resuscitation is in progress, and probably reflect movement of the bed and/or the patient being resuscitated.

Despite the slow rate, the QRS complex is narrow! This makes it unlikely that the rhythm arises from a ventricular focus. Sinus mechanism is precluded by the fact that atrial activity is absent in this lead II monitoring lead. Thus, Figure 3A-18 probably represents an *escape rhythm* that arises from somewhere in the conduction system.

> The combination of the exceedingly slow rate in Figure 3A-18, the lack of atrial activity, and the narrow QRS complex suggests that the escape focus for this arrhythmia is likely to arise from *low down* in the conduction system (in the His or bundle branches). Regardless of where the escape focus arises, however, treatment will be the same—acceleration of the heart rate in an attempt to improve hemodynamic status.

Atrial Activity

Let us now concentrate on the presence of P waves and their meaning.

PROBLEM   **Examine the rhythms shown in *Figures 3A-19, 3A-20,* and *3A-21*. What is the mechanism for each of these arrhythmias? Are P waves present? Are they related to the QRS complex?**

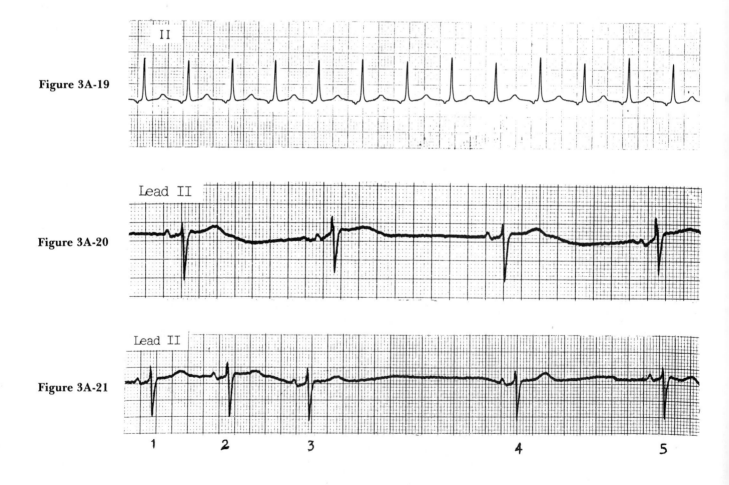

Figure 3A-19

Figure 3A-20

Figure 3A-21

ANSWER TO FIGURE 3A-19   The rhythm is regular at a rate of 105 beats/min. The QRS complex is narrow. Although P waves with a constant PR interval are present, these P waves are *negative* in this standard lead II monitoring lead. This means that *the rhythm cannot be arising from the sinus node*. It must be either a *junctional* or *low atrial rhythm*.

Because the heart rate of the rhythm in Figure 3A-19 is over 100 beats/min, *tachycardia* is present. Thus the rhythm is either junctional or low atrial tachycardia. It is impossible to distinguish between these two entities from this rhythm strip alone. Clinically, this distinction is of little importance.

ANSWER TO FIGURE 3A-20   A slow, slightly irregular rhythm is present with a heart rate of about 35 beats/min (the R-R interval is between eight and nine boxes; $300 \div 8.5 \approx 35$). The QRS complex is not widened (i.e., it is not *greater* than half a large box). An upright P wave with a constant PR interval precedes each QRS complex, indicating sinus mechanism. This is *sinus bradycardia* and *sinus arrhythmia*.

Despite the slow rate, the key to diagnosing this arrhythmia lies with recognition of consistent atrial activity preceding each QRS complex with a constant PR interval. The PR interval in this example is about 0.19 second. This is still within normal limits. For *1° AV block* to be present, the PR interval must clearly be *greater* than 0.20 second.

ANSWER TO FIGURE 3A-21   The tracing in Figure 3A-21 was obtained from the same patient as was the tracing in Figure 3A-20. Sinus rhythm at a rate of about 60 beats/min is seen for the first three beats, after which long pauses precede the next two QRS complexes. However, the QRS configuration of beats #4 and #5 is identical to that of the first three beats, and sinus P waves with a constant PR interval precede all five QRS complexes in the rhythm strip. The basic rhythm is therefore still of a *sinus* mechanism. *Sinus pauses* follow beats #3 and #4. The pause following beat #3 is *over 2.6 seconds* (13 little boxes) in duration. The combination of sinus arrhythmia, bradycardia, and sinus pauses seen in Figures 3A-20 and 3A-21 suggest that this patient has *sick sinus syndrome*.

Sick Sinus Syndrome

Sick sinus syndrome (SSS) is a commonly encountered entity among the elderly. The syndrome encompasses a wide variety of cardiac arrhythmias that result from progressive deterioration of sinoatrial (SA) node function. These include persistent *sinus bradycardia* (which is the most common and often the earliest manifestation of SSS), *sinus arrhythmia*, and *sinus pauses*. As the disease develops, sinus pauses may become progressively more prolonged, until eventually sinus node activity ceases *(sinus arrest)*. When this happens, some other escape focus must take over or asystole will result. Escape rhythms may arise from elsewhere in the atria (ectopic or low atrial rhythm), from the AV node (junctional rhythm), or from the ventricles (AIVR). Alternatively, atrial fibrillation (which we will discuss in the next section) may supervene. Because patients with SSS frequently have AV nodal disease, the ventricular response to atrial fibrillation is often slow.

In addition to the bradyarrhythmias noted above, many patients with SSS intermittently manifest tachyarrhythmias (hence the alternative name, *tachycardia-bradycardia syndrome*). Tachyarrhythmias may include paroxysmal supraventricular tachycardia (PSVT), atrial fibrillation or flutter, and ventricular tachycardia.

The course of SSS is highly variable. Development of the full electrocardiographic picture often takes years. Despite extremely slow heart rates, symptoms are minimal or absent in a surprising number of individuals. Underlying etiologies of SSS include myocardial infarction and coronary artery disease, degenerative disease of the conduction system, and hypothyroidism. Iatrogenic causes of the disorder (e.g., excessive use of medications such as digoxin, β-blockers, or verapamil) must be ruled out. Permanent pacemaker implantation is recommended once patients become symptomatic.

PROBLEM   **We conclude Section A with the rhythm shown in *Figure 3A-22*, which was taken from another patient with SSS. Can you explain the irregularity in the rhythm?**

ANSWER TO FIGURE 3A-22   The QRS complex remains narrow (≤0.10 second) throughout this rhythm strip, suggesting that all five beats arise at or above the AV node. Beats #4 and #5 are clearly sinus conducted. Each is preceded by a P wave with a fixed PR interval of 0.16 second. In contrast, no P wave precedes beats #1 and #2. These are *junctional (AV nodal) escape beats* that (fortunately) arise in response to the lack of atrial activity.

MCL-1

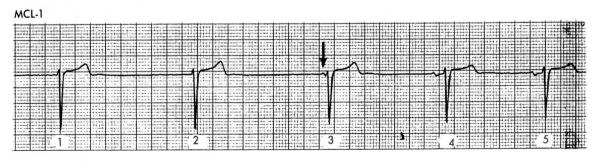

Figure 3A-22

Note that the rhythm strip shown in Figure 3A-22 was not obtained from lead II. Nevertheless, we can assume that beats #4 and #5 are sinus conducted because each is preceded by a P wave with a normal PR interval.

PROBLEM   **What is the rate of the AV nodal escape pacemaker in this example?**

ANSWER   One can determine the rate of the AV nodal escape pacemaker by calculating the R-R interval between successive junctional beats. Approximately nine boxes separate beats #1 and #2. Therefore, the AV nodal rate is about 33 beats/min ($300 \div 9$) in this example.

PROBLEM   **A P wave is seen immediately preceding beat #3 (arrow). Do you suppose it is conducted?**

ANSWER   The PR interval of the P wave preceding beat #3 is exceedingly short. Normally, *at least* 0.12 second is required for normal conduction (from the SA node through the AV node) to occur. In this particular example, we know from beats #4 and #5 that 0.16 second is needed for normal conduction (since this is the PR interval of these sinus conducted beats). Therefore, *the P wave that precedes beat #3 is too short to conduct*!

PROBLEM   **Then what type of beat *(sinus? junctional? ventricular?)* is beat #3 in Figure 3A-22?**

ANSWER   Since the PR interval of beat #3 is too short to conduct, it cannot be coming from the SA node. Beat #3 is not ventricular because the QRS complex is narrow and looks very much like the other supraventricular complexes in this rhythm strip. By the process of elimination, beat #3 must arise from the AV node.

Further support for this assumption comes from the observation that the R-R interval between beats #2 and #3 is equal to the R-R interval between beats #1 and 2. Marked sinus slowing occurred before the onset of this rhythm strip. This led to the emergence of a junctional escape rhythm (beats #1 and #2) at a rate of 33 beats/min. Atrial activity then resumed with the P wave (arrow) preceding beat #3. Acceleration of atrial activity finally leads to resumption of sinus rhythm by the end of the strip (beats #4 and #5). Thus, the complete interpretation of the arrhythmia shown in Figure 3A-22 would be sinus bradycardia and arrhythmia, with emergence of a slow, AV nodal escape pacemaker.

Appreciation of the rhythms encountered in SSS may be worthwhile for the emergency care provider since many of these same arrhythmias are frequently seen acutely during cardiac arrest.

SECTION B

PREMATURE BEATS AND TACHYARRHYTHMIAS

Premature Beats

Recognition of premature beats is an essential component of cardiac monitoring. Three different types exist:

1. Premature *atrial* contractions (**PACs**)
2. Premature *junctional* contractions (**PJCs**)
3. Premature *ventricular* contractions (**PVCs**)

Clinically, the importance in emergency cardiac care of distinguishing between these three types of premature beats lies in the fact that PVCs frequently warrant treatment, whereas premature *supraventricular* contractions (PACs and PJCs) most often do not.

Recognition of the different types of *premature* beats is usually easy. As implied in their name, PACs, PJCs, and PVCs all occur early. Under normal circumstances (as discussed in Figure 3A-11), the QRS complex of premature supraventricular beats will be narrow and identical (or nearly identical) in morphology to normal sinus beats. In contrast, the QRS complex of PVCs should be wide (≥0.12 second) and markedly different in morphology from normal sinus beats.

Theoretically, PACs should always be preceded by a premature P wave. Usually this P wave is readily apparent. Occasionally, however, it may be hard to identify and represent no more than subtle notching of the preceding T wave.

PJCs are uncommon. It is frequently difficult to distinguish them from PACs because the QRS complex looks the same for both. As noted in Figure 3A-14, P waves tend to be *inverted* in lead II with junctional beats. Inverted P waves may precede the QRS complex (usually with a short PR interval), follow the QRS complex, or be hidden within it. Because there is no difference in the clinical significance of PACs and PJCs, distinction between these two types of premature beats is primarily of academic interest.

A common mistake made by emergency care providers is to overcall PJCs, especially when the premature complex is not markedly widened or bizarre in shape. Remember—***PJCs are uncommon!*** They occur much *less* frequently than PACs.

The QRS complex of a PJC should be identical (or at least very similar) to the QRS complex of a normally conducted beat. If the QRS complex of an early beat is different from that of normally conducted beats, and is not preceded by a P wave, it is most likely a PVC!

PROBLEM   **Examine the tracing shown in *Figure 3B-1*. Beats #3, 6, and 10 all occur early. Are these premature beats likely to be PACs, PJCs, or PVCs?**

ANSWER TO FIGURE 3B-1   The underlying rhythm is sinus tachycardia at a rate of 100 beats/min. The QRS complex is narrow. As noted above, beats #3, #6, and #10 all occur early. Beat #3 is clearly a PVC. It is bizarre in shape and much wider than the normally conducted sinus beats. In contrast, beats #6 and #10 are PACs. Each is preceded by a premature P wave, and the QRS complex is virtually identical to that of the normally conducted beats.

PROBLEM   **Examine the rhythm shown in Figure 3B-2. Identify the early beats.**

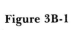
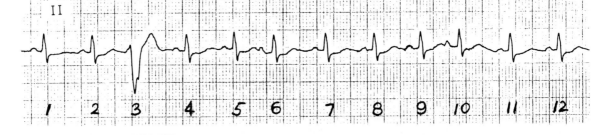

Figure 3B-1

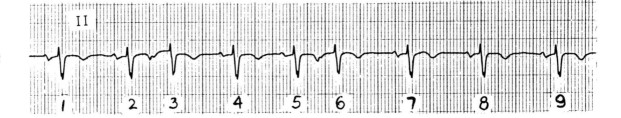

Figure 3B-2

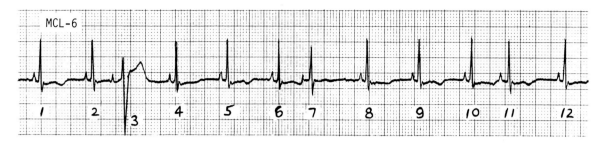

Figure 3B-3

ANSWER TO FIGURE 3B-2   The underlying rhythm is sinus (albeit with slight irregularity). Beats #3 and #6 clearly occur early. Because the QRS complex of these premature beats is narrow and virtually identical to that of the sinus conducted beats, these premature beats must be *supraventricular* (PACs or PJCs).

PROBLEM   **Do you see a premature P wave preceding beats #3 and #6?**

ANSWER   Subtle notching of the T wave preceding beats #3 and #6 is evident. This represents the premature P wave. The fact that *none* of the other T waves in this tracing are notched supports our assumption that this notching (of the T waves of beats #2 and #5) truly represents premature atrial activity.

> Although impossible to be certain, one can assume beats #3 and #6 in Figure 3B-2 are PACs rather than PJCs. As noted above, PJCs are uncommon. As a result, premature beats should probably *not* be interpreted as PJCs unless preceding atrial activity is definitely absent or the preceding P wave is clearly inverted in lead II and the PR interval is short.

PROBLEM   **Examine *Figure 3B-3*. Although beat #3 looks markedly different from the other QRS complexes, it is *not* a PVC. Why?**

ANSWER TO FIGURE 3B-3   The underlying rhythm is sinus at a rate of 85 beats/min. Beats #3, #7, and #11 all occur early. The latter two beats are clearly PACs. This is because the QRS complex of these beats is narrow, similar in morphology to the sinus beats, and preceded by a premature P wave.

Although beat #3 is wider and different in shape, it too is clearly preceded by a premature P wave. Consequently, beat #3 must also be a PAC. The reason for its different appearance is that this PAC is conducted with *aberrancy*.

Aberrant Conduction

> Immediately following depolarization of a normal sinus impulse, the conduction system becomes *refractory*. Additional impulses, no matter how strong, cannot be conducted at this time. The *absolute refractory period (ARP)* lasts only a short while. It is followed by a *relative refractory period (RRP)* during which some portions of the conduction system have recovered, whereas others have not. Additional impulses may now be

conducted, but because a part of the ventricular conduction system is still refractory, such conduction will not be normal. Instead it will be *aberrant*. QRS morphology may differ markedly from normal when premature impulses occur during the RRP. This is the case with beat #3 in Figure 3B-3.

On close inspection it can be seen that the other premature beats in this tracing (#7 and #11) are also conducted with minimal degrees of aberrancy. Although similar in morphology to the normally conducted impulses, the S waves of each of these beats are slightly deeper than normal. The reason beats #7 and #11 are *less aberrant* than beat #3 is that they are not quite as early (i.e., they occur at a time when a greater portion of the ventricular conduction system will have recovered).

The concept of aberrancy is rather complicated. For this reason we defer full discussion of this topic until Chapter 15. For now, suffice it to say that not all wide complex premature beats are PVCs. Although helpful guidelines do exist for differentiating between aberrantly conducted supraventricular beats (PACs, PJCs) and PVCs, most of these extend well beyond the scope of this chapter. However, the one finding that can be looked for is a *premature* P wave preceding the anomalous complex. When seen (as it was in beat #3 above), this finding argues strongly in favor of aberrancy. If doubt remains, *always consider a premature beat as "guilty"* (i.e., a PVC) *until proven otherwise*.

PROBLEM   **Examine *Figure 3B-4*. What would you say about beats #3 and #8?**

ANSWER TO FIGURE 3B-4   The underlying rhythm is sinus at a rate of 80 beats/min. The PR interval is at the upper limits of normal (0.20 second). Beats #3 and #8 are both premature. The former is definitely a PVC. It is wide and bizarre, and is not preceded by premature P wave. In contrast, beat #8 is not all that different in appearance from the normally conducted sinus beats. One might be tempted to call it a PAC (or PJC).

The point to remember is that when doubt exists, **a premature beat should always be considered as guilty (a PVC) until proven otherwise.** Careful inspection of the T wave preceding beat #8 does not reveal any deformity that might suggest a hidden premature P wave. One must therefore assume beat #8 is also a PVC.

> Beat #8 is *not* a PJC. As we have previously emphasized, PJCs should manifest a similar (if not identical) morphology as sinus conducted beats. Moreover, PJCs are much less common than PVCs. QRS morphology of beat #8 in Figure 3B-

Lead V₁

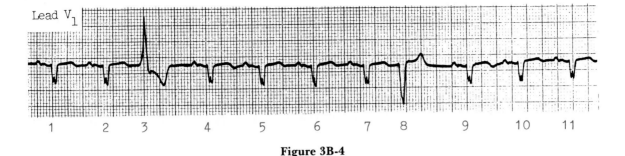

Figure 3B-4

4 differs much more from the sinus conducted beats than one would expect if this beat were a PJC.

When PVCs of differing morphologies are seen (as they are in Fig. 3B-4), they are said to be *multiform*. In the past, such PVCs were called *multifocal* since it used to be thought that different morphologies indicated different ectopic *foci*. We now know that this is not necessarily the case. PVCs may arise from the same focus (site) but use a different reentrant pathway, thus giving rise to a different morphology. As a result, it is more appropriate to use the term multiform than multifocal.

COMPLEX VENTRICULAR ECTOPY

In general, PVCs are cause for increasing concern as they become more frequent and complex in nature. Examples of *complex* forms of ventricular ectopy include:

1. *Multiform PVCs*
2. *Couplets* (two PVCs in a row)

3. *Salvos* (three PVCs in a row)
4. Longer runs of *ventricular tachycardia* (VT)

In the past it was thought that multiformity was a strong indicator of increased risk. However, numerous Holter monitor studies on otherwise healthy subjects have demonstrated that some degree of multiformity is an extremely common finding in a majority of individuals who have frequent PVCs, and that multiformity per se is really of only minimal prognostic significance. Of much greater concern clinically is the finding of *repetitive* ventricular ectopy (i.e., two or more PVCs in a row). This includes couplets, salvos, and longer runs of VT as listed above.*

PROBLEM   *Figures 3B-5* through *3B-8* were recorded sequentially from a patient with acute myocardial infarction. What is happening?*

---

*The definition of VT is a run of *three* or more PVCs in a row. Thus, a salvo is really a short run of VT.

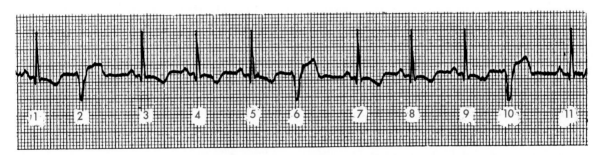

Figure 3B-5

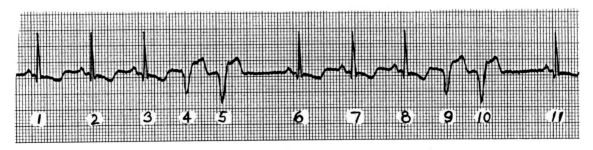

Figure 3B-6

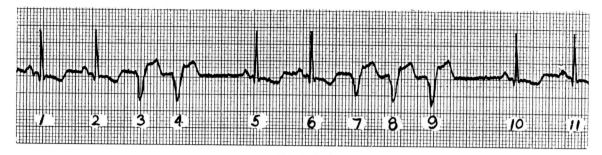

Figure 3B-7

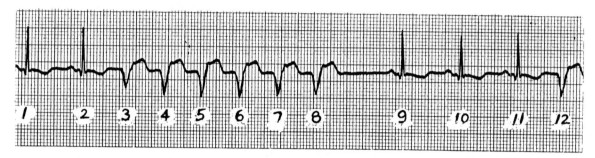

Figure 3B-8

ANSWER TO FIGURES 3B-5 THROUGH 3B-8

The underlying rhythm is sinus at a rate of 85 beats/min. Increasingly frequent and complex ventricular ectopy is noted. This is a particularly worrisome finding in the setting of acute infarction.

Single *uniform* (of similar morphology) PVCs are seen in *Figure 3B-5* (beats #2, #6, & #10). Repetitive PVCs are seen in the other rhythm strips. In *Figure 3B-6*, there are two ventricular *couplets* (beats #4 & #5, & #9 & #10). In *Figure 3B-7*, there is one couplet (beats #3 & #4) and one *salvo* (beats #7 to #9). Finally, a six-beat run of VT is seen (beats #3 to #8) in *Figure 3B-8*.

> In the acute care setting, frequent and repetitive ventricular ectopy (couplets, salvos, and *nonsustained VT*) are frequent precursors of *sustained* VT (i.e., VT lasting more than 15 seconds) and ventricular fibrillation. Aggressive treatment is indicated.
>
> With respect to PVC *frequency*, a wide range of definitions for this term have been proposed. In patients with chronic ventricular ectopy, as few as 10 PVCs per hour (which comes out to a PVC every 6 minutes) is sometimes considered "frequent", since this incidence has been associated with an increased risk of sudden death in patients with underlying heart disease. Acutely, the term *"frequent"* is usually applied when PVCs number ≥5 per minute. In either instance when deciding whether to treat, *far more important than frequency per se is consideration of the clinical setting in which the ectopy occurs.* (See Section E in Chapter 11 on Sudden Cardiac Death).
>
> In Figure 3B-5, PVCs occur every fourth beat. This is known as ventricular *quadrigeminy*. (It is ventricular *trigeminy* if PVCs occur every third beat, and ventricular *bigeminy* if they occur every other beat.)

Atrial Tachyarrhythmias

Let us now turn our attention to the atrial tachyarrhythmias.

PROBLEM   Examine *Figures 3B-9* and *3B-10.* Is there evidence of atrial activity?

ANSWER TO FIGURE 3B-9   The QRS complex is narrow. The rhythm is irregularly irregular (each R-R interval is different). Although there are undulations in the baseline, no definite P waves are present. This is *atrial fibrillation* by definition.

Atrial Fibrillation

Atrial fibrillation is recognized by the absence of P waves and the *irregular irregularity* of the rhythm. Although multiple atrial foci are firing at an extremely rapid rate (up to 600 times per minute), only a fraction of these atrial impulses are able to be conducted through the AV node.

Untreated, the ventricular response to atrial fibrillation is typically *rapid* (greater than 120 beats/min). Following treatment with digitalis, the ventricular response becomes more *"controlled"* and usually falls within the range of 60 to 110 beats/min. If too much digitalis is given (or in some cases of sick sinus syndrome or atrioventricular heart block), atrial fibrillation may manifest a *slow* ventricular response (less than 60 beats/min).

PROBLEM   What type of ventricular response is evident in *Figure 3B-9*?

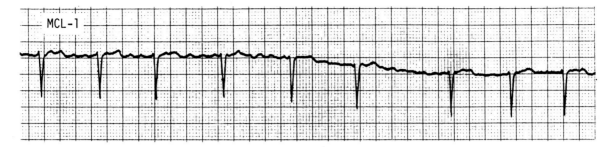

Figure 3B-9

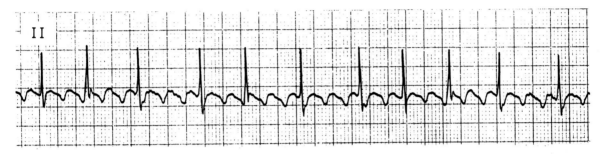

Figure 3B-10

ANSWER   The R-R interval throughout most of this rhythm strip is between three and five large boxes. Therefore the heart rate varies between 60 and 100 beats/min. This is atrial fibrillation with a *controlled ventricular response*.

ANSWER TO FIGURE 3B-10   Once again the QRS complex is narrow and the rhythm is irregularly irregular. However, as opposed to Figure 3B-9, more definite evidence of atrial activity is present. A repetitive negative deflection is seen at a rate of 280 beats/min. This is *atrial flutter*, in this case with a *variable* ventricular response. The negative deflections are flutter waves.

Atrial Flutter

Atrial flutter is an interesting arrhythmia that is characterized by regular atrial activity at a rate of around 300 beats/min in adults (range 250 to 350 beats/min). Atrial activity typically manifests a *sawtooth* (zigzag) pattern in inferior leads (such as lead II). Fortunately, the AV node is unable to conduct each atrial impulse at this rapid a rate. If 1:1 AV con-

duction were possible, the ventricular response with atrial flutter would be about 300 beats/min, which is much too fast a rate to maintain effective cardiac pumping. As a protective mechanism, the AV node limits the number of atrial impulses that are conducted to the ventricles. Usually every other impulse is conducted, so that *the most common ventricular response to untreated atrial flutter is 2:1* (atrial rate of 300 beats/min and a ventricular response of 150 beats/min). Less commonly there is 4:1 AV conduction. Least commonly there may be variable AV conduction (as in Figure 3B-10), or an odd-numbered conduction ratio (e.g., 3:1 AV conduction).

The most characteristic feature of atrial flutter is the regularity of atrial activity at a rate (in adults) that approximates 300 beats/min. Awareness of this feature is extremely helpful in making the diagnosis. It is important to realize that when the rhythm is treated medically (with antiarrhythmic agents such as quinidine or procainamide), the atrial rate of flutter may be slowed (to 200-250 beats/min, or less).

PROBLEM   The rhythm strip shown in *Figure 3B-11* is taken from another patient in atrial flutter. *How many flutter waves are present for every QRS complex?*

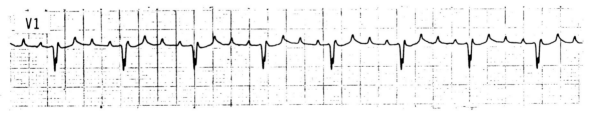

Figure 3B-11

V1

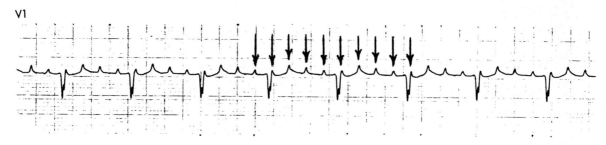

Figure 3B-12. Atrial flutter with 4:1 AV conduction. Arrows demonstrate that the fourth flutter wave is hidden in the terminal (r′) portion of the QRS complex.

ANSWER TO FIGURE 3B-11 The QRS complex is narrow, and the ventricular response is regular at a rate of about 80 beats/min. Atrial flutter waves are regular and occur in this V₁ lead as upright deflections at a rate of about 320 beats/min. There are *four* flutter waves for each QRS complex (i.e., there is 4:1 AV conduction).

If you had difficulty spotting the fourth flutter wave, it makes up the terminal r′ of the QRS complex *(Figure 3B-12).*

When the characteristic sawtooth pattern of atrial flutter (seen in Fig. 3B-10) or distinct atrial activity at a rate approximating 300 beats/min (seen in Fig. 3B-11) are present, recognition of this arrhythmia usually does not pose a problem. However, flutter waves are often much more subtle in their appearance.

PROBLEM **Examine the 12-lead ECG shown in** *Figure 3B-13.* **Focus for a moment on lead II. A regular supraventricular tachycardia at a rate of 140 beats/min is present.** *Could this possibly be sinus tachycardia?*

ANSWER TO FIGURE 3B-13 No. Since normal upright P waves are not present in lead II, sinus tachycardia can be ruled out. Instead, the rhythm in Figure 3B-

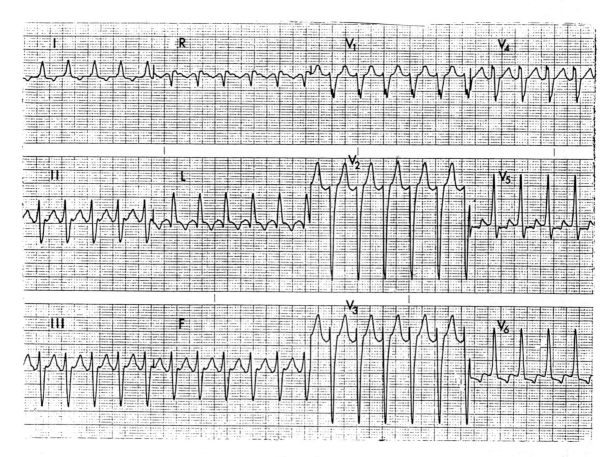

Figure 3B-13

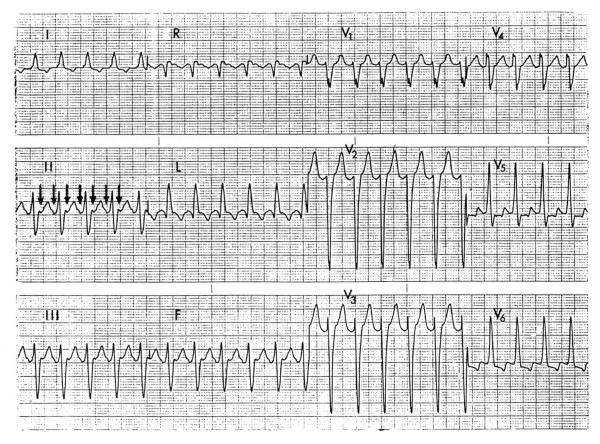

Figure 3B-14

13 is *atrial flutter*, although admittedly the diagnosis is not at all obvious from this tracing. Arrows in *Figure 3B-14* indicate that the only leads that even remotely hint at the presence of the characteristic sawtooth pattern of flutter are the inferior leads (II, III, and aVF). Note in particular that evidence of atrial activity is totally lacking from leads I, V_{1-3}, and V_6.

Because flutter waves are frequently not apparent, the diagnosis is often overlooked. In order to avoid this pitfall, one must always maintain a high index of suspicion and *strongly consider the possibility of atrial flutter in the presence of any regular supraventricular tachycardia with a rate of between 140 and 160 beats/min when normal atrial activity cannot be identified.*

PROBLEM   **Interpret the arrhythmias shown in *Figures 3B-15* and *3B-16*. Is atrial flutter likely to be present in either tracing?**

ANSWER TO FIGURE 3B-15   A regular supraventricular tachyarrhythmia at a rate of 150 beats/min is present. Although a seemingly normal P wave is seen preceding each QRS complex, notching on the upstroke of each T wave suggests that there may actually be two P waves for each QRS complex.

When definitive diagnosis of a tachyarrhythmia is not apparent from inspection of a tracing, it may sometimes be made clear by slowing the ventricular response with application of a vagal maneuver such as *carotid sinus massage*. *Figure 3B-15A*

Lead MCL₁

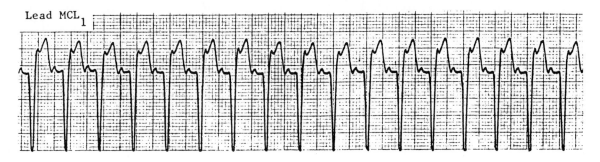

Figure 3B-15

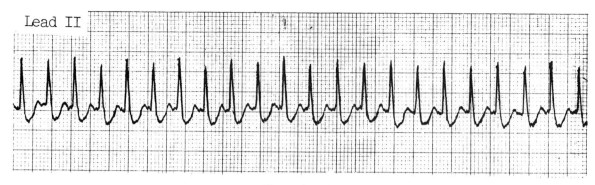

Figure 3B-16

shows the effect of carotid massage on the rhythm in Figure 3B-15. The degree of atrioventricular block has been increased by carotid massage, and atrial activity (flutter waves) at a rate of about 300 beats/min (arrows) are now evident.

> The point to emphasize is that **atrial flutter** should *always be suspected (until proven otherwise) whenever there is a regular, supraventricular tachyarrhythmia at a rate of approximately 150 beats/min, especially when normal atrial activity cannot be identified.* Failure to do so is likely to result in overlooking this arrhythmia.

ANSWER TO FIGURE 3B-16

Once again a regular supraventricular tachyarrhythmia is seen. The rate, however, is significantly faster than it was for Figure 3B-15. The R-R interval in this tracing is between one and two large boxes, making the rate between 150 and 300 beats/min. As suggested earlier (in Fig. 3A-7), when the rate is regular and this rapid, a useful technique for calculating heart rate is to measure the R-R interval of every other beat. Here, the R-R interval for every other beat (i.e., half the rate) is a little less than three large boxes. Therefore half the rate is about 110 beats/min, and the actual rate is approximately 220 beats/min.

Atrial flutter with 1:1 AV conduction would be unlikely at this rate unless the patient was being treated with a medication (such as quinidine or procainamide) that might slow the atrial response. Atrial flutter with 2:1 AV conduction would also be unlikely because this would require an atrial rate of 440 beats/min (220 × 2), which is well beyond the usual range for flutter.

PROBLEM
Does the upright deflection seen between QRS complexes in *Figure 3B-16* represent atrial activity?

ANSWER
It is impossible to determine from Figure 3B-16 whether the upright deflection between QRS complexes represents a P wave, the T wave, or both. If it were the P wave, then the rhythm in Figure 3B-16 would be sinus tachycardia at a rate of 220 beats/min. Since sinus tachycardia rarely exceeds 160 beats/min in a nonambulatory adult, this diagnosis is unlikely. Thus, the upright deflection probably represents the T wave, and the rhythm is presumed to be *paroxysmal supraventricular tachycardia (PSVT)*.

Paroxysmal Supraventricular Tachycardia

PSVT is a commonly seen, extremely regular tachyarrhythmia that usually has a rate of between 150 to 250 beats/min. In the past, distinction was made between two types of PSVT, *paroxysmal atrial tachycardia (PAT)* and *paroxysmal junctional tachy-*

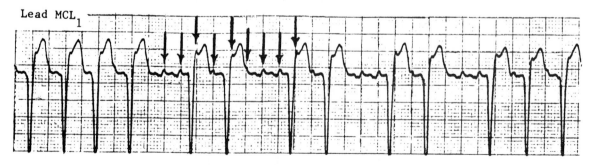

Figure 3B-15A. Application of a vagal maneuver (carotid sinus massage) slows the rhythm shown in Figure 3B-15. Arrows now demonstrate regular atrial activity (flutter) at a rate of 300 per minute.

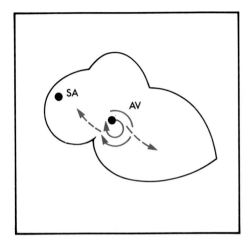

Figure 3B-17. The mechanism of PSVT in adults is usually *reentry* in which a continuous cycle is set up and perpetuated with the impulse circulating around the AV node as it is conducted down (to the ventricles) and back (to the atria).

cardia (PJT). Such differentiation was probably more of academic interest than of clinical utility, since both tachyarrhythmias are thought to be due to similar *reentry* mechanisms involving the AV node. In reentry, the impulse travels through the AV node, enters the ventricular conduction system, and then somehow is conducted back to *(reenters)* the AV node. A continuous cycle in which the impulse is conducted down (to the ventricles) and back (to the AV node) is perpetuated, and rapid heart rates are attained *(Figure 3B-17).* Conduction to the atria with PSVT is retrograde.

The QRS complex is most often narrow with PSVT, unless bundle branch block or aberrant conduction exists. P waves are usually not evident. When present, they are frequently inverted (because atrial activity is retrograde) and partially hidden in the terminal portion of the QRS complex.

A final point about PSVT should be made regarding terminology. It is important not to confuse this entity with the more generally used term, supraventricular tachycardia. By definition, a *supraventricular tachycardia* is any tachycardia (arrhythmia with a rate of ≥ 100 beats/min) in which the impulse originates at or above the AV node. Examples include:

1. Sinus tachycardia
2. Junctional tachycardia
3. Atrial fibrillation
4. Atrial flutter
5. Multifocal atrial tachycardia
6. Ectopic atrial tachycardia
7. PSVT

The term PSVT implies that the mechanism of a particular tachyarrhythmia is reentry. A better term for these arrhythmias might simply be to call them *reentry tachycardias.* Thus, the rhythm in Figure 3B-15 is a *supraventricular* tachycardia, but it is not PSVT!

Subtle Clues in Diagnosis of Tachyarrhythmias

We conclude this section with a series of illustrative arrhythmias that consolidate the concepts we have covered thus far.

PROBLEM   **Examine the tracings shown in *Figures 3B-18* through *3B-21.* Does the regularity of the rhythms and the width of the QRS complex supply clues to the etiology?**

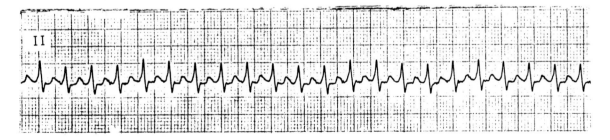

Figure 3B-18. This patient was awake, alert, and hemodynamically stable at the time this tracing was recorded.

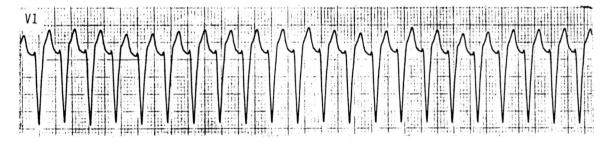

Figure 3B-19

Lead II

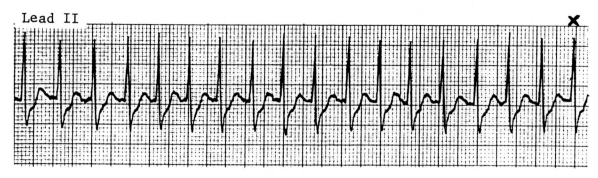

Figure 3B-20

ANSWER TO FIGURE 3B-18   The rhythm is precisely regular at a rate of 190 beats/min. The QRS complex appears wide (at least 0.12 second in duration), and no atrial activity is evident.

PROBLEM   ***Could this tachyarrhythmia possibly be of supraventricular etiology?***

ANSWER   Yes. As discussed in the response to Figure 3A-15, whenever one is confronted by a regular wide-complex tachyarrhythmia, *five* entities must always be kept in mind:

1. Ventricular tachycardia
2. VENTRICULAR TACHYCARDIA
3. **VENTRICULAR TACHYCARDIA**
4. SVT *(supraventricular tachycardia)* with preexisting bundle branch block
5. SVT with aberrant conduction

Thus, the regular wide-complex tachyarrhythmia shown in Figure 3B-18 *could* be supraventricular (with either preexisting bundle branch block or aberrant conduction). However, unless there is strong evidence to the contrary, ventricular tachycardia *must* always be assumed until proved otherwise.

> The clinical history in this example (that the patient was alert and hemodynamically stable at the time the tracing was recorded) is a "red herring." *Not all patients in ventricular tachycardia immediately decompensate.* On the contrary, selected patients may remain alert and hemodynamically stable despite persistence of this arrhythmia for minutes, hours (and *even*

days!). Thus, hemodynamic stability *cannot* be used as a diagnostic point in favor of a supraventricular etiology. As stated above, **whenever there is a regular, wide-complex tachyarrhythmia and sinus P waves are not evident, VT must always be assumed until proven otherwise!**

ANSWER TO FIGURE 3B-19   This rhythm is also precisely regular at 190 beats/min. The QRS complex appears to be narrow, and P waves seemingly precede each QRS complex. One might be lulled into thinking this was sinus tachycardia.

> Actually, the rhythms shown in Figures 3B-18 and 3B-19 were obtained *simultaneously* from the *same* patient! They emphasize the point previously stated that the QRS complex may appear deceptively narrow in certain leads when a portion of the QRS is isoelectric with the baseline. This patient was in *ventricular tachycardia* despite his stable hemodynamic status! The rate is much faster than one usually sees with sinus tachycardia in adults, and the upright deflection seen between QRS complexes in Figure 3B-19 represents the T wave, *not* the P wave. To avoid overlooking the diagnosis of ventricular tachycardia, always try to view an arrhythmia from more than one monitoring lead (whenever this is possible).

ANSWER TO FIGURE 3B-20   The QRS complex appears to be narrow in this lead, and no definite P waves are seen. At first glance, the rhythm appears to be regular. If this were the case, then the differential diagnosis of this arrhythmia would be identical to that considered for the regular narrow complex tachyarrhythmia shown in Figure 3B-16—sinus tachycardia, atrial flutter, or PSVT.

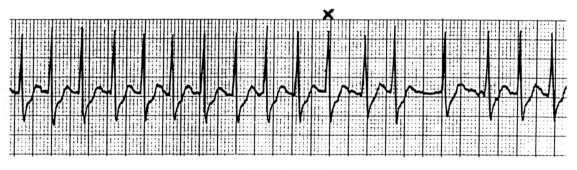

Figure 3B-20A

Lead II

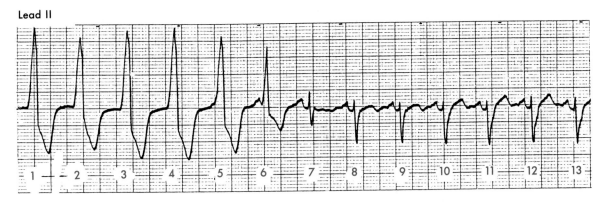

Figure 3B-21

PROBLEM   Is the rhythm in *Figure 3B-20* really regular? *Be sure to verify your answer with calipers!*

ANSWER   Careful inspection with calipers reveals slight but definite irregularity of the R-R interval in Figure 3B-20. *Figure 3B-20A* shows the continuation of this rhythm strip from the point marked **X**. The irregular irregularity of the rhythm becomes much more evident during the final beats of Figure 3B-20A. Thus the rhythm in Figure 3B-20 is *atrial fibrillation* with a *rapid ventricular response*.

> This example highlights the difficulty of recognizing the irregularity of atrial fibrillation when the ventricular response is rapid. Without careful use of calipers it would be extremely easy to mistake the rhythm shown in Figure 3B-20 as PSVT. This misdiagnosis might have important clinical implications. Although either digoxin or verapamil can be used to treat rapid atrial fibrillation and PSVT, many clinicians prefer digoxin for the former and verapamil for the latter. Recently, adenosine has become a drug of choice for treatment of PSVT in the acute care setting. Although it may temporarily slow the rhythm (and clarify the diagnosis), adenosine is *not* effective in the treatment of nonreentry mechanism tachyarrhythmias such as atrial fibrillation.

PROBLEM   Try your hand at this final example *(Figure 3B-21). Does the regularity of the rhythm and* width of the QRS complex supply clues to the etiology of the arrhythmia? *Does the regularity of the rhythm change?*

ANSWER TO FIGURE 3B-21   This is a difficult tracing. The easiest way to approach the interpretation of more difficult arrhythmias is to begin with that part of the tracing that is easiest to interpret. *Mentally block out the first seven beats on this tracing.* If all you had to worry about was the last six beats in Figure 3B-21 (beats #8 to #13), how would you interpret the arrhythmia *(Figure 3B-22)?*

ANSWER TO FIGURE 3B-22   Beats #8 to #13 are regular at a rate of 110 beats/min. The QRS complex is narrow, and each QRS is preceded by normal appearing (upright) P waves with a normal PR interval. Beats #8 to #13 represent *sinus tachycardia.*

PROBLEM   *Now mentally block out the last eight beats on this tracing.* **If all you had to worry about were the initial five beats, how would you interpret the arrhythmia *(Figure 3B-23)?***

ANSWER TO FIGURE 3B-23   Beats #1 to #5 are regular at a rate of just *over* 100 beats/min (the R-R interval is just *under* three large boxes in duration). The QRS

Lead II

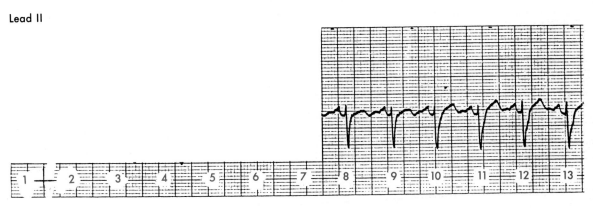

Figure 3B-22.   The first seven beats of Figure 3B-21 have been blocked out. *How would you interpret the arrhythmia represented by beats #8 to #13?*

Lead II

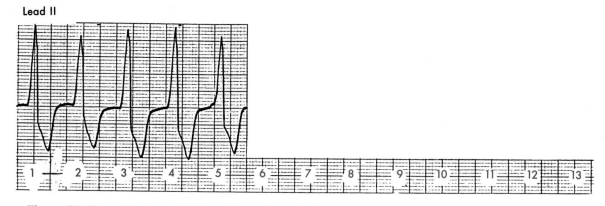

Figure 3B-23. The last eight beats (beats #6 to #13) of Figure 3B-21 have been blocked out. *How would you interpret the arrhythmia represented by beats #1 to #5?*

Lead II

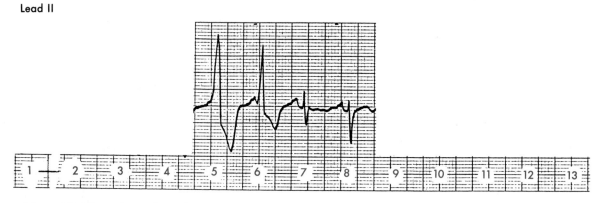

Figure 3B-24. Beats #1 to #4, and #9 to #13 of Figure 3B-21 have been blocked out. *Can you figure out what is happening with beats #5 to #8?*

complex of these beats is wide, bizarre, and not preceded by atrial activity. This suggests a ventricular etiology. Since the usual rate of an idioventricular escape rhythm is much slower (in the range of 30 to 40 beats/min), we describe the arrhythmia represented by beats #1 to #5 in Figure 3B-23 as an **a**ccelerated **i**dio**v**entricular **r**hythm (or AIVR).

PROBLEM   **Return to Figure 3B-21. Now focus on the difficult part of the tracing—beats #5 to #8 (Figure 3B-24). Can you figure out what is going on?**

HINT: Sequential consideration of the following four questions may lead you to the diagnosis:

1. What kind of beat is beat #8? *(See Answer to Fig. 3B-22)*
2. What kind of beat is beat #5? *(See Answer to Fig. 3B-23)*
3. Would you expect the P wave preceding beat #6 to be able to conduct normally? *(If not, why not?)*
4. Think of beats #5 and #8 as "parent beats." If these parent beats (#5 and #8) were to mate (i.e., combine) and "have children," *what would you expect the children to look like?*

ANSWER TO FIGURE 3B-24   Since the rhythm represented in Figure 3B-22 is sinus tachycardia, beat #8 must be a sinus conducted beat. Similarly, since the rhythm represented by Figure 3B-23 is AIVR, beat #5 must be a ventricular beat. Note that the PR interval preceding beat #6 is shorter than the PR interval preceding other sinus conducted beats (beats #8 to #13 in Fig. 3B-21). It is *too short* to conduct normally. Note also that although the QRS complex of beat #6 is entirely upright, it is not nearly as wide as the other upright (ventricular) beats (beats #1 to #5 in Fig. 3B-21). Beat #6 is a **fusion beat**.

Fusion Beats

Fusion beats occur as a result of *simultaneous* occurrence of supraventricular and ventricular impulses. This concept is illustrated in *Figure 3B-25*.

Panel A in the figure shows the pathway of normal conduction (SA node, AV node, bundle branches). This results in a sinus conducted beat **(S)** with a normal PR interval and a narrow QRS complex.

In contrast, the impulse in Panel B begins in the ventricles **(V)**. This results in a wide QRS complex without atrial activity.

The phenomenon of *fusion* is represented in Panel C, in which

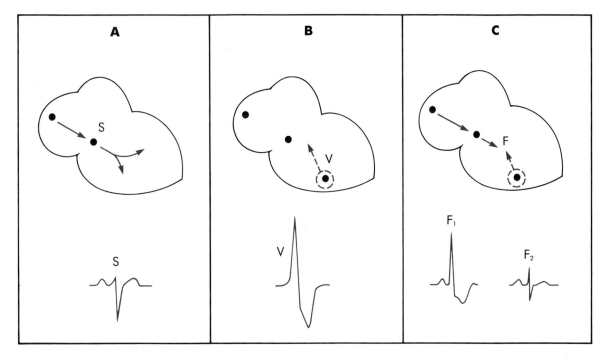

Figure 3B-25.   Illustration of the concept of fusion beats. **A,** Sinus conducted beat **(S). B,** Ventricular beat **(V). C,** Fusion beats **(F1** and **F2).**

there is simultaneous (or near simultaneous) occurrence of a supraventricular and ventricular complex. Depolarization wavefronts meet before they are able to complete their path, and the ECG appearance of the resultant **fusion beat** takes on characteristics of both the supraventricular *and* ventricular complex **(F).** Depending on whether the wavefronts meet high or low in the ventricles, the fusion beat will take on more characteristics of the supraventricular complex (F2 in Panel C) or of the ventricular complex (F1 in Panel C).

Clinically, the reason recognition of fusion beats is important is that it proves anomalous complexes in a tracing must be of ventricular etiology.

Return to Figure 3B-21. It should now be apparent that this arrhythmia begins with a five-beat run of AIVR (at 100 to 105 beats/min). Sinus tachycardia at a slightly faster rate (110 beats/min) then takes over (beats #8 to #13). Beats #6 and #7 manifest a QRS morphology *intermediate* between that of the ventricular and supraventricular complexes. Beats #6 and #7 are therefore *fusion* beats, with the former more closely resembling the morphology of ventricular beats (as was the case for **F1** in Panel C of Fig. 3B-25), and the latter most closely resembling the morphology of the QRS complex during sinus tachycardia (as was the case for **F2** in Fig. 3B-25).

The appearance of beats #6 and #7 in Figure 3B-21 is as might be anticipated considering the PR interval that precedes each of these fusion beats. That is, the very short PR interval preceding beat #6 would not be expected to allow sufficient time for deep penetration of the supraventricular impulse (P wave) into the ventricles. Thus beat #6 much more closely resembles the beats of ventricular etiology.

In contrast, the PR interval preceding beat #7 is almost normal. As a result, this supraventricular impulse (P wave)

should have had time to travel relatively far down the conduction system before fusion occurred (explaining why this beat more closely resembles the morphology of supraventricular beats).

Clinically, *recognition that beats #6 and #7 in this tracing are fusion beats confirms the ventricular etiology of beats #1 to #5.*

It should be emphasized that understanding fusion beats is an *advanced* concept. Nevertheless we chose to include it here because appreciation of this concept not only provides huge dividends in evaluation of the etiology of anomalous complexes, but also allows better understanding of the mechanism of cardiac arrhythmias.

BONUS: If the concept of fusion beats was new (and/or confusing) to you, **STOP HERE** (*and **move on to Section 3C**)!!!*

If you choose to read on, ***BE FOREWARNED!!!!!*** The answer to the BONUS PROBLEM is *exceedingly* subtle (and extends *well beyond* what you'll need to know to successfully complete the ACLS course). But if you're up to the challenge, turn the page and read on. . . . .

BONUS PROBLEM   **Return one more time to Figure 3B-21. In addition to beats #6 and #7, there are *three* more fusion beats in this tracing. *Can you spot them?***

ANSWER TO BONUS PROBLEM   Beats #5, #8, and #9 are also fusion beats! *The KEY to recognizing fusion beats is to look for the ever-so-slightly subtle differences that may be present between the beat(s) in the question and the complexes of known etiology.* Thus, careful inspection of beat #5 reveals that its R wave is not quite as tall and its T wave not quite as deep as the other ventricular beats. Note also that the very initial portion of the upstroke of this R wave is deformed. A P wave is hiding here—and accounts for the slight degree of fusion that this beat manifests.

Beats #8 and #9 are also fusion beats. Careful comparison of these beats with beats #10 to #13 reveals that they have a slightly narrower QRS complex and a T wave that is smaller and less peaked.

SECTION C

ARRHYTHMIA REVIEW (I)

As review of material covered so far, analyze the following 20 tracings. We suggest you use the systematic Four-Question approach (and a pair of calipers) in your interpretation.

Lead II

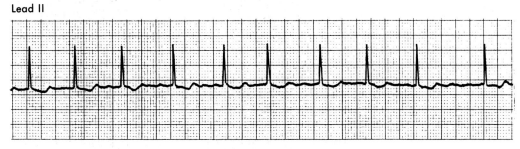

Figure 3C-1

Lead II

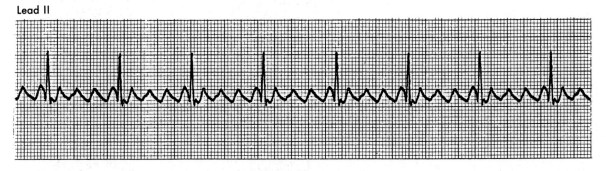

Figure 3C-2

Lead II

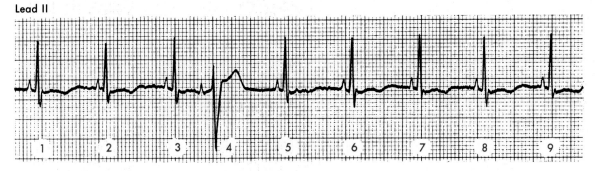

Figure 3C-3

Lead II

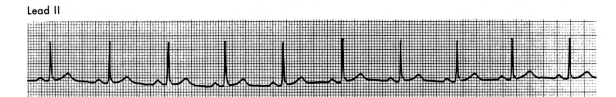

Figure 3C-4

Lead II

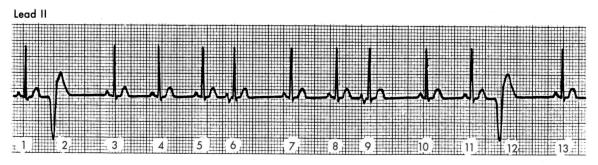

Figure 3C-5

Lead II

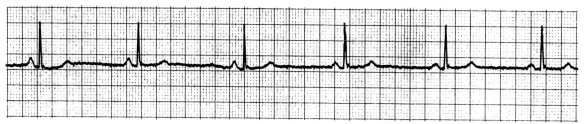

Figure 3C-6

Lead II

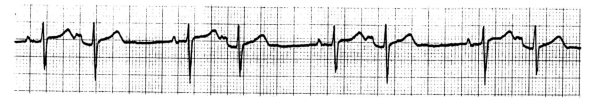

Figure 3C-7

MCL-1

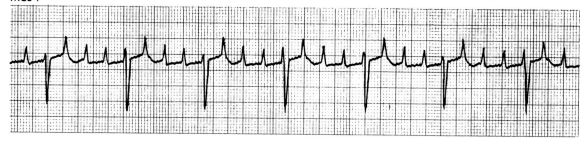

Figure 3C-8

Lead II

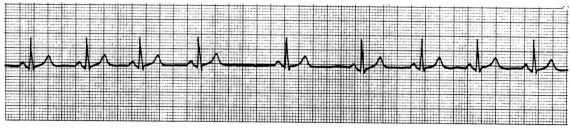

Figure 3C-9

Lead II

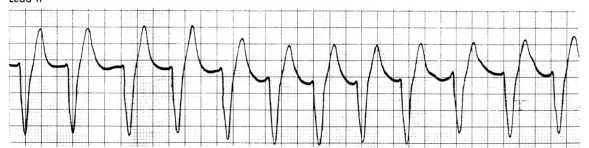

Figure 3C-10

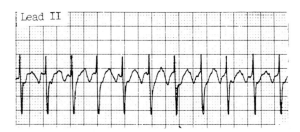

Figure 3C-11

Lead II

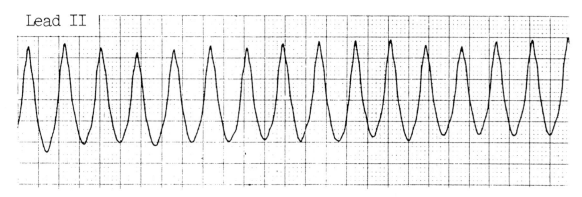

Figure 3C-12

Lead VI

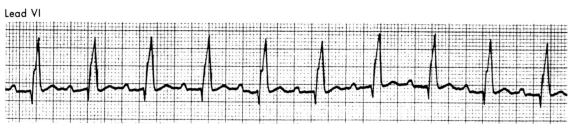

Figure 3C-13

Lead MCL-1

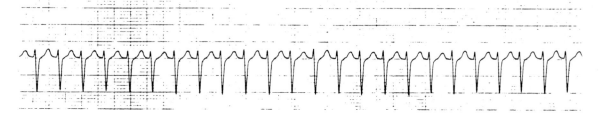

Figure 3C-14

Lead II

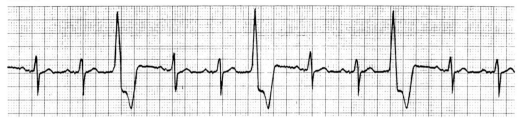

Figure 3C-15

Lead II

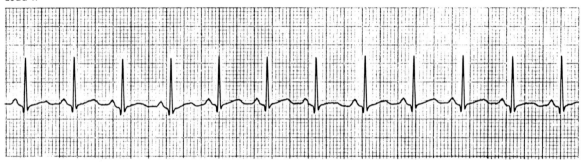

Figure 3C-16

Lead II

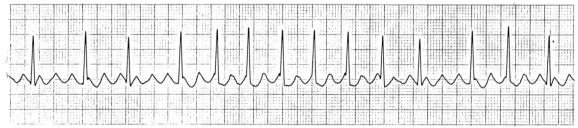

Figure 3C-17

Lead II

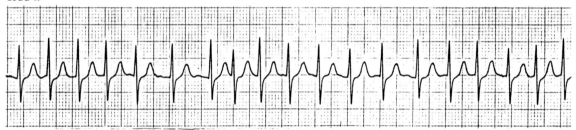

Figure 3C-18

Lead MCL-1

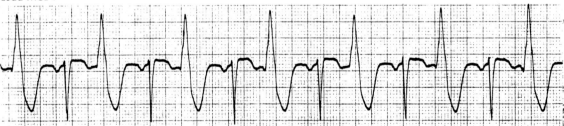

Figure 3C-19

Lead MCL-1

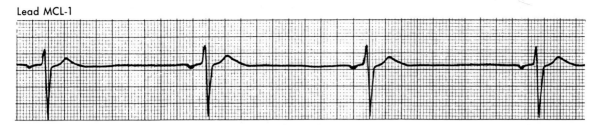

Figure 3C-20

ANSWERS TO ARRHYTHMIA REVIEW (I)

ANSWER TO FIGURE 3C-1

Rhythm—Regular
Rate—65 to 70 beats/min
PR interval—Normal (0.18 second)
QRS complex—Normal duration (≤0.10 second)
Impression: Normal sinus rhythm.

ANSWER TO FIGURE 3C-2

Rhythm—Irregularly irregular
P waves—None
QRS complex—Normal duration
Impression: Atrial fibrillation with a controlled ventricular response
Comment: Although many undulations are seen along the baseline, no consistent atrial activity is present. Atrial fibrillation is diagnosed by the finding of an irregularly irregular rhythm and the absence of definite P waves. The ventricular response averages out to be between 60 and 110 beats/min (*controlled* ventricular response). The fine undulations in the baseline are produced by the fibrillating atria (*"fib waves"*).

ANSWER TO FIGURE 3C-3

Rhythm—Regular
Atrial rate—Sawtooth flutter waves at 270 beats/min
Ventricular rate—65 to 70 beats/min
QRS complex—Normal duration
Impression: Atrial flutter with 4:1 AV conduction.
Comment: Untreated atrial flutter most commonly manifests 2:1 AV conduction (atrial rate ≈ 300 beats/min; ventricular rate ≈ 150 beats/min). The next most common conduction ratio is 4:1, as is shown here. It is uncommon to have atrial flutter with an odd number conduction ratio.

ANSWER TO FIGURE 3C-4

Rhythm—Essentially regular except for beat #4
Rate—85 beats/min
PR interval—A little short (0.10 second)
QRS complex—Normal duration
Impression: Sinus rhythm (with a short PR interval) and a PAC that conducts with aberrancy

Comment: Although beat #4 is much wider and looks quite different from the normal sinus beats, it *is* preceded by a *premature* P wave. This makes the beat a PAC that conducts with aberrancy.

ANSWER TO FIGURE 3C-5

Rhythm—Irregular
PR interval—Normal (or perhaps a little short) for the sinus conducted beats
QRS complex—Normal duration (except for beats #2 and #12)
Impression: Sinus tachycardia (at a rate of 100 beats/min) with PACs and PVCs.
Comment: There are four early-occurring (i.e., *premature*) beats in this tracing. Beats #2 and #12 are clearly PVCs. They are wide, bizarre in appearance, and very much different from normally conducted beats. In contrast, beats #6 and #9 are PACs. Both are preceded by a premature P wave, and the QRS looks identical to that for the normally conducted beats. Note that the morphology of the two premature P waves differs from that of the sinus P waves.

ANSWER TO FIGURE 3C-6

Rhythm—Slightly irregular
Rate—≈45 beats/min
PR interval—Normal
QRS complex—Normal duration
Impression: Sinus bradycardia and arrythmia. Note that P wave morphology varies slightly from beat to beat. This may reflect a changing site of the atrial pacemaker (*wandering* pacemaker). Clinically, the significance of this arrhythmia is limited.

ANSWER TO FIGURE 3C-7

Rhythm—Irregular
Atrial rate—Irregular
QRS complex—Normal duration
Impression: Atrial bigeminy
Comment: Every other beat is a PAC. Ectopic P waves are broader and notched compared to the more pointed sinus P waves. Note that QRS morphology varies

slightly from beat to beat. There is no definite pattern to this variation. It is probably artifactual in nature, and of no clinical significance.

ANSWER TO FIGURE 3C-8

Atrial rate and rhythm—Regular at about 230 beats/min

Ventricular rate and rhythm—Regular at just under 60 beats/min

QRS complex—Normal duration

Impression: Probable atrial flutter with 4:1 AV conduction (versus atrial tachycardia with 4:1 AV block)

Comment: Rapid and regular atrial activity is seen. However, the atrial rate is a little slower than the 250 to 350 beats/min usually seen with flutter, and the typical saw-tooth pattern (noted in Fig. 3C-3) is not evident in this particular lead (the baseline between P waves is isoelectric). This raises the possibility that the rhythm could be atrial tachycardia with 4:1 block. It is hard to distinguish between these two possibilities from this one rhythm strip alone.

There are four P waves (or flutter waves) for each QRS complex. However, every fourth atrial impulse is partially hidden within the QRS complex.

ANSWER TO FIGURE 3C-9

Rhythm—Irregular

P waves—Precede each QRS complex with a constant PR interval

QRS complex—Normal duration

Impression: Sinus arrhythmia

Comment: Despite fairly marked irregularity, the finding of normal-appearing P waves with a constant (and normal) PR interval in front of each QRS complex confirms that the mechanism of this arrhythmia is sinus. Sinus arrhythmia is a common normal variant in children and young adults. In the elderly it may be a manifestation of sick sinus syndrome.

ANSWER TO FIGURE 3C-10

Rhythm—Slightly irregular

Rate—Varies between 85 and 110 beats/min

P waves—None evident

QRS complex—Wide (0.16 second)

Impression: Atrial fibrillation with preexisting bundle branch block (versus slow ventricular tachycardia)

Comment: It is hard to be certain of the etiology of this arrhythmia from this tracing alone. At first glance the R-R interval appears to be fairly constant. However, close inspection reveals a definite *irregular irregularity* to the rhythm. In the absence of atrial activity, this degree of irregularity suggests atrial fibrillation. Admittedly, we would feel more comfortable with this diagnosis if it were known that this patient had a preexisting bundle branch block with similar QRS morphology on a baseline 12-lead ECG.

The other possibility to consider is an accelerated idioventricular rhythm ("slow VT"), although a greater degree of regularity is usually seen with this arrhythmia.

ANSWER TO FIGURE 3C-11

Rhythm—Regular

Rate—155 beats/min

QRS complex—Normal duration

Impression: Regular supraventricular tachycardia (SVT) at a rate of 155 beats/min. The rhythm is probably atrial flutter with 2:1 AV conduction.

Comment: One should always maintain a high index of suspicion for atrial flutter in the presence of any regular SVT with a rate of about 150 (140 to 160) beats/min. In this particular tracing, normal atrial activity is *not* present because P waves are *not* upright in this lead II. If one sets a pair of calipers at precisely half the R-R interval, the negative deflection that precedes the QRS complex can be seen to notch the ST segment, further supporting flutter. Confirmation is forthcoming with application of a vagal maneuver *(Fig. 3C-21)*.

Lead II

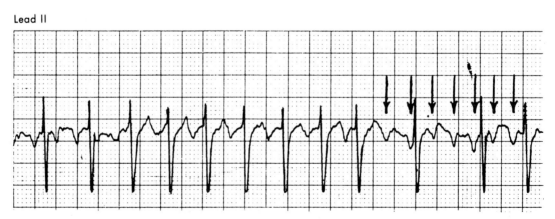

Figure 3C-21. Application of a vagal maneuver to the rhythm shown in Figure 3C-11.

The vagal maneuver slows AV conduction, permitting flutter waves (at a rate of approximately 300 beats/min) to become more evident (arrows in *Figure 3C-21*).

ANSWER TO FIGURE 3C-12

Rhythm—Regular
Rate—170 beats/min
P waves—None
QRS complex—Wide!
Impression: Ventricular tachycardia
Comment: A regular wide-complex tachycardia is seen. Although the differential includes SVT with either preexisting bundle branch block or aberrant conduction, ventricular tachycardia must always be assumed until proved otherwise.

ANSWER TO FIGURE 3C-13

Rhythm—Regular
Rate—90 beats/min
PR interval—Prolonged (0.24 second)
QRS complex—Wide (0.13 second)
Impression: Sinus rhythm with 1° AV block
Comment: Despite the fact that the QRS is wide, each complex is preceded by a P wave with a fixed (albeit prolonged) PR interval. Therefore the mechanism of the rhythm is sinus. QRS prolongation is due to preexisting bundle branch block.

ANSWER TO FIGURE 3C-14

Rhythm—Regular
Rate—210 beats/min
P waves—None
QRS complex—Normal duration
Impression: PSVT
Comment: A regular supraventricular tachycardia is present at a rate of 210 beats/min. The differential includes sinus tachycardia, atrial flutter, and PSVT. Sinus tachycardia is unlikely because the rate of this rhythm usually does not exceed 160 beats/min in adults. Atrial flutter is also unlikely, given that the ventricular response of flutter is almost always around 150 beats/min (unless the patient received antiarrhythmic medication). By the process of elimination, this leaves PSVT as the probable diagnosis.

ANSWER TO FIGURE 3C-15

Rhythm—Irregular
P waves—Precede each of the sinus beats
PR interval—Normal (0.20 second)
QRS complex—Normal duration (0.10) for the sinus conducted beats
Impression: Ventricular trigeminy
Comment: Every third beat is a PVC (wide QRS complex with bizarre morphology).

ANSWER TO FIGURE 3C-16

Rhythm—Regular
Rate—110 beats/min
PR interval—Normal
QRS complex—Normal duration
Impression: Sinus tachycardia

ANSWER TO FIGURE 3C-17

Rhythm—Irregularly irregular
Rate—Between 130 to 160 beats/min
P waves—None
QRS complex—Normal duration
Impression: Atrial fibrillation with a rapid ventricular response

ANSWER TO FIGURE 3C-18

Rhythm—Irregular
Rate—Between 85 and 135 beats/min
P waves—Sawtooth appearance
QRS complex—Normal duration
Impression: Atrial flutter with a variable (moderately rapid) ventricular response
Comment: As opposed to the irregular rhythm just discussed in Figure 3C-17, atrial activity *is* present in this tracing in the form of the typical sawtooth pattern characteristic of flutter. Although the ventricular response with atrial flutter most often is regular (usually with an even conduction ratio such as 2:1 or 4:1), it may occasionally be irregular as shown here.

ANSWER TO FIGURE 3C-19

Rhythm—Irregular
P waves—Precede the sinus beats
PR interval—Normal
QRS complex—Normal duration for the sinus conducted beats
Impression: Ventricular bigeminy
Comment: Every other beat is a PVC. Because two sinus beats never occur in a row, it is impossible to know the underlying sinus rate.

Clinically, PVCs that can be palpated in the peripheral pulse contribute to cardiac output. This explains why many patients with persistent ventricular bigeminy are able to tolerate this arrhythmia for extended periods of time.

ANSWER TO FIGURE 3C-20

Rhythm—fairly regular
Rate—about 30 beats/min
P waves—precede each QRS complex with a constant PR interval
PR interval—normal
QRS complex—normal duration
Impression: Marked sinus bradycardia (and slight sinus arrhythmia)

SECTION D

AV BLOCKS (BASIC CONCEPTS)

Diagnosis of the AV blocks is a common source of confusion for the emergency care provider not accustomed to dealing with these rhythm disturbances on a daily basis. Confusion begins with terminology, encompasses diagnosis, and extends into therapeutic implications.

To facilitate understanding, we have divided the topic of the AV blocks into two parts. In this introductory chapter on Basic Concepts, we define the three degrees of AV block, point out their clinical significance, and present some basic examples of each type. We also introduce the concept of AV dissociation. A more in-depth discussion of the AV blocks including a number of subtleties in diagnosis (and sprinkled with pearls and pitfalls along the way) will follow in Section B of Chapter 16).

Classification of the AV Blocks

Table 3D-1 indicates the traditional classification of the AV blocks. Implicit in division of these blocks into three degrees is the tacit assumption that 2° AV block portends a more ominous prognosis than 1° AV block, and that 3° AV block portends the poorest prognosis of all. This is *not* necessarily the case.

Table 3D-1

Traditional Classification of the AV Blocks

1° AV block
2° AV block
  • Mobitz type I (Wenckebach)
  • Mobitz type II
3° (complete) AV block

"Unclaimed" Terms
  • AV dissociation?
  • High-grade heart block?
  • High-degree block?

Imagine the case of a patient who "only" has 1° AV block (PR interval prolongation), but who has marked bradycardia (say, a heart rate of 20 beats/min), resultant hypotension, and severe chest pain. Compare this scenario to that of another patient who has complete (and presumably "more severe") AV block in association with an AV nodal rhythm with an appropriate escape rate of 45 beats/min (which is well within the usual 40 to 60 beat/min range for AV nodal rhythm), who is asymptomatic and able to maintain a normal blood pressure of 120/80 mm Hg. *Which patient is better off?* The one who "only" has 1° AV block (but a heart rate of 20 beats/min, marked hypotension, and severe chest pain), or the second patient with "more severe" (complete) AV block who is asymptomatic and has normal hemodynamics?

An additional problem stemming from use of the traditional classification is the issue of "unclaimed" (i.e., "left over") terms such as *high-degree* or *high-grade heart block* and AV *dissociation*. Although in common use, these terms frequently hold different meanings to different emergency care providers. Particularly misunderstood is the concept of AV dissociation, which is often interchanged (used synonymously) with 3° AV block. The two terms are very different, as we shall see momentarily.

> From the above, it should already be apparent that simple description of an AV conduction disturbance according to the "traditional classification" *without explicit reference* to the patient's associated hemodynamic status is inadequate. Thus, a complete description of the first patient in our imagined scenario would be:
>
> "Sinus bradycardia at a heart rate of 20 beats/min with 1° AV block, in association with severe chest pain and resultant hypotension."
>
> Despite the trivial conduction disturbance, the need for immediate intervention is clear from this description. In contrast, description of the second patient's conduction disturbance would be:
>
> "Complete AV block with a junctional escape pacemaker at 45 beats/min with normal hemodynamic status and no symptoms."

Overview

In Section A of this chapter we discussed how with normal sinus rhythm all QRS complexes are preceded by P waves with a *constant* PR interval. Each atrial impulse is conducted to the ventricles, and the PR interval is ≤0.20 second. With **1° AV block,** atrial impulses are still conducted to the ventricles with a constant PR interval, but AV conduction is delayed (to ≥0.21 second).

With more severe impairment of AV conduction (with **2° AV block**), conduction of one or more atrial impulses to the ventricles is prevented *("blocked")*. P waves may precede and be related to at least some of the QRS complexes, but their relationship may not be readily apparent. This type of block is broken down further into **Mobitz I** and **Mobitz II** varieties (Table 3D-1).

Finally, with complete block of AV conduction (**3°** or **complete AV block**), none of the atrial impulses are conducted to the ventricles. In this case, both the atria and ventricles discharge at their own inherent rate. P waves may precede QRS complexes, but they are totally unrelated to them, and the PR interval continually changes.

Approach to Diagnosis

Application of the systematic Four-Question approach to arrhythmia analysis that was presented earlier is all that is needed to diagnose the AV blocks. Thus one looks for:

1. Regularity of the rhythm
2. Evidence of atrial activity (P waves)
3. QRS widening
4. The relationship (if any) between P waves and the QRS complex

Not all conduction disturbances will fall "neatly" into the three categories of AV block that are listed in Table 3D-1. However, even when the type of AV block is not readily apparent, attention to each of the above four factors will usually narrow down the diagnostic possibilities, as well as assist in describing the characteristics of the conduction disturbance in question.

The diagnostic approach for determining the type (degree) of AV block may be simplified into the following deductive process:
1. Look first to see if 1° AV block is present. *This is usually easy to recognize.*
2. Look next to see if 3° AV block is present. *This is also usually easy to recognize.*
3. If the block is neither 1° or 3°, but beats are being dropped (nonconducted) as a result of AV block, the block *must* be 2°!

First-Degree AV Block

As alluded to above, *1° AV block* is usually very easy to recognize. It is simply a sinus rhythm in which the PR interval is prolonged. All atrial impulses are conducted to the ventricles—they just take a little longer to arrive.

PROBLEM   **Examine *Figure 3D-1*. Does it appear that the P waves in this rhythm strip are conducted?**

ANSWER TO FIGURE 3D-1   The atrial and ventricular rates in this example are regular at 65 beats/min. The QRS complex is borderline prolonged (it appears to be half of a large box in duration, or about 0.10 second). Each QRS is preceded by a P wave. These P waves appear to be conducting because the PR interval preceding each QRS complex is constant. *First-degree AV block* is present because this PR interval is prolonged (to 0.34 second).

> Criteria for defining a normal PR interval are age dependent. This becomes readily apparent with our discussion of Pediatric Arrhythmias in Section D of Chapter 17. For example, a PR interval of 0.17 second in a 3-year-old child is definitely *prolonged* and constitutes 1° AV block for this age group.
> At the other extreme, older individuals often normally demonstrate slight prolongation in AV conduction. Thus, although 0.20 second is usually taken as the upper limit of normal for the PR interval in adults, a slightly longer interval is probably still normal for many older individuals. Practically speaking, the isolated occurrence of 1° AV block is rarely of clinical importance. As a result, *we prefer* **not** *to call 1° AV block unless the PR interval is clearly prolonged to* **at least** *0.22 second*. For a similar reason we tend to avoid the term *borderline* 1° AV block (for PR intervals of 0.19 to 0.21 second), as this connotation rarely adds useful clinical information.*

Third-Degree AV Block

Surprisingly, *3° (complete) AV block* is also *usually* an easy conduction disturbance to recognize. Because none of the atrial impulses are able to penetrate through to the ventricles, atrial activity is separated from what occurs in the rest of the heart. As a result, the atria beat at their own inherent rate, an escape pacemaker (from the AV node or a site below) does the same, and "n'er the twain shall meet."

PROBLEM   **Analyze *Figure 3D-2* by the Four-Question approach. Is there any apparent relationship between P waves and the QRS complex?**

---

*Reflect for a moment. If one describes the isolated finding of a PR interval of 0.19 (or even 0.20 second) in an adult as "borderline" 1° block, all one is saying is that you *almost* have a finding that, even if it were present, would not have any significant clinical meaning.

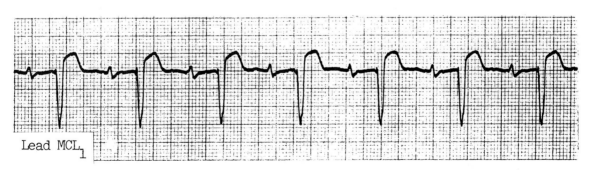

Lead MCL₁

Figure 3D-1

Lead II

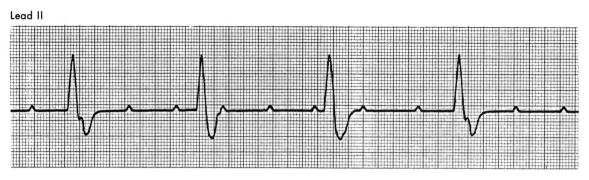

Figure 3D-2

ANSWER TO FIGURE 3D-2   Although both atrial and ventricular rates are fairly regular, P waves appear *unrelated* to (i.e., they "march through") the QRS complex. We describe this lack of relationship between atrial and ventricular activity as ***AV dissociation.*** It is easily recognized in this example by looking in front of each QRS complex and noting the *varying PR interval*.

This patient is in *3° AV block*. Despite the fact that P waves are given ample opportunity to conduct (they occur at every possible point in the R-R interval), they fail to do so.

With **3° AV block,** then one expects to see:
1. A regular atrial rate (constant P-P interval)
2. A regular ventricular rate (constant R-R interval)
3. No relationship between the two (*complete* AV dissociation).

Most of the time the ventricular response will be regular with 3° AV block. This is an extremely helpful point to keep in mind when sorting out AV conduction disturbances, since recognition of R-R irregularity makes it much less likely that complete AV block is present.

We have already alluded to the fact that 3° AV block may occur at two levels: *at* the AV node or *below* the AV node.

PROBLEM   **What would you expect the escape pacemaker to look like if the level of 3° AV block was *at* the AV node? What if it were *below* the AV node? (What is the probable level of block for the example shown in *Fig. 3D-2?*)**

ANSWER   If the level of 3° AV block was at the AV node, an AV *nodal* pacemaker should take over. One would therefore expect the QRS complex of the escape pacemaker to be narrow, very similar (or identical) in morphology to the QRS of normally conducted beats, and occurring at a rate of between 40 and 60 beats/min.

If on the other hand the level of 3° AV block was below the AV node, an *idioventricular* escape pacemaker should take over. In this case the QRS complex would be wide, very different in morphology from the sinus conducted beats, and occurring at a much slower rate (usually between 30 to 40 beats/min).

The fact that the QRS complex in Figure 3D-2 is markedly widened and the rate exceedingly slow (34 beats/min) suggests that the block occurs at a low level (*below* the AV node) in the conduction system.

PROBLEM   *Figure 3D-3* **is taken from the same patient who was shown to be in 1° AV block in Figure 3D-1. Initially in this tracing the P waves appear to be totally unrelated to the QRS complex.** *Has the patient gone into 3° AV block?*

ANSWER TO FIGURE 3D-3   *Resist the urge to comment on the dropped beats until you have systematically analyzed*

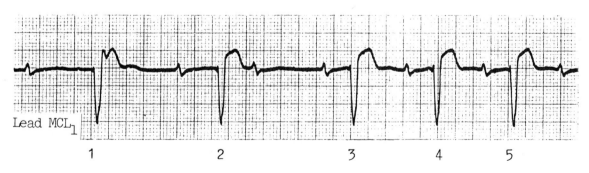

Lead MCL₁

1   2   3   4   5

Figure 3D-3

Lead II

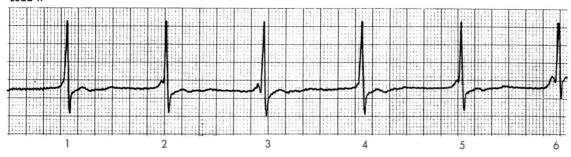

Figure 3D-4

the tracing! The QRS complex is at the upper limit of normal (0.10 second), and the atrial rate is fairly regular. The last three beats of the tracing very much resemble the rhythm shown previously in Figure 3D-1 (i.e., P waves precede the QRS complex of beats #3, #4, and #5 with a fixed [albeit prolonged] PR interval). These P waves appear to be conducting—so 3° AV block *cannot* be present! Instead there is *transient AV dissociation*. At least momentarily, atrial activity appears totally unrelated to the QRS complexes of beats #1 and #2.

> An easy way to tell *at a glance* that 3° AV block is probably *not* present in Figure 3D-3 is to note that the ventricular rate does not remain constant!

> In *most* cases, **the ventricular response with 3° AV block will be regular.** This is because none of the supraventricular (sinus) impulses will be conducted to the ventricles if the heart block is complete, and *most* of the time escape rhythms (be they junctional or idioventricular) are regular. It follows that, *if AV block is present, but the ventricular response is not regular, the conduction disturbance is likely to be something other than 3° AV block* (i.e., a more complicated form of 2° AV block in which there may be transient AV dissociation, escape beats, and the like)!!!

Return to Figure 3D-3. Note that the atrial rate is *not* perfectly regular. Occasionally in the setting of AV block or AV dissociation with a slow escape rhythm, the atrial rate will vary slightly (**ventriculophasic sinus arrhythmia**). The mechanism of this is not clear. However, consistent P wave morphology throughout the rhythm strip strongly supports our assumption that the slight atrial irregularity is due to ventriculophasic sinus arrhythmia, and not ectopic/premature atrial beats.

PROBLEM   Now examine *Figure 3D-4. Is there evidence of atrial activity? If so, how many P waves can you identify? Are P waves related to the QRS complex?*

ANSWER TO FIGURE 3D-4   The QRS complex appears to be narrow and the ventricular rate regular at 53 beats/min. Atrial activity *is* present! P waves precede each QRS complex and deform its initial upstroke (see arrows in *Fig. 3D-5*). However, none of the P waves are related in any consistent manner to the QRS complex (i.e., the PR interval is extremely short and keeps changing). *Complete AV dissociation* therefore is present.

> Identification of atrial activity in Figure 3D-4 is exceedingly subtle! The best clue to its presence lies with analysis of beat #3 (and to a lesser extent beat #6), in which a definite P wave *can* be seen to precede (and be separate from) the QRS complex. This tells us that the initial portion of the QRS has a *very straight upslope*, and that rounding of the initial portion of the QRS complex in beats #1, #2, #4, and #5 is likely to be the result of an occult P wave.

Lead II

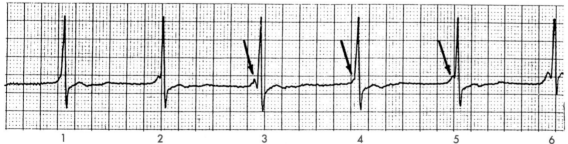

Figure 3D-5.   Arrows indicate that atrial activity is present in Figure 3D-4. P waves precede *each* QRS complex and deform its initial upslope.

PROBLEM   **Is there also 3° AV block in Figure 3D-5?**

> HINT: Is there any way to tell from this rhythm strip alone if there is 3° AV block?

ANSWER TO FIGURE 3D-5   Although there *may* be 3° AV block, there is no way to tell this from the rhythm strip shown in Figure 3D-5. Thus, despite the presence of complete AV dissociation, the reason 3° AV block cannot be diagnosed is that *none of the P waves are ever given a reasonable opportunity to conduct*. The PR interval throughout the rhythm strip simply remains too short to allow conduction. Without more information (i.e., a longer rhythm strip), there is no way to know if P waves could conduct were they given the chance.

We might therefore restate our criteria for diagnosing **3° AV block** as the following:
1. Atrial regularity
2. Ventricular regularity (usually)
3. Complete AV dissociation (*despite adequate opportunity for normal conduction to occur*)

This last condition implies that the ventricular rate must be slow enough (and the rhythm strip long enough) for P waves to occur at all points of the R-R interval so as to provide maximal opportunity for conduction to occur. *Usually this requires a ventricular rate of 45 beats/min or less.* Inclusion of this rate criterion helps avoid overdiagnosing cases of transient or rate-related AV dissociation as complete AV block.

Thus, the final criterion for diagnosing **3° AV block** is:
4. A sufficiently slow heart rate (*usually 45 beats/min or less*) to ensure adequate opportunity for normal conduction to occur

---

PROBLEM   **Return to *Figure 3D-2*. Does it meet *all* of these criteria for diagnosing 3° AV block?**

ANSWER   Yes. Atrial and ventricular rates are regular (for practical purposes),* complete AV dissociation is present, and the ventricular response is *less* than 45 beats/min. None of the P waves conduct *despite having adequate opportunity to do so.*

---

*We acknowledge that there *is* slight variability in the atrial rate in Figure 3D-2. This probably represents the ventriculophasic sinus arrhythmia discussed previously (since the degree of irregularity is minimal and all P waves manifest a similar morphology). As we have already indicated, *slight* variability in the atrial rate is common in patients with 2° or 3° AV block and a slow ventricular response.

Second-Degree AV Block

Let us now turn our attention to the 2° AV blocks. If the atrial rate is *regular* (or at least *almost* regular) and some atrial impulses are conducted to the ventricles but others are not, a type of 2° AV block (Mobitz I or II) is present.

> It is important to emphasize the need for *regularity of the atrial rate* in this definition. Awareness of this point helps differentiate 2° AV blocks from mimics such as blocked PACs and sinus pauses (in which there is definite and often abrupt variation from the usual atrial rate).
>
> In addition, consideration must be given to the appropriateness of the failed conduction. For example, the usual atrial rate in flutter is 300 beats/min. One-to-one ventricular conduction under these circumstances would be incompatible with life (since it would produce a ventricular rate of 300 beats/min). Fortunately, the AV node is able to protect the ventricles by limiting the number of atrial impulses it allows to pass through. Much of the time this entails conduction of every other atrial impulse. The result is that the most common ventricular response to atrial flutter in adults is 2:1 AV conduction with a ventricular rate of approximately 150 beats/min (300 ÷ 2). This rhythm should *not* be misclassified as 2:1 AV "block" because it represents a *physiologic* phenomenon (in which we are happy conduction is 2:1 instead of 1:1).

MOBITZ I (WENCKEBACH) 2° AV BLOCK

Mobitz I 2° AV block is characterized by progressive lengthening of the PR interval until a beat is dropped. This conduction disturbance is most often associated with acute inferior infarction. Anatomically, it is located at the level of the AV node. This accounts for the fact that QRS duration tends to be normal. The PR interval may be prolonged (1° AV block). The junctional pacemaker is usually reliable with Mobitz I 2° AV block, and observation of the patient until the conduction disturbance spontaneously resolves is often all that is needed. If hemodynamic status is compromised (due to marked bradycardia), atropine will often be effective in improving AV conduction (since the anatomic level of the conduction disturbance is at the AV node). Pacemaker therapy is rarely needed *(Table 3D-2)*.

MOBITZ II 2° AV BLOCK

In contrast, *Mobitz II 2° AV block* is associated with anterior or anteroseptal myocardial infarction. The level of this block is anatomically lower in the conduction system (it is *always* infranodal) than the level of Mobitz I block. As a result, the QRS complex is most often wide, and the escape focus much less reliable. In addition, Mobitz II has a disturbing tendency to progress to complete AV block (or even ventricular standstill), often with little (or no) warning. *Immediate* consideration of pacemaker therapy is therefore essential as soon as this conduction disturbance is recognized. This is in contrast to Mobitz I 2° AV block which tends to progress in an orderly fashion (from 1° to

Table 3D-2

Comparison of Mobitz I and Mobitz II 2° AV Block		
	Mobitz I	**Mobitz II**
Clinical occurrence and course	Usually associated with *inferior* infarction	Usually associated with *anterior* or *anteroseptal* infarction
	Relatively frequent	Uncommon
	Usually transient (and often spontaneously resolving)	Often *progresses* (sometimes abruptly) to complete AV block or ventricular standstill
Anatomic level	At the level of the AV node	Below the AV node
ECG characteristics	Gradually lengthening PR interval until a beat is dropped: • 1° AV block is common • QRS is usually narrow	Constant PR interval until one or more beats are dropped: • PR interval is usually normal • QRS is usually wide
Treatment	Observation usually suffices (provided that the ventricular response is adequate) Atropine (if there is hemodynamic compromise)	Pacemaker standby and/or insertion is required (since progression to complete AV block may be abrupt) Atropine may be tried (while awaiting pacemaker therapy), but it is unlikely to improve the ventricular response

2° to 3° AV block) in those cases in which complete AV block does develop. Because of the low (infranodal) anatomic level of the conduction disturbance with Mobitz II, atropine will rarely be effective in improving the ventricular response.

Electrocardiographically, Mobitz II 2° AV block is recognized by nonconduction of one or more atrial impulses despite maintenance of a constant PR interval. As for Mobitz I, the atrial rate remains fairly regular throughout (Table 3D-2).

Clinically, Mobitz II 2° AV block is a much, much *less* common conduction disturbance than Mobitz I. Nevertheless, because of its potential for rapid progression to complete heart block and/or ventricular standstill, it is important to remain on the lookout for Mobitz II (especially in patients with large, acute anterior infarctions). Active consideration of pacemaker therapy should receive top priority as soon as Mobitz II is identified.

PROBLEM Examine *Figure 3D-6*. What type of AV block is present—Mobitz I or Mobitz II? *(Are the P waves in some way related to the QRS?)*

ANSWER TO FIGURE 3D-6 The atrial rate is regular at 65 to 70 beats/min. The QRS complex is narrow, and each QRS is preceded by a P wave. Even though the PR interval is not constant, P waves *are* related to the QRS complex (by progressive PR interval lengthening in each sequence [from 0.25 to 0.48 second] until a beat is

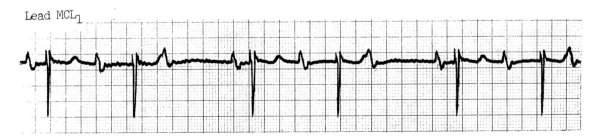

Lead MCL₁

Figure 3D-6

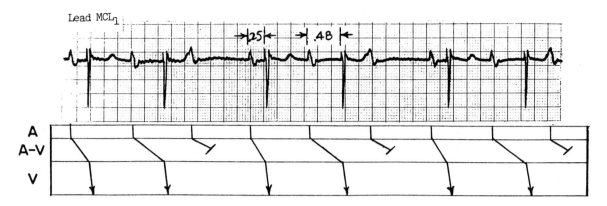

Figure 3D-7.   Demonstration that the rhythm presented in Figure 3D-6 is 2° AV block, Mobitz type I. The laddergram shows that the PR interval in each sequence progressively lengthens (from 0.25 to 0.48 second) until a beat is dropped.

dropped) *(Figure 3D-7)*. Therefore this is *Mobitz I* 2° AV block.

Several features characterize Mobitz I 2° AV block. Marriott has colorfully labeled these the "footprints of Wenckebach." They include:

1. Regularity of the atrial rate
2. Group beating
3. Progressive lengthening of the PR interval until a beat is dropped
4. Duration of the pause (that contains the dropped beat) of less than twice the shortest R-R interval

All of these features are present in Figure 3D-7.

> The finding of **group beating** is deserving of special mention. Note in Figure 3D-6 (and in Fig. 3D-7) that there is a *regular irregularity* to the rhythm (alternating short-long-short-long segments of the R-R interval). *Whenever a repetitive cadence to the R-R interval (group beating) is noted, one should suspect that a Wenckebach block may be operative.*

As noted previously, other features commonly associated with Mobitz I are normal QRS duration, 1° AV block, and accompanying acute inferior infarction.

> Figure 3D-7 illustrates the features of Mobitz I 2° AV block by means of a **laddergram.** We introduced this extremely helpful teaching tool during our discussion of junctional rhythm in Section A of this chapter (see Fig. 3A-14). As we have already emphasized, appreciable time and prowess in

arrhythmia interpretation is needed to learn how to construct laddergrams. However, understanding laddergrams that are already drawn is surprisingly easy, and tremendously facilitates explanation of even complicated rhythm disorders (which is why we choose to use them often throughout this book for illustrative purposes).

Thus, in Figure 3D-7, the **atrial tier** (labeled **A**) shows regular atrial activity. The **AV nodal tier** (labeled **A-V**) shows *progressive delay* in conduction, with every third beat being blocked. Impulses that do make it out of the A-V nodal tier are then conducted normally to the **ventricles** (through the tier labeled **V**).

PROBLEM   **Examine *Figure 3D-8*. Note the pause between beat #8 and #9. *Is this due to Wenckebach?***

ANSWER TO FIGURE 3D-8   Yes, although the diagnosis of Mobitz I in this example is not nearly as evident as it was in Figure 3D-6. Eight consecutive beats are conducted (with 1° AV block) in this tracing until a beat is finally dropped. However, if one merely compared consecutive PR intervals during these eight conducted beats, it would not be at all apparent that the PR interval was progressively lengthening. *Only by comparing the last PR interval just before the dropped beat* (the PR interval of beat #8) *with the PR interval at the start of the rhythm strip* (the PR interval of beat #1) *can this relationship be established.* With the onset of the next Wenckebach cycle (beat #9), the PR interval has again shortened.

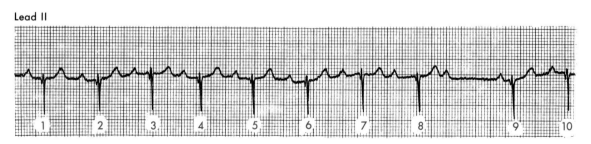

Figure 3D-8

Lead MCL₁

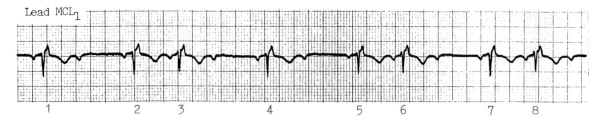

Figure 3D-9

Figure 3D-8 effectively illustrates how with Wenckebach *the pause containing the dropped beat* (the R-R interval between beats #8 and #9) *is less than twice the shortest R-R interval*. This finding is especially helpful in differentiating Wenckebach blocks from Mobitz II 2° AV block (in which the pause is precisely twice the regular R-R interval) and from sinus pauses (in which the interval including the dropped beat is often more than twice the regular R-R interval).

PROBLEM **What type of conduction disturbance is present in *Figure 3D-9?***

ANSWER TO FIGURE 3D-9 The atrial rate is fairly regular at 98 to 100 beats/min. Several atrial impulses are not conducted (the P waves following beats #1, #3, #4, #6, and #8). The QRS appears to be wide and P waves precede each complex. In contrast to the case with Mobitz I 2° AV block, the PR interval remains *constant* for beats that are conducted *(Figure 3D-10)*. This is *Mobitz II 2° AV block.*

Even though *group beating* is present in Figure 3D-9, this is one case in which group beating is *not* due to Wenckebach. Note again how nicely the laddergram in Figure 3D-10 illustrates what happens with Mobitz II 2° AV block. Atrial activity is regular, but some of the atrial impulses again fail to make it through the AV nodal tier. As opposed to the case for Mobitz I 2° AV block (Fig. 3D-7), atrial impulses that do make it through the AV nodal tier are conducted normally (*without* progressive delay).

Second-Degree AV Block with 2:1 AV Conduction

The presence of 2° AV block with 2:1 AV conduction poses an additional problem.

PROBLEM **Consider *Figure 3D-11,* in which every other beat is conducted. *Is this likely to represent the Mobitz I or Mobitz II type of 2° AV block?***

Lead MCL₁

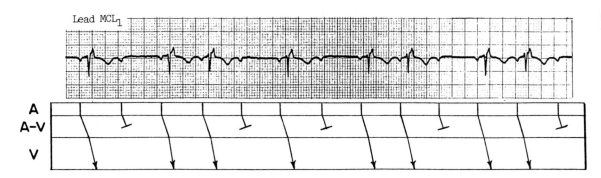

Figure 3D-10. Demonstration that the rhythm presented in Figure 3D-9 is 2° AV block, Mobitz type II. The laddergram shows that the PR interval remains *constant* (and AV conduction does *not* become prolonged) for the beats that are conducted.

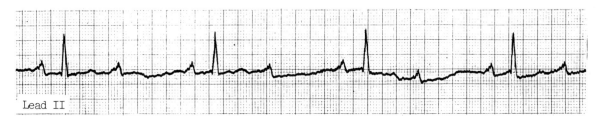

Lead II

Figure 3D-11

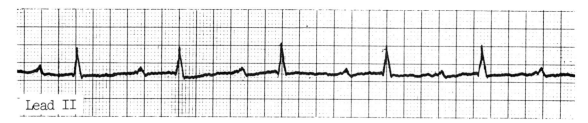

Figure 3D-12.   Rhythm developing from Figure 3D-11 after administration of 0.5 mg of atropine.

ANSWER TO FIGURE 3D-11   Both atrial and ventricular rates are regular (at 58 and 29 beats/min, respectively). Each QRS complex is preceded by a P wave with a constant PR interval, but only half of the atrial impulses are conducted to the ventricles. This is *2° AV block with 2:1 AV conduction* (since every other atrial impulse is blocked). The problem with 2:1 AV conduction is that it may result from *either* Mobitz I or Mobitz II 2° AV block. Because of the constant PR interval, one's natural inclination may be to suspect that the rhythm in Figure 3D-11 is Mobitz II. However, this is not necessarily the case. Since only one QRS complex at a time is conducted, *the opportunity for the PR interval to lengthen before dropping a beat does not exist.* There is therefore no way from this rhythm strip alone to rule out the possibility of Mobitz I 2° AV block.

PROBLEM   **There are two hints on the ECG shown in Figure 3D-11 that suggest the conduction disturbance is the result of Mobitz I rather than Mobitz II. *What are they?* (Feel free to refer back to Table 3D-2 for assistance.)**

ANSWER   The two ECG characteristics in favor of a Mobitz I etiology are:

1. The normal duration of the QRS complex
2. The presence of 1° AV block.

PROBLEM   **What else in the clinical history might further support a Mobitz I etiology for this arrhythmia? (Again, feel free to refer back to Table 3D-2 for assistance.)**

ANSWER   Knowledge of the clinical setting in which the conduction disturbance occurred could prove insightful. Further support for a Mobitz I etiology of the arrhythmia would be forthcoming if it were known that the patient was having an acute *inferior* infarction.

One might also look through the patient's chart for prior (recent) tracings. **It is distinctly unusual for Mobitz I and Mobitz II conduction to alternate in any given patient.** Therefore, documentation of definite Mobitz I on previous tracings would be strong presumptive evidence of its presence with 2:1 AV conduction.

PROBLEM   **Because of the slow heart rate, the patient was medicated with 0.5 mg of atropine. Shortly thereafter the rhythm shown in *Figure 3D-12* was observed. *What has happened?* Does this further support our suspicion of a Mobitz I etiology for the arrhythmia?**

ANSWER TO FIGURE 3D-12   Second-degree AV block is no longer present since each P wave is now conducted (albeit with a markedly prolonged PR interval). Thus, the rhythm is now *sinus bradycardia* with *1° AV block.* This further supports our suspicion that Figure 3D-11 was the result of Mobitz I 2° AV block, since one would not expect Mobitz II to respond favorably (and so easily) to medical treatment.

In view of the difficulty sometimes encountered in distinguishing between Mobitz I and Mobitz II 2° AV block, we prefer a modified classification of the AV blocks (*Table 3D-3*).

Table 3D-3

Modified * Classification of the AV Blocks
1° AV block
2° AV block
• Mobitz type I (Wenckebach)
• Mobitz type II
• **2° AV block with 2:1 AV conduction**
3° (complete) AV block
*Table 3D-1 (which we presented in the beginning of this section) has been modified by addition of **2:1 conduction** as a *third* category for the types of 2° AV block.

We explore additional intricacies involved in interpretation of the AV blocks in Sections D and E of Chapter 16. For now, suffice it to say that *it will not always be possible to distinguish between Mobitz I and Mobitz II 2° AV block when there is 2:1 AV conduction.* In such cases,

Mobitz I *is more likely* if:
• The QRS complex is narrow
• There is 1° AV block
• The patient is having an acute *inferior* infarction

- Prior tracings show definite evidence of Mobitz I
- The conduction disturbance readily resolves with atropine

Mobitz II *is more likely* if:
- The QRS complex is wide *(although bundle branch block may also occur with Mobitz I)*
- The PR interval is normal *(although the PR interval may also be normal with Mobitz I)*
- The patient is having an acute *anterior* infarction
- Prior tracings show definite evidence of Mobitz II

Practically speaking, it is helpful to remember that *Mobitz I is a much more common conduction disturbance than Mobitz II.* However, as we have emphasized, the importance of promptly recognizing Mobitz II is that it signals the need for strong consideration of prophylactic pacemaker therapy.

In the event that clinical characteristics do not provide sufficient information to determine the etiology of the conduction disturbance, treatment considerations should be based on the hemodynamic consequences of the arrhythmia. Thus, despite the fact that the conduction disturbance shown in Figure 3D-11 is probably "only" Mobitz I, *it may still produce serious hemodynamic consequences as a result of the exceedingly slow ventricular response.* As a result, treatment (with atropine, a pressor agent, and/or a pacemaker) may be needed. In contrast, a patient with 3° (complete) AV block and an appropriate junctional escape pacemaker (at a rate of between 40 to 60 beats/min) may be hemodynamically stable and not require any immediate therapy.

It should be clear that *much more important than the "degree" of AV block per se is the ventricular response and the patient's hemodynamic status.* A patient with 1° AV block and a sinus rate of 20 beats/min will need a pacemaker (if there is no response to medical therapy), whereas one with 2° (or even 3°) AV block may not if there are no symptoms, the ventricular response is adequate, and the patient is hemodynamically stable.

Practice

Apply the material covered up to this point in evaluating the arrhythmias that follow. Use the systematic approach in your interpretation. (**HINT:** AV block is *not* necessarily present in each of these tracings!)

PROBLEM   *Figure 3D-13*

ANSWER TO FIGURE 3D-13   The most striking finding about this tracing is *group beating* (initially groups of three beats [#1, #2, #3, and #4, #5, #6] followed by groups of two beats [#7, #8, and #9, #10]). The presence of group beating should immediately increase one's suspicion that a Wenckebach block may be present.

Although the ventricular rate is variable (with the *regular irregularity* of group beating), regular P waves continue throughout the tracing. The QRS complex is narrow and always preceded by a P wave. If one focuses on one of the groups (e.g., beats #4 to #6), it becomes apparent that the PR interval progressively lengthens until a beat is dropped (the P wave following beat #6 is not conducted). The cycle then resumes with beat #7. This is Mobitz I (Wenckebach) 2° AV block.

> For the groups represented by beats #1 to #3, and #4 to #6, *four* P waves are present but only *three* are conducted. This is termed 4:3 AV conduction. For the other two groups (beats #7 and #8, and #9 and #10), three P waves are present but only two conduct (3:2 AV conduction).

Figure 3D-13 is not an easy tracing to interpret. Nevertheless it is an excellent example of how helpful recognizing group beating can be in leading up to the correct diagnosis.

Another point well illustrated by this tracing is how *calipers* can facilitate the task of dysrhythmia interpretation. There is no better way to rapidly determine that the atrial rate in Figure 3D-13 is regular!

PROBLEM   *Figure 3D-14*

ANSWER TO FIGURE 3D-14   Although group beating is again present in this tracing, the other *footprints* of a Wenckebach block are missing. Most notably, the atrial rate is not regular. Instead, beats #3 and #6 occur early—they are *premature* atrial contractions (PACs). The

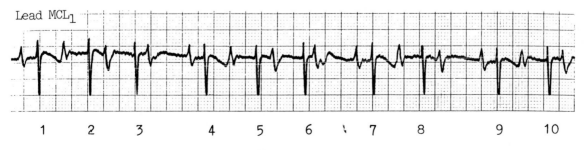

Lead MCL₁

1   2   3   4   5   6   7   8   9   10

Figure 3D-13

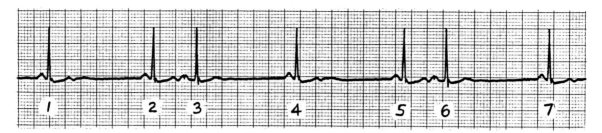

Figure 3D-14

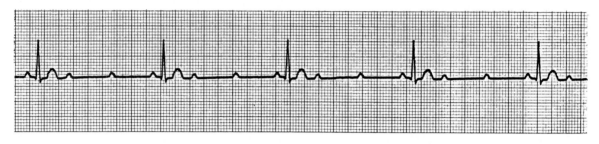

Figure 3D-15

rhythm is therefore sinus bradycardia (at a rate of about 45 beats/min) with PACs. The QRS complex is normal in duration.

In addition to occurring early, note the subtle difference in morphology of the P waves preceding beats #3 and #6 (these P waves are notched), indicating their origin from a different atrial focus.

PROBLEM   *Figure 3D-15*

ANSWER TO FIGURE 3D-15   Despite the fact that there are many more P waves than QRS complexes, 3° AV block is not present in this tracing. Both atrial and ventricular rates are regular (at 105 and 35 beats/min, respectively). Each QRS complex is preceded by a P wave with a *constant* PR interval. This rules out 3° AV block because it means that P waves *are* related to the QRS complex. By the process of elimination (since neither 1° nor 3° AV block is present), the rhythm in Figure 3D-15 must be a form of 2° AV block. We refer to this type of conduction disturbance in which multiple beats are dropped as *high-grade* (or *high-degree*) AV block. In this particular case, only one out of every three atrial impulses is conducted to the ventricles.

High-grade AV block is most often the result of a Mobitz II block. This may not be the case in Figure 3D-15, however, considering that the QRS complex is narrow, whereas it should be wide with Mobitz II. There are two possibilities:

1. A portion of the QRS complex may lie on the baseline in this particular monitoring lead (accounting for its narrow appearance), and the expected QRS widening may be readily apparent in other leads.
2. This could be Mobitz I with 3:1 AV conduction.

The dilemma presented by the conduction disturbances shown in Figures 3D-11 and 3D-15 is due to the absence of **consecutively** *conducted complexes* on each tracing. In order to diagnose the type of 2° AV block with certainty, *one must see* **at least** *two QRS complexes in a row before the dropped beat.* This is the problem with 2° AV block and 2:1 AV conduction. Because two consecutively conducted complexes are *never* seen, it is impossible to tell if the PR interval increases (as it should with Mobitz I) or remains constant (as it would with Mobitz II).

From a clinical perspective, even though the specific type of treatment may vary, the urgent need for increasing the ventricular response in Figures 3D-11 and 3D-15 is the same regardless of whether the conduction disturbance is due to Mobitz I or Mobitz II.

PROBLEM   *Figure 3D-16*

ANSWER TO FIGURE 3D-16   The QRS complex in this tracing is narrow, and the ventricular response slightly irregular. Although atrial activity precedes the last four beats, it is absent from the first four. Thus *AV nodal rhythm* is present at the start of the tracing. As the junctional pacemaker slows down ever so slightly, P waves can be seen to emerge from the QRS complex (beginning with the P wave that deforms the upstroke of the QRS complex of beat #5). This atrial pacemaker is set at 68 beats/min. Although it ultimately takes over, it is initially unrelated to the more rapid junctional pacemaker (i.e., the PR interval of beat #5 is *definitely* too short to conduct). Thus there is *transient AV dissociation,* in this case due to acceleration of the AV nodal pacemaker to 70 beats/min during the first portion of this rhythm strip.

Lead II

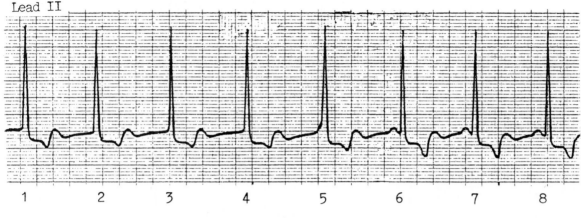

Figure 3D-16

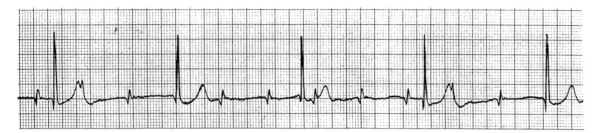

Figure 3D-17

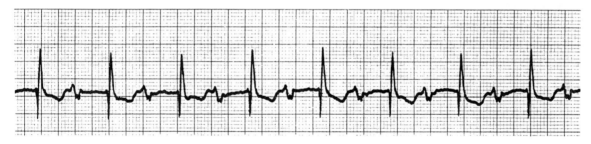

Figure 3D-18

This tracing reemphasizes the point made earlier when discussing the rhythm shown in Figure 3D-4. That is, even though AV dissociation is present (transiently in this case), diagnosis of 3° AV block (or any degree of AV block for that matter) is *not* possible here, because P waves never occur at a point in the R-R interval when they would be expected to conduct.

PROBLEM *Figure 3D-17*

ANSWER TO FIGURE 3D-17   The ventricular rate is regular at about 34 beats/min. The atrial rate is also fairly regular. However, P waves are totally unrelated to the ventricular response (i.e., P waves "march" through the QRS). Thus there is *complete AV dissociation*. In addition, there is *complete AV block*. We can diagnose this with certainty because the ventricular response is slow enough (*less than* 45 beats/min) and the rhythm strip long enough to

demonstrate P waves occurring at many points in the R-R interval when conduction should be expected to occur (but doesn't).

Note that the QRS complex does not really appear to be wide. This suggests that the level of the block occurs somewhere within the conduction system (and not at the idioventricular level). Regardless of the level at which the block occurs, treatment must still be directed at increasing the heart rate.

PROBLEM *Figure 3D-18*

ANSWER TO FIGURE 3D-18   The rhythm is regular at 70 beats/min. The QRS complex appears slightly widened. It is regularly preceded by a P wave with a constant (albeit markedly prolonged) PR interval (0.41 second). This is sinus rhythm with 1° AV block.

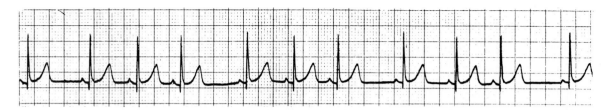

Figure 3D-19

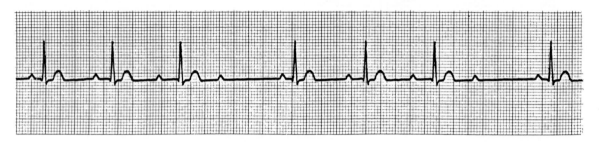

Figure 3D-20

PROBLEM   *Figure 3D-19*

ANSWER TO FIGURE 3D-19   The QRS complex is narrow. The rhythm is irregular and group beating is present. However, this is not Wenckebach since the PR interval remains constant instead of lengthening. P waves *are* related to QRS complexes in this example, and they conduct with a normal PR interval. This is *sinus arrhythmia*—in this case with marked respiratory variation producing the group beating.

> *Not every arrhythmia with group beating is Wenckebach.* This point is well illustrated by the examples shown in Figures 3D-14 and 3D-19. Nevertheless, recognition of the phenomenon of group beating is still extremely helpful in providing an initial overview impression of the arrhythmia before specifically focusing attention on the interpretive (Four-Question) approach. Having identified group beating, it is often much easier to assess the tracing for other "footprints of Wenckebach" to determine if this conduction disturbance is present.

PROBLEM   *Figure 3D-20*

ANSWER TO FIGURE 3D-20   In this final example of group beating, Mobitz I (Wenckebach) 2° AV block (with 4:3 AV conduction) is present. All of the characteristic "footprints" are here:

1. Group beating
2. Regularity of the atrial rate
3. Progressive lengthening of the PR interval until a beat is dropped
4. Duration of the pause containing the dropped beat being *less* than twice the shortest R-R interval.

The QRS complex is narrow (as expected with Mobitz I). However, the PR interval of the first conducted beat in each cycle is not prolonged (i.e., 1° AV block is not present).

Clinical Significance of the AV Blocks

Let us conclude this section by briefly reviewing the clinical significance of the conduction disturbances we have diagnosed. Hemodynamic status (as well as survival) of patients with 1° AV block and Mobitz I 2° AV block is generally not jeopardized by the conduction disturbance itself. As a result, no treatment other than observation is generally needed. In contrast, consideration of pacemaker therapy (insertion of a transvenous pacemaker, or at least ready availability of an external pacemaker) is strongly recommended for patients with Mobitz II 2° AV block because of the disturbing tendency of this conduction defect to rapidly (and suddenly) develop complete AV block.

The situation with **3° (complete) AV block** is somewhat more complicated. Pacemaker insertion is routinely performed in patients who develop complete AV block as the result of acute *anterior* infarction. As previously discussed, the escape pacemaker tends to be idioventricular (wide QRS complex) and is often associated with a slow heart rate and signs of hemodynamic compromise. On the other hand, complete AV block that develops with acute *inferior* infarction may occur with a stable junctional escape rhythm (narrow QRS complex) that is able to maintain the patient's hemodynamic status. The mechanism of AV block in this setting may simply reflect increased parasympathetic tone and/or ischemia of the AV node rather than irreversible myocardial damage. Third-degree AV block that occurs in association with acute inferior infarction is often transient. If the heart rate remains close to 60 beats/min, no treatment at all may be needed. With slower heart rates, atropine may effectively accelerate the ventricular response and/or improve AV conduction. Transvenous pacemaker insertion is not uniformly needed,

Table 3D-4

Clinical Implications of 3° AV Block with Acute Myocardial Infarction		
		Inferior Infarction
	Anterior Infarction	**Junctional escape focus (narrow QRS)**	**Idioventricular escape focus (wide QRS)**
Rate of ventricular response	• 30 to 60 beats/min (depending on the site of the escape pacemaker)	• 40 to 60 beats/min	• 30 to 40 beats/min
Usual duration of conduction disturbance	• Long term	• Transient	• Long term
Response to atropine	• Poor	• Usually good	• Poor

Recommended treatment	• Transvenous pacemaker insertion	• Observation (if hemodynamically stable)
		 • Treat symptomatic bradycardia and/or hypotension with:
		   1. Atropine
		   2a. External pacemaker
		      or
		   2b. A pressor agent (dopamine, epinephrine, or isoproterenol)
		   3. Transvenous pacemaker insertion
			• Transvenous pacemaker insertion, or at least ready (backup) availability of an external pacemaker

especially when there is ready (backup) availability of an external pacemaker *(Table 3D-4)*.

Although patients with acute inferior infarction are generally thought of as having a much better prognosis than patients with acute anterior infarction, this is not necessarily the case. Complete AV block develops in more than 10% of patients with acute inferior infarction, and is associated with a surprisingly high in-hospital mortality of at least 20% (Berger and Ryan, 1990; Clemmensen et al, 1991). The cause of mortality in these patients is *not* believed to be due to the heart block per se, but rather to the fact that development of complete AV block during the course of acute inferior infarction is a marker for increased infarct size (Berger and Ryan, 1990).

As emphasized earlier, an important exception to the generalities we suggest for treatment considerations is illustrated by the example shown in Figure 3D-11. Despite the fact that this conduction disturbance is "only" a Mobitz I 2° AV block, the accompanying marked bradycardia would be likely to jeopardize the patient's hemodynamic status if it had not responded to atropine. *Clinical significance of the AV blocks generally depends much more on the ventricular re-* *sponse and hemodynamic status of the patient than on the "degree" of the AV block per se.*

The final concept we emphasize is that of **AV dissociation.** The rhythm shown in Figure 3D-16 is *not* due to 3° AV block. Instead it simply reflects what may happen when a previously silent AV nodal escape pacemaker *accelerates* to a rate that exceeds that of the underlying sinus rhythm. Pacemaker therapy is generally *not* indicated for this arrhythmia (because the resultant ventricular response is usually *more than* adequate to maintain hemodynamic stability).

Clinically, accelerated junctional rhythms (and resultant AV dissociation) are commonly encountered in two settings:

1. Acute inferior infarction
2. Digitalis toxicity

Recognition of the difference between AV dissociation and 3° AV block is essential for avoiding unnecessary treatment with pacemaker insertion.

Additional subtleties involved in differentiating between AV dissociation and 3° (complete) AV block are deferred until Section D in Chapter 16. For now, suffice it to say that:

1. AV dissociation is *not* the same as 3° AV block.
2. 3° AV block should probably *not* be diagnosed unless the heart rate is slow enough (usually 45 beats/min or less) and the rhythm strip long enough to demonstrate consistent failure of atrial conduction despite more than adequate opportunity for conduction to occur.

3. The ventricular rate will usually be *regular* with 3° AV block. If beats are dropped but the ventricular rate is not regular, it is likely that some other conduction disturbance is present (i.e., Mobitz I, Mobitz II, *or a more complicated form of 2° AV block with escape beats from transient AV dissociation*—as shown in the very beginning of this section in Fig. 3D-3!).

You are now armed with sufficient information to attack the gamut of arrhythmias likely to be encountered in a cardiac arrest. *Are you up to the challenge?* If so, move on to Section E . . .

SECTION E

RHYTHMS OF CARDIAC ARREST

It's time to apply the techniques we have covered up to now to diagnosing the arrhythmias that are commonly encountered during a cardiac arrest. The patient in question is a middle-aged man admitted for acute myocardial infarction. Imagine **yourself** as the emergency care provider **assigned to watch the ECG monitor.** At the time you arrive, the patient is awake but complaining of chest pain. His extremities are cold and clammy, and a systolic blood pressure of 90 mm Hg is recorded. Two sublingual nitroglycerin tablets and 5 mg of morphine sulfate have already been given.

PROBLEM   **The code director asks you to describe the rhythm (Figure 3E-1). How do you respond?**

ANSWER TO FIGURE 3E-1   The underlying rhythm is sinus tachycardia at a rate of 100 beats/min. Two PVCs (beats #2 and #10) and a PAC (beat #7) are seen.

Although beats #2 and #10 are not quite as wide as one expects PVCs to be (they are not ≥0.12 seconds in duration), these beats are clearly much wider than the normally conducted sinus beats and are definitely very different in morphology. They must be considered PVCs. (It is possible that

if other monitoring leads were obtained these beats might appear "wider.")

The other early beat (beat #7) is identical in morphology to the normally conducted sinus beats and is preceded by a premature P wave. This is a PAC.

The patient suddenly becomes unresponsive.

PROBLEM   **What has happened (Figure 3E-2)?**

ANSWER TO FIGURE 3E-2   Sinus tachycardia continues for the first three beats of Figure 3E-2. This is followed by a PVC (beat #4), another sinus beat, and then the abrupt onset of *ventricular fibrillation*.

Ventricular Fibrillation

Ventricular fibrillation is an extremely common inciting mechanism of cardiac arrest. Electrocardiographically, this rhythm is totally chaotic. The P wave, QRS complex, and T wave are all absent. Instead, an irregular zig-zag pattern is seen in which electrical waveforms continuously vary in size and shape. There is no meaningful perfusion with this arrhythmia.

The patient is immediately defibrillated with 200 joules.

Lead II

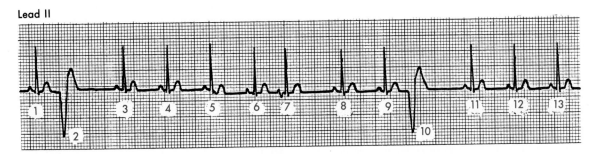

Figure 3E-1.   Initial rhythm. The patient is complaining of chest pain. His extremities are cold and clammy, and he has a systolic blood pressure of 90 mm Hg.

Lead II

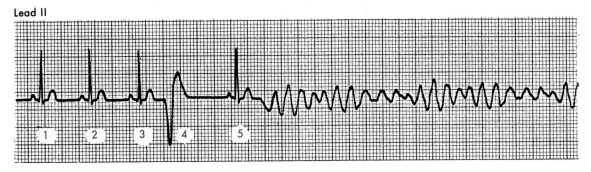

Figure 3E-2.   The patient suddenly becomes unresponsive.

Lead II

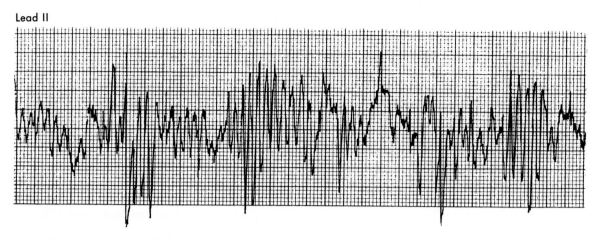

Figure 3E-3.   Defibrillation with 200 joules results in this rhythm. A rapid but definite pulse is palpated.

This results in the rhythm shown in *Figure 3E-3*. A rapid but definite pulse is palpated at the bedside.

PROBLEM   **How would you interpret the rhythm shown in *Figure 3E-3*? Would you want to ask members of the code team who are at the bedside to do anything?**

ANSWER TO FIGURE 3E-3   A bizarre series of vertical lines at an extremely rapid rate is noted. This rhythm is incompatible with the physical finding of a palpable pulse, and one should strongly suspect *artifact*. Ask team members who are at the bedside to see if a monitor lead has fallen off.

Artifact

Artifactual rhythms are very commonly seen during cardiopulmonary resuscitation. This should not be unexpected considering the usual scenario in which a large number of health care providers are feverishly working at the bedside. Potential *artifact-generating* tasks performed include CPR, intubation, ventilation, defibrillation, intravenous cannulation, and drawing of arterial blood gases. In addition, monitor leads may frequently be knocked off. For all of these reasons one should always check for the presence of a pulse and patient responsiveness *before* defibrillating a patient thought to be in ventricular fibrillation from the reading of the ECG monitor.*

---

*This is the reason we ask *"Annie, Annie! Are you OK?"* before initiating CPR. If Annie responds, *"Yes"*–then you shouldn't do CPR!

The disconnected monitor lead is reapplied. The rhythm shown in *Figure 3E-4* now flashes across the monitor. A rapid pulse is still palpated.

PROBLEM   *What is the rhythm?*

ANSWER TO FIGURE 3E-4   A *supraventricular tachycardia* at a rate of 150 beats/min is seen. The rhythm is regular. Although hard to be sure, P waves appear to be present (arrow). This suggests that the rhythm is probably *sinus tachycardia*.

The usual differential for *regular* supraventricular tachyarrhythmias with a rate in the range of 150 beats/min is sinus tachycardia, atrial flutter, and PSVT. We have already emphasized the need to maintain a high index of suspicion for atrial flutter in such cases. However clinically, of much greater concern at this point in the code than the differential diagnosis of the arrhythmia is the patient's hemodynamic status. Even if the rhythm was atrial flutter (or PSVT), immediate treatment would not necessarily be needed if the patient was not compromised hemodynamically.

A normal blood pressure is obtained momentarily. Then the rhythm on the monitor suddenly changes *(Figure 3E-5)*.

PROBLEM   **What has happened? (What would you want to know *most* about the patient?)**

Lead II

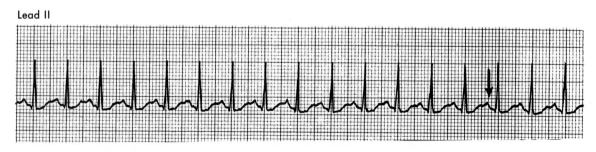

Figure 3E-4.   ECG rhythm seen after the disconnected monitoring lead is reapplied.

Lead II

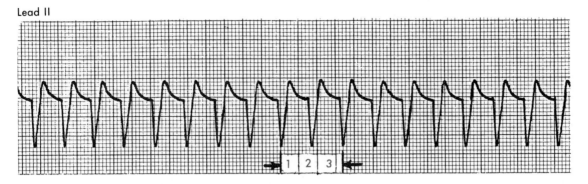

Figure 3E-5. The rhythm shown in Figure 3E-4 suddenly changes to this rhythm.

ANSWER TO FIGURE 3E-5   A regular, wide-complex tachycardia is now seen at a rate of about 170 beats/min. This is *ventricular tachycardia.*

> That the rate is approximately 170 beats/min can be determined by the ***every-other-beat method*** suggested earlier. Select a QRS complex that peaks on a heavy line. Then calculate the R-R interval for two beats. This is just over three boxes in this example (Fig. 3E-5). *Half the rate* is, therefore, about 85 beats/min. The actual rate must be twice this, or 170 beats/min.
>
> Although the QRS complex of the tachycardia in this figure is not as wide as one might normally expect for ventricular tachycardia (it is not ≥0.12 second), it is clearly wider and dramatically different in morphology from the supraventricular rhythm that was just seen in Figure 3E-4. While one cannot absolutely rule out the sudden development of aberrant conduction, *ventricular tachycardia must be assumed until proven otherwise (and treatment must be based accordingly)!*
>
> An additional point in favor of VT as the etiology of this tachyarrhythmia is that the morphology of the QRS complex in Figure 3E-5 is *identical* to that of the PVCs identified earlier in Figure 3E-1.

The thing you would want to know *most* about this patient is their hemodynamic status (because this information will dictate the optimal therapeutic course). It's important to appreciate that despite persistence of ventricular tachycardia, some patients may remain alert and/or hemodynamically stable for extended periods of time.

In this particular case, however, a systolic blood pressure of only 70 mm Hg "palp" is obtained in association with the rhythm shown in Figure 3E-5. Synchronized cardioversion is ordered.

PROBLEM   **Synchronized cardioversion with 200 joules is delivered at the point designated by the arrow in *Figure 3E-6. What is the result?***

ANSWER TO FIGURE 3E-6   Synchronized cardioversion results in *ventricular fibrillation.*
There is no longer any pulse.
The patient is immediately defibrillated with 200 joules.

PROBLEM   **Defibrillation results in a rapidly changing sequence of events *(Fig. 3E-7).* How would you interpret the rhythm for the code director?**

ANSWER TO FIGURE 3E-7   The rhythm begins with four beats of what appears to be VT at an extremely rapid rate. This is followed by a 10-beat run of a supraventricular tachycardia (at a rate of about 210 beats/min), which then deteriorates to ventricular fibrillation.
The pulse is lost. Defibrillation is again ordered.

PROBLEM   **Defibrillation with 300 joules is delivered at the point designated by the arrow in *Figure 3E-8. What does this lead to?***

Lead II

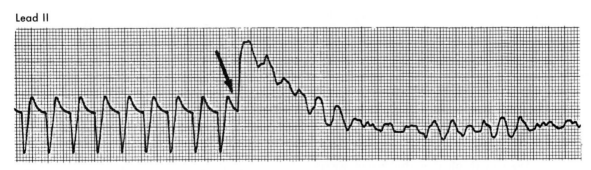

Figure 3E-6. The rhythm shown in Figure 3E-5 is electrically cardioverted with 200 joules (at the point designated by the *arrow*).

Lead II

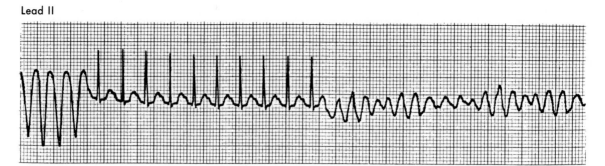

Figure 3E-7. Defibrillation of the rhythm shown in Figure 3E-6 results in a rapidly changing sequence of events.

Lead II

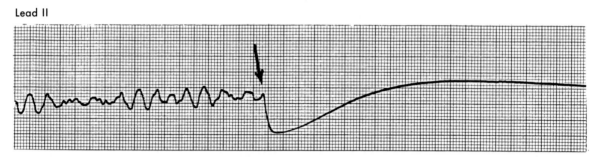

Figure 3E-8. The patient is defibrillated with 300 joules (at the point designated by the *arrow*).

Lead II

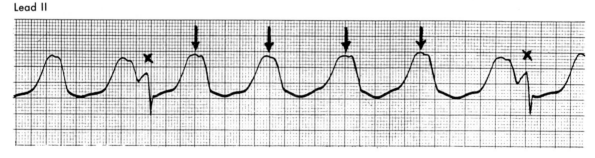

Figure 3E-9. Defibrillation of the rhythm shown in Figure 3E-8 resulted in asystole. CPR was resumed.

ANSWER TO FIGURE 3E-8 Defibrillation leads to *asystole*.

There is no pulse.

CPR is resumed and the patient is intubated. The code director asks you if there is any change in the rhythm?

PROBLEM **What do you now see on the monitor (Figure 3E-9)?**

ANSWER TO FIGURE 3E-9 Extremely broad waveforms (arrows) are seen separating rare *idioventricular complexes* (labeled **X** in the figure).

PROBLEM **Do you think that the broad waveforms in *Figure 3E-9* might be due to CPR? *Is there a way to tell?***

ANSWER TO FIGURE 3E-9 Yes. Stop CPR.

CPR is stopped and the rhythm shown in *Figure 3E-10* results. This confirms your previous suspicion.

PROBLEM **Could Figure 3E-10 possibly represent *fine ventricular fibrillation?* Is there a way to tell?**

ANSWER TO FIGURE 3E-10 Yes! Switch the ECG monitor to several other leads to see whether a flat line is still recorded.

The "Flat Line" Recording: Asystole or Ventricular Fibrillation?

On rare occasions, ventricular fibrillation may "masquerade" as asystole. Like any other electrocardiographic complex, the undulations of ventricular fibrillation possess a predomi-

Lead II

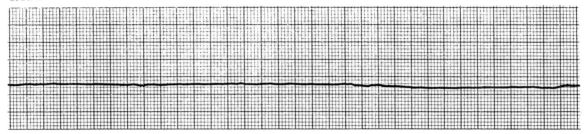

Figure 3E-10.   In response to the rhythm shown in Figure 3E-9, CPR is stopped.

Lead II

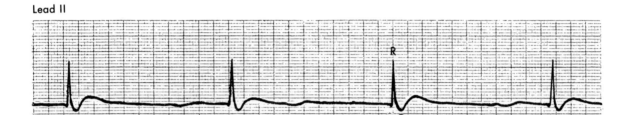

Figure 3E-11.   Rhythm developing after asystole (shown in Fig. 3E-10) is treated with epinephrine.

nant vector of electrical activity. Should this vector be *perpendicular* to the electrical axis of the monitor lead being recorded, a flat line will be observed. As a result, many clinicians advocate countershocking asystole on the remote chance that the rhythm may really be ventricular fibrillation in disguise. While it is hard to fault this practice (since realistically there is little to lose by shocking the patient at this point even if the rhythm is asystole), a simpler (although less dramatic) way to determine if ventricular fibrillation is masquerading as asystole is to switch the ECG monitor to several other monitoring leads. If ventricular fibrillation is present, this should be clearly evident in the other leads. On the other hand, if all other leads demonstrate a flat line recording, one can be confident that the rhythm is truly asystole.

PROBLEM   Was CPR being performed *correctly* in *Figure 3E-9?*

ANSWER TO FIGURE 3E-9   No. The R-R interval of the broad waveforms in Figure 3E-9 is about five large boxes. This corresponds to a rate of 1 waveform (or external chest compression) per second, and 60 compressions per minute. This is significantly *slower* than the recommended rate (of 80 to 100 compressions per minute).

At this point (Fig. 3E-10), there is no pulse and the patient's rhythm is asystole. CPR is resumed (with a faster compression rate), and epinephrine is given by the intravenous route. A minute passes.

PROBLEM   How would you describe the rhythm now seen on the monitor *(Fig. 3E-11)?*

ANSWER TO FIGURE 3E-11   The rhythm is fairly regular, and the rate is just under 30 beats/min. P

waves are absent, and the QRS complex appears to be wide. This is a slow *idioventricular escape rhythm.*

The R-R interval measures approximately 11 large boxes. If it were exactly 10 large boxes, the rate would be 30 beats/min (300 ÷ 10). The rate must therefore be a little slower, or about 28 beats/min.

If one includes the deep S wave in measurement of QRS duration in this example, there is no question that the QRS is wide. The problem lies in determining where the QRS really ends and the ST segment begins. There is really no way to be sure from this single monitoring lead alone. Clinically, however, regardless of whether the QRS is wide, the escape rhythm is exceedingly slow and the treatment priority is the same— *speed up the rate!*

Slow Idioventricular Rhythm (IVR)

Slow IVR is a rhythm that is commonly encountered during cardiac arrest. It is seen more often than the AV blocks in this setting. As discussed earlier, the SA node usually acts as the principal pacemaker of the heart. With normal sinus rhythm, it fires at a rate of between 60 and 100 beats/min. Should something happen to the SA node's pacesetting ability, other areas of the heart with inherent automaticity must take over. With an inherent rate of 40 to 60 beats/min, the AV node is usually next in line. However, should the AV nodal pacemaker also fail, the pacesetting function then falls to the ventricles. Hopefully an idioventricular escape rhythm will arise and be able to take over.

The inherent automaticity of slow IVR in adults is usually between 30 and 40 beats/min (although it may occasionally be as slow as 20 beats/min). Electrocardiographically, this rhythm is recognized as a fairly regular wide-complex bradyarrhythmia. P waves are absent. Supportive treatment with positive chronotropic and inotropic agents is needed until pacemaker therapy can be employed.

Lead II

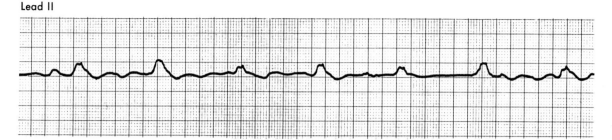

Figure 3E-12.   Deterioration of the rhythm shown in Figure 3E-11 after administration of additional epinephrine.

Lead II

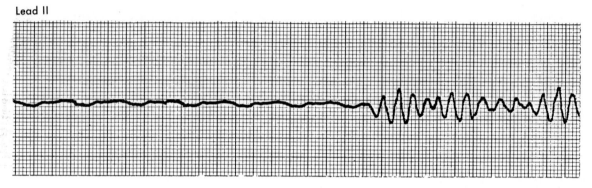

Figure 3E-13.   Rhythm developing after more epinephrine is given.

Lead II

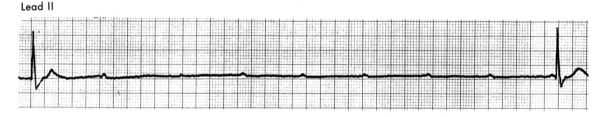

Figure 3E-14.   Rhythm developing after defibrillation with 360 joules.

Additional epinephrine is given for the rhythm shown in Figure 3E-11. Unfortunately, deterioration to the rhythm shown in *Figure 3E-12* results.

PROBLEM   **Given that CPR is *not* being performed at the time Figure 3E-12 is recorded, how would you interpret this tracing?**

ANSWER TO FIGURE 3E-12   The complexes in this rhythm are extremely wide (over 0.20 second in duration) and totally amorphous. This is an *agonal rhythm.*

Agonal Rhythm

In general, agonal rhythm (as its name implies) is a manifestation of a dying heart. Surprisingly, this sporadic electrical activity may continue for minutes (and sometimes even hours) after meaningful cardiac function has ceased. Isolated and grouped idioventricular complexes (or the amorphous waveforms seen in Fig. 3E-12) may appear, be interrupted by periods of asystole, and then reappear on the monitor. Clinically,

the significance of an agonal rhythm is similar to that of asystole.

CPR is continued. More epinephrine is given.

PROBLEM   **Is there any change *(Figure 3E-13)*?**

ANSWER TO FIGURE 3E-13   Midway through the rhythm strip shown in Figure 3E-13, ventricular fibrillation develops.

This is one occasion when development of ventricular fibrillation should be viewed as a favorable response! The chance for potential reversibility is much greater for this rhythm than for agonal rhythm or asystole.

The patient is defibrillated with 360 joules. The rhythm shown in *Figure 3E-14* results.

PROBLEM   ***What has happened?***

Lead II

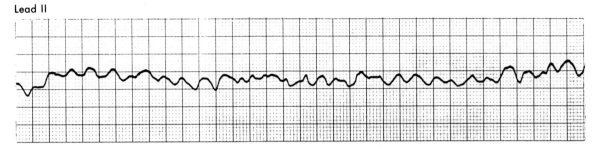

Figure 3E-15. Rhythm developing after more epinephrine is given.

Lead II

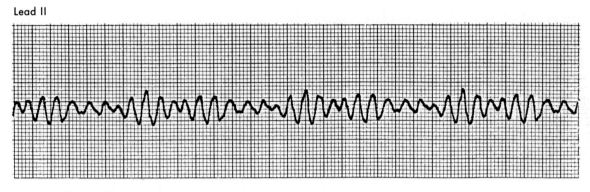

Figure 3E-16. Rhythm developing (from Fig. 3E-15) after additional epinephrine is given.

ANSWER TO FIGURE 3E-14 Idioventricular complexes begin and end this rhythm strip. In between, there is a long period of *ventricular standstill*. Slightly irregular atrial activity at a rate of about 70 beats/min continues throughout.

> None of the atrial impulses seen in this rhythm strip conduct, suggesting 3° (complete) AV block. However, more than heart block, the problem is the absence of an appropriate escape focus.

CPR is resumed. Arterial blood gases are drawn, and more epinephrine is administered.

PROBLEM **The monitor changes again (Figure 3E-15). What has happened?**

ANSWER TO FIGURE 3E-15 The patient has gone back into ventricular fibrillation. Waveform undulations are of small amplitude—this is *fine* ventricular fibrillation.

More epinephrine is given.

PROBLEM **Was the epinephrine successful (Figure 3E-16)?**

ANSWER TO FIGURE 3E-16 The fine ventricular fibrillation of Figure 3E-15 has now become *coarse*. Many clinicians view such coarsening as a beneficial therapeutic response to epinephrine (thought to facilitate subsequent conversion to sinus rhythm when countershock is applied).

Realize that "coarsening" may be artificially produced by manipulating the amplitude of the ECG monitor. In the same manner, "fine ventricular fibrillation" can be made to appear as asystole if the amplitude dial is turned all the way down. This is one reason we believe it is advantageous to always hook up a 12-lead ECG machine at the bedside as soon as possible during any code.

Following defibrillation, the rhythm shown in *Figure 3E-17* is seen. This is associated with a slow, weak pulse.

PROBLEM **Is this another slow IVR?**

ANSWER TO FIGURE 3E-17 No. The rhythm shown in Figure 3E-17 is regular and exceedingly slow. With an R-R interval of just under 12 large boxes, the heart rate is approximately 25 beats/min (300 ÷ 12). However, this is not a slow IVR because P waves *are* present. P waves precede each QRS complex with a constant PR interval. The rhythm is therefore *sinus bradycardia* with an extremely slow ventricular response.

> The PR interval in Figure 3E-17 is 0.20 second, which is still within the normal range. For 1° AV block to be present, the PR interval must clearly *exceed* 0.20 second.

Moments later, the pulse is again lost.

PROBLEM **What happened (Fig. 3E-18)?**

ANSWER TO FIGURE 3E-18 An 11-beat run of ventricular tachycardia (at a rate of 210 beats/min) begins

Lead II

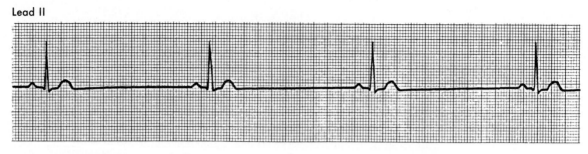

Figure 3E-17.   Rhythm developing after defibrillation of the rhythm shown in Figure 3E-16.

Lead II

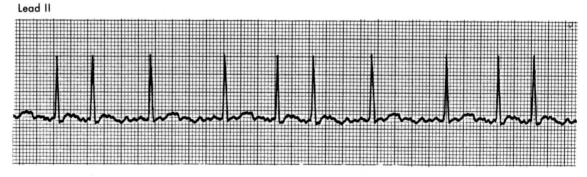

Figure 3E-18.   The pulse that was present in association with the rhythm shown in Figure 3E-17 has been lost.

Lead II

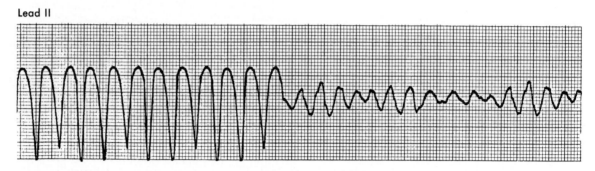

Figure 3E-19.   Rhythm developing after defibrillation of the rhythm shown in Figure 3E-18.

this rhythm strip. This deteriorates into ventricular fibrillation.

A *precordial thump* is delivered as the paddles are charged. The patient remains pulseless. Countershock with maximal energy is repeated.

A strong but irregular pulse is now palpable and associated with a blood pressure of 120/80 mm Hg. A bolus of lidocaine is given, and an intravenous infusion of this drug is started. The patient begins to wake up.

PROBLEM   **How would you interpret the rhythm** *(Figure 3E-19)?*

ANSWER TO FIGURE 3E-19   The rhythm is irregularly irregular. Atrial activity is evident (there are undulations in the baseline), but there are no clear P waves. This is *atrial fibrillation* with a *controlled* ventricular response.

> Even though normal sinus rhythm has not been restored, the patient's hemodynamic status has stabilized and resuscitation is successful.

This sequence of events is probably as complicated as any you will encounter in a real-life setting. Appreciation of the rationale presented here for arrhythmia recognition should make you much more comfortable performing both at the MEGA CODE station, as well as in actual code situations.

ARRHYTHMIA OR DYSRHYTHMIA?
. . . .AND OTHER CONFUSING TERMS

A number of years ago, a Task Force was appointed with the specific goal of trying to standardize the terminology used in electrocardiographic interpretation (Surawicz et al, 1978). Controversy began with the attempt to define "normality" and persisted throughout the entire conference. Even among experts, wide discrepancies in the use of certain electrocardiographic terms are still prevalent (Julian, 1987; Marriott, 1987; Grauer et al, 1987, 1989).

Examples of confusing terminology abound in the field of arrhythmia interpretation and advanced cardiac life support. Before delving any further into description of the various cardiac arrhythmias, it may therefore be helpful to clarify a number of points about terminology that come up in discussion of cardiopulmonary resuscitation and emergency cardiac care.

The opinions expressed in this section are our own. We fully acknowledge that they may not be shared by others in the field.

Arrhythmia versus Dysrhythmia

The two terms that have probably generated the most controversy are *arrhythmia* and *dysrhythmia*. Which one should be used?

The purist undoubtedly favors *dysrhythmia*, despite the fact that this word lacks both the tradition and phonetic facility of arrhythmia. He/she would contend that *arrhythmia* should literally mean "no rhythm" (or asystole), since attachment of the prefix *"a"* to any word implies an "absence of" the entity in question. These individuals prefer to add the prefix *"dys"* (meaning "a disorder of") to the word stem "rhythm." The result—**dys***rhythmia*—"properly" connotes a disturbance of rhythm.

This line of reasoning is faulty. The prefix *"a"* is *not* limited to meaning an "absence of" the entity in question, but may also be used to imply an *imperfection* of the entity. Furthermore, the root "rhythmos" is not restricted to meaning "a regular recurring motion," but instead has also been used to describe "an arrangement, a symmetry, or order"—and *"What could be more disorderly than atrial fibrillation?"* (Marriott, 1984).

Were one to restrict words to their derivations and/or original meanings, much of the color and richness of the English language would be lost. Similarly, the evolutionary importance accrued from usage over the years would also

be lost. We believe the dictionary definition of *arrhythmia*—"a variation from the normal rhythm, especially of the heart beat"—has withstood the test of time. We do not ascribe any difference to the meaning of arrhythmia and dysrhythmia and favor using these terms interchangeably.

Characteristics of Ideal Terminology:

The ideal term should be *easily* pronounced, spelled, written, and remembered. It should not be ambiguous or likely to engender confusion in interpretation (i.e., it should be widely applicable in electrical and mechanical senses, at the bedside, on the ECG, and during regular and irregular rhythms). If subject to abbreviation, the letters chosen for this should not be the same as other commonly used abbreviations. Finally, the term should not be one that promotes fear or panic when overheard by a patient with the disorder (Constant, 1978; Marriott, 1986; Marriott, 1987).

Heart Block versus AV Block

"Heart block" is a poor term that disregards several of the above ground rules. One can easily imagine a patient becoming unduly alarmed on learning that his/her heart is "blocked." Technically, the term lacks specificity, and fails to differentiate between the various types of heart block: atrioventricular (AV) block, bundle branch block, and fascicular (hemi-) block. When used to indicate a defect in atrioventricular conduction, it doesn't offer the listener the slightest clue as to whether 1°, 2°, or 3° AV block is present.

Classification of the types of AV blocks was discussed in detail in Section D of this chapter. Let us reemphasize the need for clearly defining conduction disturbances in as complete and specific a manner as possible. Referral to a disorder as "2° AV block, Mobitz Type I" is decidedly better (and more accurate) than simply describing a rhythm as "Wenckebach."

PVCs, VPDs, and Ventricular Extrasystoles

Numerous terms have been used to define early-occurring beats of ventricular origin. These include:

1. PVC (Premature ventricular contraction)
2. VPC (Ventricular premature complex)
3. VPD (Ventricular premature depolarization)
4. VPB (Ventricular premature beat)
5. VEC (Ventricular ectopic complex)
6. Ventricular extrasystole
7. Ectopic beat

Which of these connotations is chosen depends less on any inherent benefits of the term than on how one was taught and what general custom prevails in one's area of practice. Semantic problems can be found with the use of *each* of these terms (Marriott, 1986; Marriott, 1987). For example, a shortcoming of the term *VPD* is that a "depolarization" is really only *half* a beat (Spodick, 1981; Marriott, 1987)! Thus, the more proper connotation using this term would have to be a VPD-R (ventricular premature "depolarization-repolarization"). Use of "ectopic beat" is far too general and encompasses PACs, escape beats, parasystolic beats, and the like. Ventricular "extrasystole" may well be the preferred term from a purely technical standpoint (Schamroth, 1987), but as Marriott states, the word *extrasystole* is a "quinquepedalian sequence of sibilants, and as such is a daunting tongue twister." *It is hard to imagine the cry "Extrasystoles!" going up in a coronary care unit* (Marriott, 1987).

The problem with the term PVC (premature ventricular *contraction*) is that the word "contraction" implies a mechanical event, whereas the electrocardiographic manifestation of the phenomenon in question is purely electrical. Despite legitimate concerns about the appropriateness of this term, years of usage have accustomed us to "the PVC," and we use this connotation exclusively throughout this book.

Supraventricular Tachycardia, PAT, PJT, or PSVT?

As discussed in Section B of this chapter, the term *supraventricular tachycardia (SVT)* is a general one that encompasses all tachyarrhythmias (rhythms with a heart rate of 100 beats/min or faster) in which the impulse originates at or above the AV node. Unless aberrant conduction or preexisting bundle branch block is present, the QRS complex will be narrow. Entities included within this definition are:

1. Sinus tachycardia
2. Junctional tachycardia
3. Atrial fibrillation or flutter with a moderately rapid or rapid ventricular response
4. Multifocal atrial tachycardia (MAT or chaotic atrial mechanism)
5. Ectopic atrial tachycardia

6. Paroxysmal atrial or junctional tachycardia (PAT or PJT)
7. Paroxysmal supraventricular tachycardia (PSVT)

In the past, the term SVT was used synonymously with either PAT or PJT. This practice is potentially misleading since arrhythmias such as sinus tachycardia constitute a form of SVT that is very different from ectopic atrial tachycardia, PAT, or PJT. Normal atrial activity (upright P waves in lead II) is seen with sinus tachycardia. In contrast, with ectopic atrial tachycardia, another atrial focus (often recognized by unusual-looking P waves in lead II) takes over with enhanced automaticity. Finally, with PAT or PJT, the tachyarrhythmia is *paroxysmal* (of sudden onset) and is due to a *reentry* phenomenon involving the AV node.

The usage we favor is to apply *supraventricular tachycardia* as the generic, all-encompassing term for any narrow QRS complex tachyarrhythmia (e.g., sinus tachycardia, atrial fibrillation or flutter). We tend to minimize use of the abbreviation *SVT* because it is too easily confused with PSVT. We use this latter abbreviation *(PSVT)* to connote those regular supraventricular tachycardias that appear to operate by a *reentry* mechanism involving the AV node. This contrasts with the situation in which ectopic P waves can be clearly identified. In such cases the rhythm is most appropriately termed *atrial tachycardia* (with or without associated block at the AV node). Finally, we have discarded the terms *PAT* and *PJT* since these abbreviations imply more than we know about the mechanism and site of origin of the arrhythmia.

Surprising Origin of the P-QRS-T

We close this section by commenting on the derivation of the lettering used to describe electrocardiographic morphology. Impetus for selecting the sequence of letters **P-Q-R-S-T-U** to denote various waveforms on the electrocardiogram actually has *nothing* to do with electrocardiography (Henson, 1971). Instead it dates back to the time of the great mathematician René Descartes, who lived in the mid-1600s. Descartes opted to choose the letter "P" as a convenient starting place in many of his mathematical series primarily because of its alliterative and mnemonic effects (i.e., starting at the *"point P"*). These effects were operative in the Latin, French, Dutch, and German languages. Willem Einthoven (1860-1927), trained as a physician at the University of Utrecht in Holland, was heavily schooled in mathematics and physiology. It is thought that he adopted this sequence of letters as the nomenclature for electrocardiography in follow-up to Descartes and as a result of his *mathematical* training!

SECTION G

ARRHYTHMIA REVIEW (II)

As additional review, interpret the following 30 tracings.

Lead II

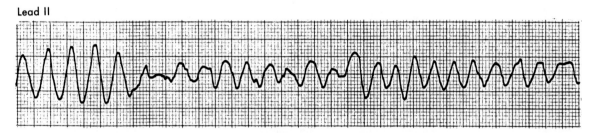

Figure 3G-1

Lead II

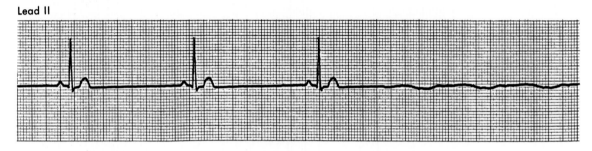

Figure 3G-2

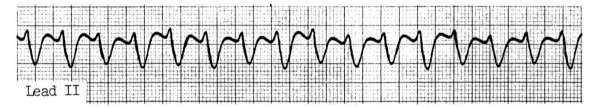

Lead II

Figure 3G-3

Lead MCL$_6$

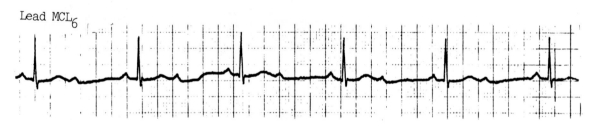

Figure 3G-4

Lead II

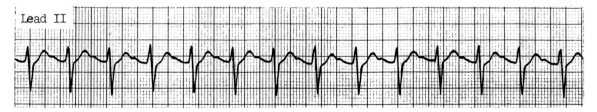

Figure 3G-5

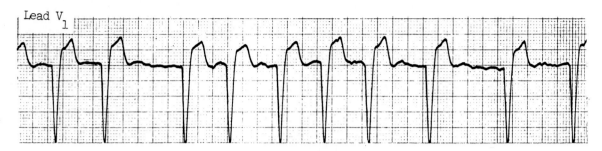

Figure 3G-6

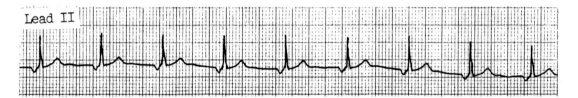

Figure 3G-7

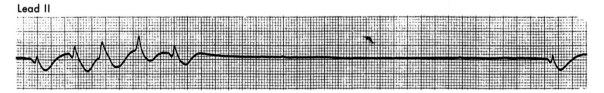

Figure 3G-8

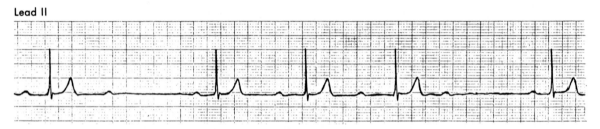

Figure 3G-9

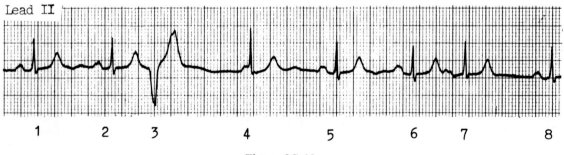

Figure 3G-10

Lead II

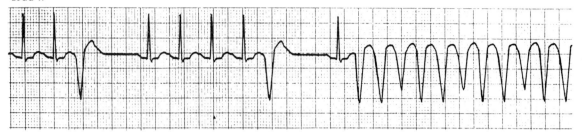

Figure 3G-11

Lead II

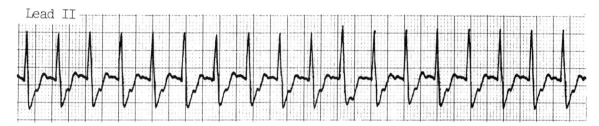

Figure 3G-12

Lead II

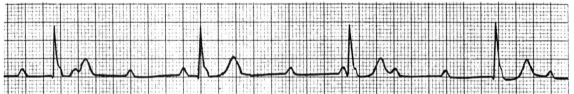

Figure 3G-13

Lead V₁

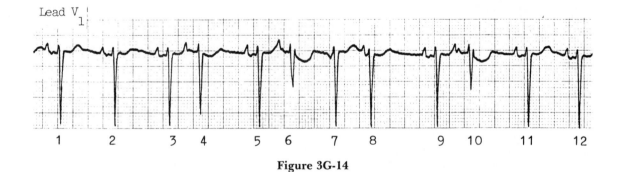

Figure 3G-14

Lead II

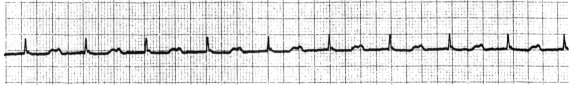

Figure 3G-15

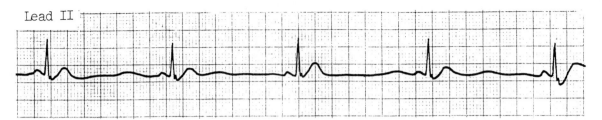

Figure 3G-16

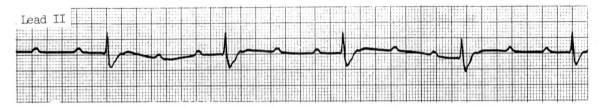

Figure 3G-17

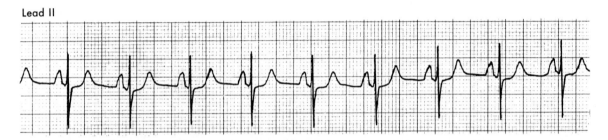

Figure 3G-18

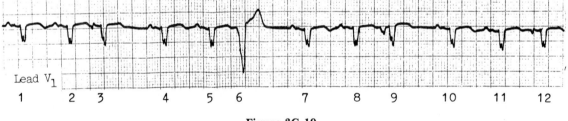

Figure 3G-19

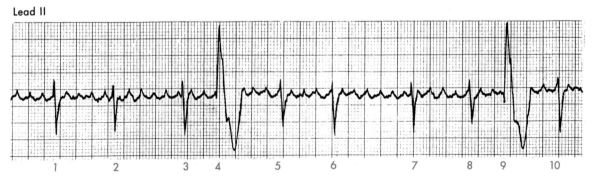

Figure 3G-20

Lead MCL₁

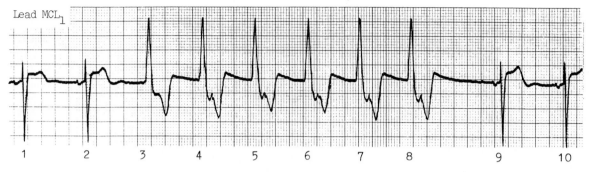

Figure 3G-21

Lead II

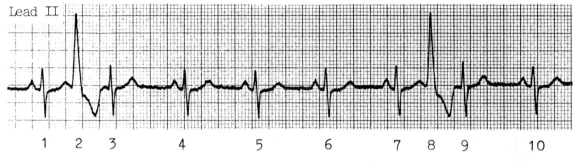

Figure 3G-22

Lead II

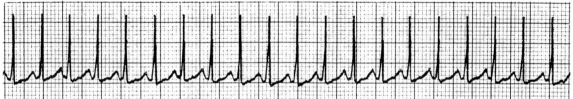

Figure 3G-23

Lead II

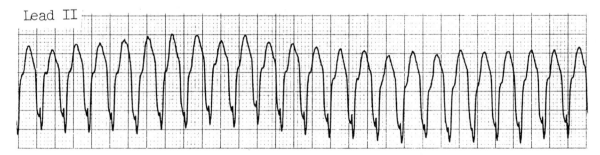

Figure 3G-24

Lead II

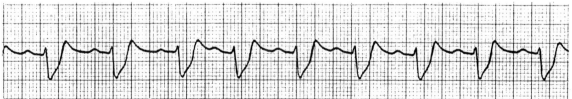

Figure 3G-25

Lead II

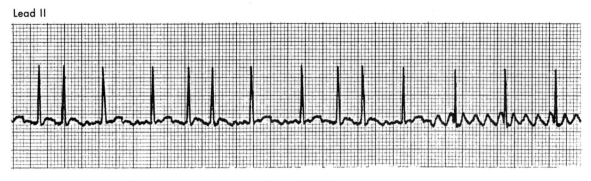

Figure 3G-26

Lead II

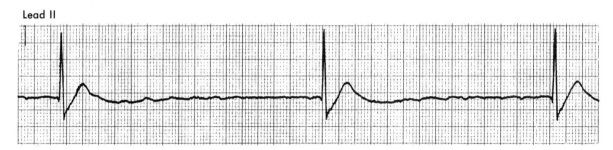

Figure 3G-27

Lead II

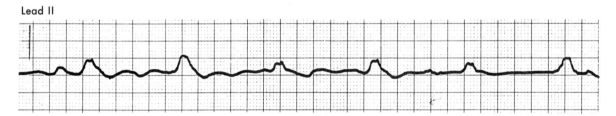

Figure 3G-28

Lead II

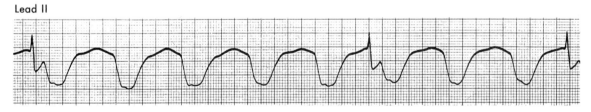

Figure 3G-29

Lead MCL₁

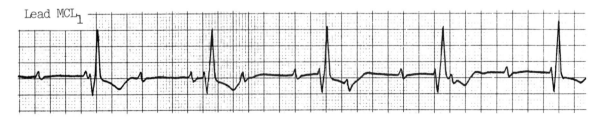

Figure 3G-30

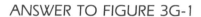

ANSWERS TO ARRHYTHMIA REVIEW (II)

ANSWER TO FIGURE 3G-1

Rhythm—Irregular

Impression: Ventricular flutter rapidly degenerating to coarse ventricular fibrillation

Although not universally accepted, we use the term *ventricular flutter* to describe the sinusoid pattern arrhythmia seen for the first five beats of this tracing. Ventricular flutter is a short-lived nonperfusing rhythm that is almost invariably followed by ventricular fibrillation. Electrocardiographic distinction between these two entities is often *not* clear, and simple description of the arrhythmia in Figure 3G-1 as ventricular fibrillation (or as "coarse" ventricular fibrillation) is equally correct (and all that need be said for the ACLS course).

ANSWER TO FIGURE 3G-2

Rhythm—Regular for the first three beats, then flat line

Rate—35 beats/min initially

PR interval—Normal

QRS complex—Normal duration

Impression: Sinus bradycardia initially, then asystole

ANSWER TO FIGURE 3G-3

Rhythm—Regular

Rate—155 beats/min

P waves—None evident

QRS complex—Wide

Impression: Ventricular tachycardia

Comment: It is impossible to know for sure where the QRS complex ends and the ST segment begins from this rhythm strip alone. Regardless, it is clear that the QRS complex is significantly widened, and that atrial activity is not evident in this lead II monitoring lead. Admittedly, this rhythm could possibly represent a supraventricular tachycardia with either aberrant conduction or preexisting bundle branch block, however, ventricular tachycardia *must* be assumed until proved otherwise.

ANSWER TO FIGURE 3G-4

Rhythm—Regular

P waves—An extra P wave is seen to follow each T wave, so that there are *two* P waves for each QRS complex

PR interval—Constant and of normal duration (for those P waves that do conduct)

Atrial rate—90 beats/min

Ventricular rate—45 beats/min

QRS complex—Normal duration

Impression: 2° AV block with 2:1 AV conduction, either Mobitz I or Mobitz II

Comment: One cannot absolutely differentiate between Mobitz I and II 2° AV block in the presence of 2:1 AV conduction. However, the normal QRS duration *strongly* favors Mobitz I.

ANSWER TO FIGURE 3G-5

Rhythm—Regular

Rate—112 beats/min

PR interval—Probably normal (0.20 second)

QRS complex—Borderline prolongation (0.11 second)

Impression: Sinus tachycardia

Comment: Although not obvious, P waves follow each T wave (arrows in *Fig. 3G-31* below). Thus, a P wave *does* precede each QRS complex with a fixed (and normal) PR interval. Were the rate to speed up any more, it is easy to imagine how these P waves would become completely buried in the T wave.

Given the difficulty of recognizing P waves in this tracing, the following interpretation would be equally correct:

"Supraventricular tachycardia–probably sinus tachycardia–but more information (i.e., additional monitoring leads that show better definition of atrial activity) is needed to be sure."

ANSWER TO FIGURE 3G-6

Rhythm—Irregularly irregular

P waves—None evident

QRS complex—Wide (0.12 second)

Impression: Atrial fibrillation with a controlled ventricular response

Comment: Although low-amplitude undulations are seen along the baseline, no consistent atrial activity is present. The QRS prolongation is caused by a preexisting left bundle branch block (LBBB).

Lead II

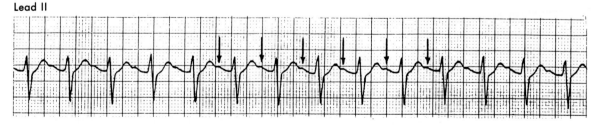

Figure 3G-31

ANSWER TO FIGURE 3G-7

Rhythm—Regular
Rate—80 beats/min
P waves—*Inverted* (and precede each QRS complex with a short PR interval in this lead II monitoring lead)
QRS complex—Normal (≤0.10 second)
Impression: Accelerated junctional (AV nodal) rhythm.
Comment: With junctional rhythm, P waves may precede the QRS complex as shown here, follow the QRS complex, or be hidden by their simultaneous occurrence with the QRS complex. Because activation of the atria from a junctional focus is *retrograde*, P waves will be *inverted* in lead II. A low atrial rhythm may also manifest negative P waves in lead II, but the PR interval is usually longer than is shown here.

The heart rate in this tracing is somewhat faster than the 40 to 60 beat/min range typically seen with junctional rhythm. If the patient was on digitalis, toxicity should be suspected.

A final possibility should be considered in this tracing. It is impossible to be sure from this one monitoring lead alone that the negative deflection preceding each QRS complex is really a P wave. *It could be part of the QRS.* If this were the case, then the QRS complex would be wide, and this would be an accelerated idioventricular rhythm (AIVR). *The importance of having (using) more than one monitoring lead for diagnosing arrhythmias cannot be overstated.*

ANSWER TO FIGURE 3G-8

Rhythm—Irregular
Atrial rate and rhythm—Fairly regular (at 45 to 50 beats/min)
P waves and PR interval—P waves precede each QRS complex with a PR interval that progressively increases until a beat is dropped
QRS complex—Normal duration
Impression: 2° AV block, Mobitz type I (Wenckebach).
Comment: For the most part, the typical "footprints of Wenckebach" are all here:

1. Regularity (or in this case, near regularity) of the atrial rate
2. Suggestion of group beating (although admittedly this finding would be more evident with a longer rhythm strip)
3. Progressive lengthening of the PR interval until a beat is dropped
4. Duration of the pause (that contains the dropped beat) of *less* than twice the shortest R-R interval.

In addition, the QRS complex is narrow and the PR interval of the first conducted beat in each sequence prolonged.

The tracing was taken from an elderly patient who presented with syncopal spells. There was no acute infarction, and the patient was not on any cardioactive drugs. Despite the fact

that the rhythm is "only Mobitz I," a permanent pacemaker was justifiably implanted because of the slow ventricular response and associated symptoms (syncope). *Much more important than the degree of AV block per se are the ventricular response and hemodynamic status of the patient in the context of the clinical setting in which the conduction disturbance occurs.*

ANSWER TO FIGURE 3G-9

Rhythm—Irregular
P waves—None
QRS complex—Wide
Impression: *Agonal rhythm* with a long period of asystole. This is usually a preterminal rhythm.

ANSWER TO FIGURE 3G-10

Rhythm—Irregular
PR interval—Normal (not *greater* than 0.20 second) for the sinus conducted beats
QRS complex—Normal duration (except for beat #3)
Impression and Comment: The first two beats are sinus. Beat #3 is a PVC. It is wide, bizarre in shape, and demonstrates a QRS configuration that is oppositely directed to the normally conducted beats.

The P wave preceding beat #4 occurs on time, but the PR interval of this beat is simply too short to conduct. Although beat #4 differs slightly in configuration from other sinus conducted beats, it has a similar initial deflection, a similar T wave, and it is not really widened. It is a *junctional escape beat* that occurred before the P wave preceding it could be conducted to the ventricles.

Beat #7 is a PAC. The QRS complex of this beat is narrow (and very similar in morphology to that of the sinus conducted beats on this tracing), and it is preceded by an early *(premature)* P wave of different morphology.

This tracing nicely illustrates the difference between *premature* beats which occur earlier than expected in the cycle (i.e., beats #3 and #7) and *escape* beats that occur later than expected (beat #4).

ANSWER TO FIGURE 3G-11

Rhythm—Irregular
QRS complex—Narrow initially. Then QRS morphology changes and the complex widens
Impression: Sinus tachycardia with PVCs. The third PVC exhibits the "R-on-T" phenomenon and precipitates ventricular tachycardia at a rate of 210 beats/min.
Comment: The underlying rhythm is sinus tachycardia at a rate of 140 beats/min. P waves are not well seen during the supraventricular tachycardia (they are probably "notching" the terminal portion of the T wave) but become more apparent in front of QRS complexes that terminate the postectopic pauses.

Note how QRS morphology of the two PVCs is the same as that during the run of ventricular tachycardia.

ANSWER TO FIGURE 3G-12

Rhythm—Regular
Rate—155 beats/min
P waves—No well-defined P waves are seen, although notching of the baseline may represent atrial activity, possibly flutter
QRS complex—Probably of normal duration, although one cannot be certain of where the QRS complex ends and the ST segment begins
Impression: Regular tachyarrhythmia at 155 beats/min
Comment: *This is a difficult tracing.* Although the occurrence of a tachyarrhythmia at a rate of about 150 beats/min and the notching in the baseline suggest the possibility of atrial flutter, it would be presumptive (and potentially dangerous) to make a definitive diagnosis based on this one tracing alone. The notching could be part of the QRS complex itself, in which case the rhythm might be ventricular tachycardia.

Assuming that the patient was hemodynamically stable, obtaining a 12-lead ECG might be helpful in resolving the issue. If the QRS complex was clearly of normal duration in other leads, then the differential diagnosis would be that of supraventricular tachycardia (PSVT, sinus tachycardia, or atrial flutter). Maneuvers to better elicit atrial activity (obtaining additional monitoring leads, carotid massage) might then prove diagnostic.

On the other hand, if the QRS complex appeared consistently wide in other leads of a 12-lead ECG, one would again be faced with having to differentiate between ventricular tachycardia and supraventricular tachycardia with either preexisting bundle branch block or aberrant conduction. Clearly, more information is needed.

> This tracing again emphasizes the point that it will *not* always be possible to make a definitive diagnosis from a single monitoring lead. In such cases, it is best to acknowledge the limits of our diagnostic ability and to indicate our need for additional information (i.e., more rhythm strips and/or monitoring leads) as allowed by the patient's clinical condition.

ANSWER TO FIGURE 3G-13

Atrial rate and rhythm—Regular at 100 beats/min (with some P waves being hidden within or notching the T waves)
Ventricular rate and rhythm—Regular at 37 beats/min
PR interval—Variable (P waves "march" through the QRS complex)
QRS complex—Wide (0.12 second)
Impression: Complete (3°) AV block.
Comment: The diagnosis of 3° AV block can be confidently made here because the ventricular rate is slow enough (*less than* 45 beats/min) to ensure that P waves consistently fail to conduct despite being given more than adequate opportunity to do so.

This tracing illustrates how easy diagnosis of 3° AV block may be. Third-degree AV block is present when:

1. The atrial and ventricular rates are regular.
2. P waves are completely unrelated to (*dissociated* from) QRS complexes.
3. The heart rate is slow enough (45 beats/min or less) and the rhythm strip long enough to ensure that none of the P waves conduct despite having adequate opportunity to do so.

ANSWER TO FIGURE 3G-14

Rhythm—Irregular
PR interval—Normal
QRS complex—Normal duration
Impression: Sinus rhythm with frequent PACs (most of which conduct with some degree of aberration)
Comment: The first three beats demonstrate an underlying sinus rhythm at 80 beats/min. Beats #4, #6, #8, and #10 are all PACs.

Note that despite variability in the PR interval in this rhythm strip, we describe it as "normal" (i.e., of constant duration and not greater than 0.20 second). We do so because the PR interval is constant and of normal duration for *each* of the normally conducted beats (beats #1, #2, #3, #5, #9, #11, and #12). It *only* changes (becoming shorter or longer) in front of the *premature* beats.

The only beat we have not described is beat #7. To be honest, *we are not sure what type of beat this is!* It is clearly supraventricular (because the QRS complex is narrow and identical in morphology to the normally conducted beats). However, it is hard to be sure if this beat is early, and it is preceded by a different appearing (negative) P wave with a short PR interval. Clinically, in the context of the remainder of this rhythm strip, it matters little whether beat #7 is a PAC, a PJC, or some type of supraventricular escape beat.

ANSWER TO FIGURE 3G-15

Rhythm—Regular
Rate—75 beats/min
PR interval—Markedly prolonged (0.39 second)
QRS complex—Normal duration
Impression: Sinus rhythm with 1° AV block
Comment: Although one might be tempted to interpret this as a junctional rhythm, the notch in the T wave is most likely the result of a P wave with a markedly prolonged PR interval, suggesting that the rhythm is probably sinus with 1° AV block.

ANSWER TO FIGURE 3G-16

Rhythm—Regular
Rate—40 beats/min
PR interval—Normal
QRS complex—Normal duration
  Impression: Sinus bradycardia

ANSWER TO FIGURE 3G-17

Atrial rate and rhythm—110 beats/min and fairly regular (with every third P wave subtly notching the terminal portion of the QRS complex)

Ventricular rate and rhythm—38 beats/min and fairly regular.
QRS complex—Wide (0.13 second), although admittedly it is difficult to be sure where the QRS complex ends and the ST segment begins
Impression: *High-grade* 2° AV block, Mobitz type II
Comment: Although severe impairment of AV conduction is clearly present, each QRS complex *is* preceded by a P wave with a *constant* PR interval. Thus P waves *are* related to the QRS, and therefore this *cannot* be 3° AV block.

> Although high-grade block could theoretically be due to Mobitz I, it much more commonly is the result of Mobitz II. The QRS widening seen here strongly suggests this to be the case.

ANSWER TO FIGURE 3G-18

Rhythm—Regular
Rate—85 beats/min
PR interval—Normal
QRS complex—Normal duration
Impression: Sinus rhythm
Comment: On the surface, this rhythm strip appears to be a simple example of normal sinus rhythm. *If this was your impression, you are completely correct and need not read further.*

> Some of you, however, may have suspected the possibility of extra (hidden) atrial activity because the shape of the T wave seems to resemble that of the P wave. This suggests that 2:1 AV conduction might exist. Use of calipers to measure the P-T interval reveals that it *differs* from the T-P interval. This is strong evidence *against* the presence of an extra *(hidden)* P wave, and suggests that the rhythm is simply normal sinus.

ANSWER TO FIGURE 3G-19

Rhythm—Irregular
PR interval—Normal (0.20 second) for sinus conducted beats
QRS complex—Normal duration (i.e., not *greater* than half a large box)
Impression: Sinus rhythm with PACs and a PVC
Comment: Beats #3, #9, and #12 are clearly PACs. They occur early, are preceded by P waves, and manifest a QRS configuration which is very similar to that of the normally conducted beats.

Beat #6 is a PVC. It is wider, more bizarre in shape, and has an oppositely directed initial deflection to that of the normally conducted beats. The QRS complex of each of the normally conducted beats begins with an admittedly subtle but definite tiny positive deflection. Beat #6 does *not* have this initial small r wave, but instead manifests a deep QS morphology.

> Although the PR interval of sinus conducted beats measures 0.20 second, this is still within the *upper limits* of normal. As discussed in Section D of this chapter, we prefer not to define

1° AV block unless the PR interval is clearly prolonged to at least 0.21 to 0.22 second (i.e., the PR interval should be clearly *greater* than a large box in duration).

> Similarly, although the QRS complex in this example may appear somewhat wider than is usually seen, it does not measure more than 0.10 second (i.e., it is not greater than half a large box). Therefore, QRS duration (at least in this particular monitoring lead) should be considered normal.

ANSWER TO FIGURE 3G-20

Rhythm—Irregular
Atrial rate—Sawtooth flutter waves at 350 to 400 beats/min
QRS Complex—Normal duration (except for beats #4 and #9)
Impression: Atrial flutter with a *variable* ventricular response. Uniform PVCs (beats #4 and #9).
Comment: —The atrial rate in this example is somewhat faster than one usually sees with atrial flutter. Atrial flutter most often demonstrates an even-numbered conduction ratio (2:1 or 4:1 AV conduction), although occasionally the conduction ratio is variable as is the case here.

ANSWER TO FIGURE 3G-21

Rhythm—Irregular
Impression: —Sinus rhythm interrupted by a run of accelerated idioventricular rhythm or AIVR (beats #3 to #8).
Comment: Following two sinus beats, the QRS configuration changes with beat #3. This beat is *not* premature. Instead it is an *escape beat* that arises because of the slight slowing of the sinus pacemaker. Retrograde P waves notch the T waves of beats #4 to #8. After a short pause, sinus rhythm resumes with beat #9.

> The easiest way to approach more complicated rhythms such as the one shown in Figure 3G-21 is to start with what is known (or readily determined). Beats #1 and #2, as well as #9 and #10, are clearly normal sinus conducted beats. QRS morphology changes dramatically with beat #3. This should suggest a ventricular etiology for this beat and the run that follows (beats #3 to #8).
>
> Beats #3 to #8 are *not* the result of aberration. There is no reason for these beats to conduct aberrantly because they occur so long after the refractory period of beat #2 (at a time when the conduction system should have recovered its responsiveness).
>
> Beats #3 to #8 are *not* junctional. AV nodal beats are *supraventricular* impulses that are usually narrow and identical to (or at least *closely resemble*) the morphology of sinus conducted beats. Sudden emergence of an escape junctional pacemaker with new development of bundle branch block is so rare that for practical purposes a ventricular etiology can be assumed for 99% of cases in which an escape rhythm with new QRS widening (and a different morphology) is seen.
>
> The ventricular rhythm in Figure 3G-21 (beats #3 to #8) is said to be "accelerated" because it is faster than the usual 30 to 40 beats/min rate of an idioventricular escape rhythm.

ANSWER TO FIGURE 3G-22

Rhythm—Regular except for beats #2 and #8
Rate—70 beats/min
PR interval—Normal
QRS complex—Normal duration
Impression: Sinus rhythm with two *(interpolated)* PVCs
Comment: Beats #2 and #8 are PVCs since they are wide, bizarre, and are not preceded by a premature P wave. These PVCs are somewhat unusual in that they are "sandwiched" between two normally occurring QRS complexes without producing any postectopic pause (i.e., they are "interpolated").

The reason why PVCs are almost always followed by at least a brief (compensatory) pause is that they temporarily render the conduction system refractory to the next sinus impulse. On rare occasions (i.e., if the timing is just right), the conduction system may recover soon enough to allow the next sinus impulse to be conducted on time. This is the case here. Clinically, the significance of interpolated PVCs is the same as that of other PVCs.

Two additional *subtle* comments can be made about this tracing. The upright deflection that precedes each of the PVCs is not a P wave. Instead, it is the T wave of the preceding beat (i.e., the T wave of beats #1 and #7). Finally, note that we do not see any P wave in front of beats #3 and #9. We might surmise that these P waves are probably hidden within the T wave of each PVC.

ANSWER TO FIGURE 3G-23

Rhythm—Regular
Rate—210 beats/min
P waves—Impossible to determine if the positive deflection preceding each QRS complex is a P wave, a T wave, or both
QRS complex—Normal duration
Impression: PSVT
Comment: The rhythm is a regular, supraventricular tachycardia. Although the complete differential should include PSVT, sinus tachycardia, and atrial flutter, the rate of the tachycardia provides a strong clue that these latter two possibilities are unlikely. Sinus tachycardia rarely exceeds 160 beats/min in an adult who is not exercising. With regard to flutter, the atrial rate is almost always around 300 beats/min (range 250 to 350 beats/min) in adults who are not on antiarrhythmic medication. A rate of 210 beats/min would therefore be slower than expected if there were 1:1 AV conduction, and faster than expected if there were 2:1 AV conduction. By the process of elimination, this leaves PSVT as the most likely possibility.

The age of the patient is not provided. This information is important diagnostically because *none* of the generalities stated above for heart rate ranges of different arrhythmias hold true for children. Heart rate ranges for both sinus tachycardia and atrial flutter may be much more rapid in children than in adults.

ANSWER TO FIGURE 3G-24

Rhythm—Regular
Rate—230 beats/min
P waves—None
QRS complex—Wide (0.14 second)
Impression: Ventricular tachycardia
Comment: Once again, the presence of a wide complex tachyarrhythmia without identifiable atrial activity should suggest five possibilities:

1. Ventricular tachycardia
2. Ventricular tachycardia
3. Ventricular tachycardia
4. SVT with aberration
5. SVT with preexisting bundle branch block

Ventricular tachycardia must always be assumed until proven otherwise.

ANSWER TO FIGURE 3G-25

Rhythm—Fairly regular
Rate—85 beats/min
PR interval—Prolonged (0.22 second)
QRS complex—Very wide (0.19 second)
Impression: Sinus rhythm with 1° AV block
Comment: Despite marked widening of the QRS complex, well-defined P waves precede each beat with a constant (albeit prolonged) PR interval, identifying the rhythm as sinus. Preexisting bundle branch block explains the QRS widening.

ANSWER TO FIGURE 3G-26

Rhythm—Irregular
P waves—None, although a sawtooth pattern of atrial activity is evident toward the end of the tracing
QRS complex—Normal duration
Impression: Atrial flutter/fibrillation with a controlled (or perhaps moderately rapid) ventricular response
Comment: The rhythm is irregularly irregular. Low-amplitude undulations of the baseline (consistent with atrial fibrillation) give way to the sawtooth pattern characteristic of atrial flutter. To acknowledge that the pattern of both of these atrial arrhythmias is seen, some clinicians prefer to designate the rhythm as *atrial flutter/fibrillation*. Others contend that atrial fibrillation and atrial flutter cannot be present at the same time. They would label the relatively large amplitude undulations seen toward the end of this tracing as "coarse" atrial fib waves. We believe that either of these descriptions—or more simply interpreting the rhythm shown in Figure 3G-26 as "atrial fibrillation—should be considered correct answers.

The ventricular response in Figure 3G-26 may be described as either *controlled* or *moderately rapid*, since the average heart rate is between 100 to 130 beats/min.

ANSWER TO FIGURE 3G-27

Rhythm—Slightly irregular
Rate—≈20 beats/min
P waves—None
QRS complex—Probably wide, although one cannot be certain where the QRS complex ends and the ST segment begins
Impression: Slow *idioventricular rhythm*
Comment: Slow idioventricular rhythm is a commonly encountered rhythm in cardiac arrest. It usually portends a poor prognosis.

> Another conceivable interpretation of the rhythm shown in Figure 3G-27 could be atrial fibrillation with an exceedingly slow ventricular response. As noted above, it is hard to be sure where the QRS complex ends, so that the beats in this tracing could be supraventricular in etiology. One might then argue that the irregularity of the R-R interval would be consistent with atrial fibrillation. Clearly, a longer rhythm strip (and additional monitoring leads) would be needed to be sure. Regardless, clinical implications and therapeutic priorities of this bradyarrhythmia are the same—*the rate must be sped up!*

ANSWER TO FIGURE 3G-28

Rhythm—Irregular
P waves—None
QRS complex—Very wide (up to 0.30 second)!
Impression: *Agonal rhythm*
Comment: Although this tracing superficially resembles an idioventricular rhythm, QRS complexes are exceedingly wide and formless, suggesting a preterminal state. This is why the rhythm is described as "agonal." Clinical implications and therapeutic priorities are the same as for asystole.

ANSWER TO FIGURE 3G-29

Rhythm—Irregular
P waves—None
QRS complex—The three QRS complexes seen appear to be of normal duration
Impression: *CPR rhythm* (with underlying agonal or very slow idioventricular rhythm)
Comment: Apart from an occasional agonal complex, one is struck by the regular, rounded (broad-based) negative deflections in the baseline. These occur at a frequency of about 60/min and reflect ongoing CPR. (This tracing is *dated*—current standards recommend a chest compression rate of 80 to 100 times/min in adults!)

ANSWER TO FIGURE 3G-30

Atrial rate and rhythm—Fairly regular at 85 to 90 beats/min
Ventricular rate and rhythm—40 beats/min and regular
QRS complex—Wide (0.16 second)
Impression: Complete (3°) AV block
Comment: In contrast to Figure 3G-17, the PR interval in this tracing continuously varies (i.e., the P wave "marches" through the QRS complex and is *totally dissociated* from it). Moreover, P waves have more than adequate opportunity to conduct (i.e., they occur at all phases of the R-R interval), yet they still fail to do so. The ventricular rhythm is regular and slow. The degree of AV block is therefore complete.

SECTION H

CHALLENGE ARRHYTHMIA REVIEW (III)

As a final review, interpret the following 25 tracings. In addition to the basic concepts covered in this chapter, we go one step further in a number of tracings and **challenge** your interpretation skills. *Do not expect to identify all of the subtleties we point out.* Many of them admittedly extend well *beyond* the core content for basic arrhythmia interpretation. Mastery of such subtleties is definitely *not* essential for being able to perform well on the ACLS arrhythmia test. Nevertheless, we choose to include some of these more advanced concepts here in the hope that doing so will sharpen your skills, provide insight, and help to crystallize the fundamental approach to arrhythmia interpretation.

HINT: *Recognition of arrhythmia subtleties (and understanding of our explanations) will be tremendously facilitated by use of* **calipers.**

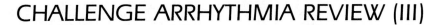

Lead II

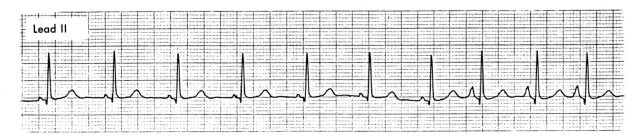

Figure 3H-1

Lead II

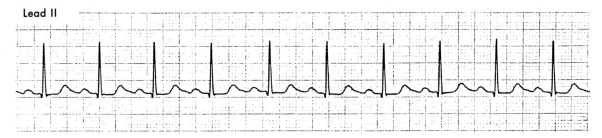

Figure 3H-2

Lead II

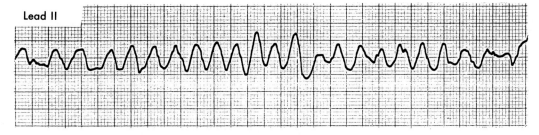

Figure 3H-3

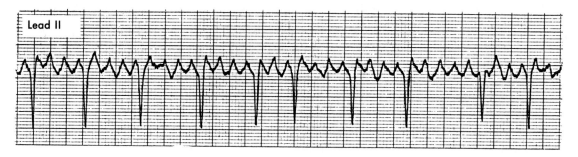

Figure 3H-4

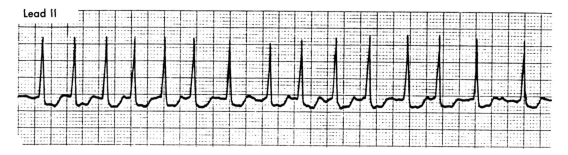

Figure 3H-5

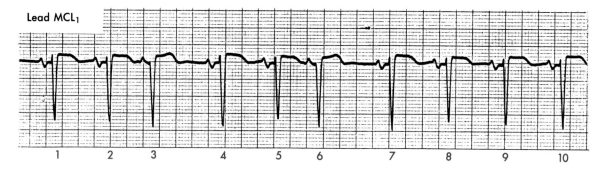

Figure 3H-6

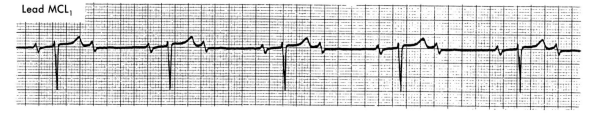

Figure 3H-7

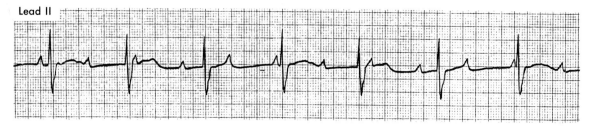

Figure 3H-8

Lead V₁

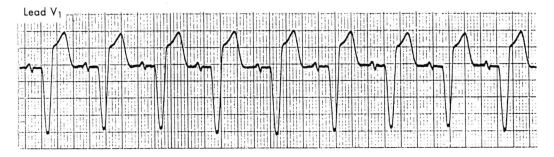

Figure 3H-9

Lead II

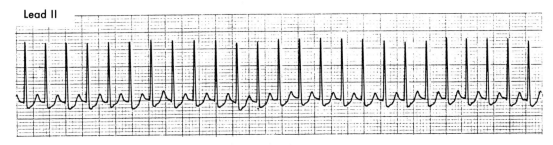

Figure 3H-10

Lead II

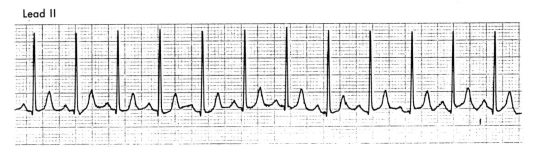

Figure 3H-11

Lead II

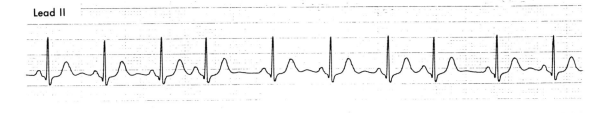

Figure 3H-12

Lead II

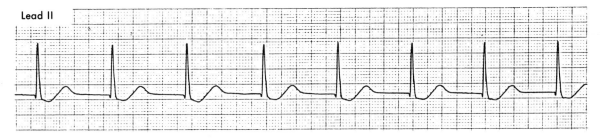

Figure 3H-13

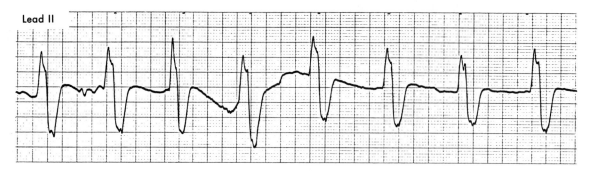

Figure 3H-14

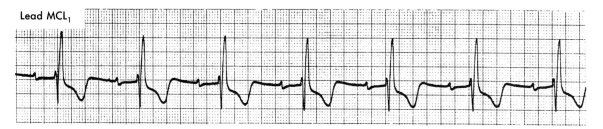

Figure 3H-15

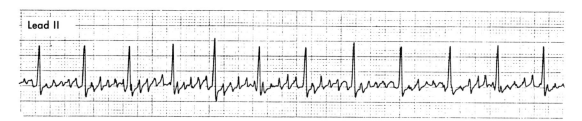

Figure 3H-16

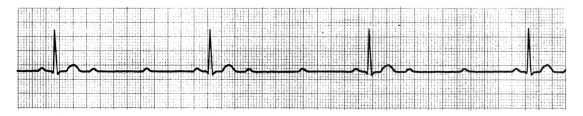

Figure 3H-17

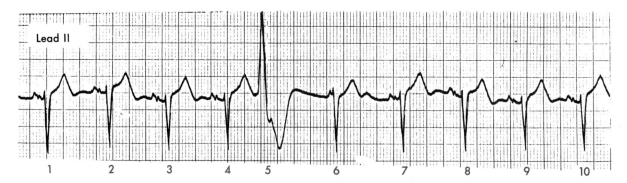

Figure 3H-18

Lead MCL$_1$

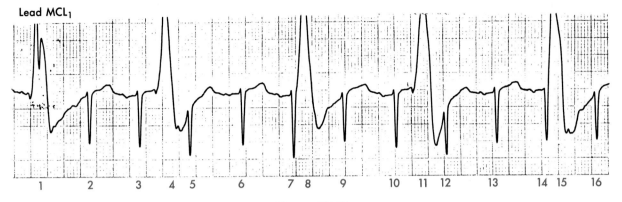

Figure 3H-19

Lead MCL$_1$

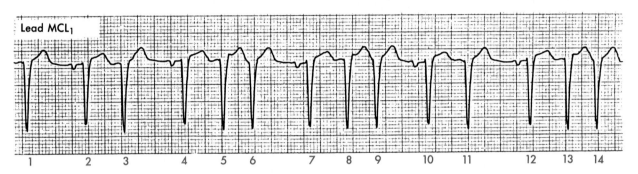

Figure 3H-20

Lead MCL$_6$

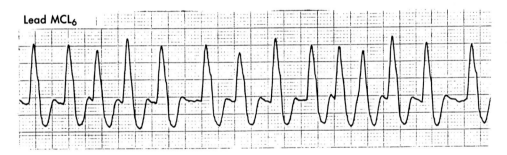

Figure 3H-21

Lead II

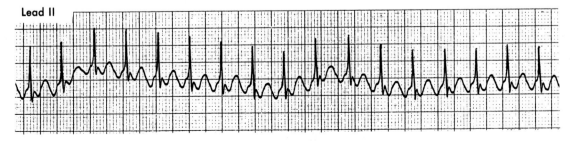

Figure 3H-22

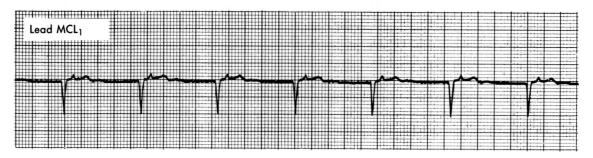

Figure 3H-23

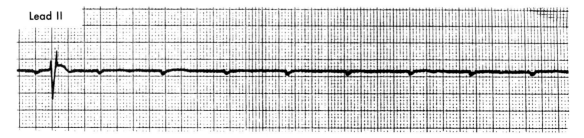

Figure 3H-24

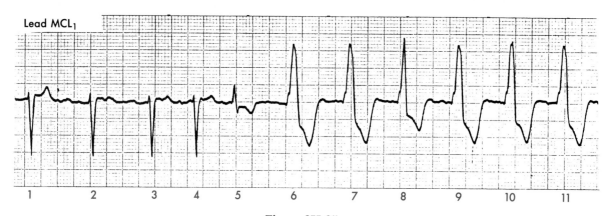

Figure 3H-25

Answers to Arrhythmia Review (III)

ANSWER TO FIGURE 3H-1

Rhythm—Regular
Rate—≈ 85 beats/min
PR interval—Normal (0.20 second)
QRS complex—Normal duration (≤0.10 second)
Impression: Normal sinus rhythm
Comment: A PR interval of 0.20 second is at the upper limit of normal for an adult. However, because the isolated finding of 1° AV block is rarely of clinical significance, and because this degree of PR interval prolongation appears to be a normal finding in many older individuals, we prefer not to call a 1° AV block unless the PR interval is clearly prolonged to *at least* 0.22 sec-

ond. For a similar reason, we tend to avoid the term *"borderline"* 1° AV block (for PR intervals of between 0.19 to 0.21 second), as this connotation rarely adds useful clinical information. Thus, all we would say about the rhythm shown in Figure 3H-1 is that there is normal sinus rhythm.

ANSWER TO FIGURE 3H-2

Rhythm—Initially fairly regular at a rate of between 75 to 80 beats/min. The rate speeds up for the last few beats in the tracing as P wave morphology changes
PR interval—Somewhat short (<0.12 second in lead II) for the initial part of the tracing, and of normal duration for the last three beats

QRS complex—Normal duration

Impression and Comment: At first glance, this rhythm may appear to be no more than another example of normal sinus rhythm. Closer inspection reveals that P wave morphology definitely changes for the last three beats in the tracing. Although a longer rhythm strip would be needed to be sure, this probably represents a *wandering atrial pacemaker* in which the site of impulse formation arises from different supraventricular locations (which explains the changing PR interval and P wave morphology). As with most other arrhythmias, its significance depends on the clinical setting in which it occurs. Wandering atrial pacemaker is usually a normal variant, especially when it occurs in otherwise healthy and young individuals without evidence of underlying heart disease.

> The fact that the PR interval is short (*less* than 0.12 second in this lead II monitoring lead) for the initial part of the tracing suggests that these P waves arise from somewhere in the atria *other than* the SA node.

ANSWER TO FIGURE 3H-3

Rhythm—Irregular

Impression and Comment: The rhythm is totally chaotic without any semblance of organized activity. This is coarse ventricular fibrillation.

ANSWER TO FIGURE 3H-4

Rhythm—Irregular

Atrial rate—A fairly regular sawtooth pattern throughout the tracing at a rate of just over 300 beats/min

QRS complex—Normal duration

Impression: Atrial flutter with a variable ventricular response

Comment: Although atrial flutter is most commonly associated with regular even-numbered AV conduction ratios (especially 2:1 and 4:1 AV conduction), odd numbered AV conduction ratios (such as 3:1) and variable AV conduction (as is the case here) may also occur.

> Note that QRS morphology changes slightly in this example, especially for the second to last beat. This probably reflects superposition of the QRS complex on a different portion of the flutter wave (rather than an alteration in conduction such as aberration).

ANSWER TO FIGURE 3H-5

Rhythm—Irregularly irregular

P waves—None

QRS complex—Normal duration

Impression: Atrial fibrillation with a moderately rapid ventricular response.

Comment: Although low-amplitude undulations are seen along the baseline, no consistent atrial activity is present in this lead II monitoring lead. Thus the rhythm must be atrial fibrillation.

Regarding the rate, the R-R interval varies between 2 and 2½ boxes throughout most of the tracing. This corresponds to a ventricular rate of between 120 to 150 beats/min, which is a fairly rapid ventricular response.

ANSWER TO FIGURE 3H-6

Rhythm—Irregular

PR interval—Normal

QRS complex—Normal duration

Impression: Sinus rhythm with PACs

Comment: Beats #3 and #6 occur early and are PACs. Note that QRS morphology changes slightly in this tracing. Although the reason for this is not apparent (? patient movement), it is unlikely to be of any clinical significance.

ANSWER TO FIGURE 3H-7

Ventricular rhythm—Fairly regular at a rate of between 35 and 40 beats/min

P waves—Precede each QRS complex with a fixed (albeit prolonged) PR interval. In addition, an extra P wave is seen to follow each T wave, so that there are two P waves for each QRS complex.

Atrial rate—Fairly regular at a rate of about 72 beats/min

QRS complex—Normal duration

Impression: Sinus rhythm with 2° AV block and 2:1 AV conduction, representing either Mobitz I or II

Comment: One cannot absolutely differentiate between Mobitz I and II 2° AV block in the presence of 2:1 AV conduction. However, the normal QRS duration and PR interval prolongation both favor Mobitz I.

ANSWER TO FIGURE 3H-8

Ventricular rate and rhythm—Fairly regular at just under 50 beats/min.

P waves—More numerous than the QRS complex. The PR interval preceding each QRS complex varies continuously.

Atrial rate—Regular at a rate of 80 beats/min

QRS complex—Probably wide (although it is hard to be sure where the QRS complex ends and the ST segment begins)

Impression: *Probable* 3° (complete) AV block

Comment: Atrial and ventricular rhythms appear to be completely independent of (i.e., *dissociated* from) each other. That is, *none of the P waves appear to conduct*, despite seemingly having more than adequate opportunity to do so (i.e., P waves *appear* to occur at all points in the R-R interval). Ideally, a slightly slower heart rate (of 45 beats/min or less) or a longer rhythm strip would be needed to ensure that the block is truly complete (which is why we qualify our answer with the word "probable").

ANSWER TO FIGURE 3H-9

Rhythm—Regular

Rate—85 beats/min

PR interval—Normal
QRS complex—Wide
Impression: Normal sinus rhythm
Comment: Despite the fact that the QRS complex is wide, each QRS complex is preceded by a P wave with a fixed PR interval. Therefore the rhythm is sinus. QRS prolongation is due to preexisting bundle branch block.

ANSWER TO FIGURE 3H-10

Rhythm—Regular
Rate—230 beats/min
P waves—Probably absent (although it is admittedly difficult to determine if the upright deflection occurring in the middle of the R-R interval is a T wave, P wave, or both).
QRS complex—Normal duration
Impression: PSVT
Comment: Heart rate is sometimes difficult to calculate when the rhythm is this fast. The **every-other-beat method** may be invaluable for estimating heart rate when the rhythm is rapid and regular. All one does is determine the R-R interval of every other beat (i.e., of *half* of the rate). In this case, the third QRS complex begins on a heavy line. Counting over, it appears that the R-R interval of every other beat is about 2½ boxes (which corresponds to a heart rate of about 115 beats/min). If *half* of the rate is 115 beats/min, the actual rate must be about 230 beats/min (115 × 2).

Thus, the rhythm shown in Figure 3H-10 is a regular, supraventricular tachycardia at a rate of 230 beats/min. The differential includes sinus tachycardia, atrial flutter, and PSVT. Sinus tachycardia usually does not exceed 160 beats/min in adults who are not exercising. Atrial flutter is also unlikely, given that the ventricular response with this arrhythmia most commonly is about 150 beats/min. This leaves PSVT as the probable diagnosis.

ANSWER TO FIGURE 3H-11

Rhythm—Regular
Rate—115 beats/min
PR interval—Normal
QRS complex—Normal duration
Impression: Sinus tachycardia

> Note the slight variation in P wave morphology. Since the R-R interval remains constant throughout this rhythm strip, it is likely that this variation is artifactual, and of no clinical significance.

ANSWER TO FIGURE 3H-12

Rhythm—Irregular
PR interval—Normal
QRS complex—Normal duration
Impression: Sinus rhythm (at a rate of 75 beats/min) with PACs
Comment: Interpretation of this rhythm is actually a bit trickier than one might at first imagine. All P waves are upright and appear to have a similar morphology and identical PR interval. Thus one might be tempted to interpret the rhythm as sinus arrhythmia (which would explain the irregularity in the rhythm). *We could not argue with this interpretation.*

The reason we favor sinus rhythm with PACs as the interpretation is that the basic underlying R-R interval is extremely regular (four large boxes), whereas sinus arrhythmia usually manifests some irregularity throughout the tracing. The fourth and eighth beats occur early, and the P waves preceding each of these beats appears to be ever so slightly wider than other P waves in the tracing, suggesting to us that these beats are PACs.

Several points are illustrated by this tracing. First, *it is sometimes exceedingly difficult (if not impossible) to be completely sure of an interpretation.* Fortunately in this case, it is unlikely to matter clinically whether the true interpretation is sinus rhythm with PACs or sinus arrhythmia.

Finally, it is well to remember that P wave morphology of PACs in any given lead may sometimes look amazingly similar to the P waves of normally conducted beats.

ANSWER TO FIGURE 3H-13

Rhythm—Regular
Rate—58 beats/min
P waves—Absent!
QRS complex—Borderline (i.e., about *half* a large box [=0.10 second] in duration), but probably *not* prolonged
Impression: Junctional (AV nodal) rhythm
Comment: A rate of 58 beats/min is within the usual expected range (i.e., between 40 to 60 beats/min) for an AV nodal escape rhythm in an adult.

ANSWER TO FIGURE 3H-14

Rhythm—Slightly irregular
Rate—60 to 65 beats/min
P waves—Absent
QRS complex—Wide
Impression: AIVR (accelerated idioventricular rhythm)
Comment: The main difference between this tracing and the last one (Fig. 3H-13) is the definite QRS widening. Although it is hard to determine the end of the S wave and the beginning of the ST segment in Figure 3H-14, it is clear that the QRS complex is markedly widened. This fact, and the absence of atrial activity suggest a ventricular origin for the site of the escape pacemaker. Because the usual idioventricular escape rate in adults is slower (i.e., between 30 to 40 beats/min), the rhythm in Figure 3H-14 is described as an *accelerated* idioventricular rhythm (AIVR).

Note that there is much artifact on this tracing. This is because the patient was being resuscitated at the time the tracing was recorded, and probably accounts for the unstable baseline as well as the small biphasic deflection between the first two complexes. Although this deflection simulates a P wave, it probably does not represent atrial activity considering the artifact and the absence of similar deflections elsewhere on the tracing.

ANSWER TO FIGURE 3H-15

Rhythm—Almost regular
Rate—50 beats/min
PR interval—Prolonged (to 0.31 second)
QRS complex—Wide
Impression: Sinus bradycardia with 1° AV block
Comment: Although the QRS complex is wide, each complex is preceded by a P wave with a fixed (albeit prolonged) PR interval. QRS morphology in this example is consistent with RBBB (right bundle branch block) in that there is an rSR′ pattern in this right-sided (MCL-1) lead. Thus, in addition to the bradycardia there is *bifascicular* block (i.e., RBBB *plus* 1° AV block).

A little later, this same patient was found to be in the rhythm below (*Figure 3H-26*). *What has happened?*

ANSWER TO FIGURE 3H-26

Rhythm—Irregular. The ventricular rhythm is punctuated by a relatively long pause between beats #2 and #3. The atrial rhythm is also slightly irregular.
P waves—Do precede each QRS complex; however, the PR interval varies. The P wave that follows beat #2 is not conducted
QRS complex—Still wide in a pattern consistent with RBBB (i.e., there is an rSR′ in this right-sided lead)
Impression: Sinus bradycardia and arrhythmia with 2° AV block, Mobitz type I (Wenckebach)
Comment: Irregularity in the atrial rhythm (in this case due to sinus arrhythmia) makes it more difficult to determine the true nature of the conduction abnormality. Nevertheless, P waves *do* precede each QRS complex, and the PR interval progressively lengthens until a beat is dropped. Thus, there is 2° AV block, Mobitz type I (Wenckebach).

QUESTION: Do you think that the P wave that precedes beat #3 in Figure 3H-26 is conducting?

> HINT #1: In view of the fact that the rhythms shown in Figures 3H-15 and 3H-26 are from the same patient, and considering the PR interval in Figure 3H-15, how much time would you expect to be needed for a P wave to be able to conduct in Figure 3H-26?
>
> HINT #2: If beat #3 did not result from conduction of the P wave that precedes it, what kind of beat is it likely to be (i.e., *Is it likely to arise from the AV node or the ventricles?*)

ANSWER: Although it is impossible to be sure from this short rhythm strip alone, beat #3 *may* be a junctional escape beat. Considering the markedly prolonged PR interval needed for conduction in Figure 3H-15, one might not expect a PR interval as short as the one that precedes beat #3 (=0.17 second) to be able to conduct. If this were the case, the escape focus for beat #3 would have to arise from the AV node because QRS morphology of this beat is identical to that of the normally conducted beats. (If beat #3 was a ventricular escape beat, its morphology should differ significantly.)

Alternatively, it is equally possible that the pause between beats #2 and #3 was sufficiently long to restore normal AV conduction (i.e., it is decidedly longer than the R-R interval in Fig. 3H-15), in which case the P wave preceding beat #3 *could be* conducting. Support for this theory is added by the fact that the PR interval preceding beat #4 is less than the PR interval in Figure 3H-15.

> Let us *emphasize* that determination of the etiology of beat #3 is *not* a simple task, and that the rationale we present above extends *well beyond* the core material needed for basic arrhythmia interpretation. If you simply interpreted the rhythm shown in Figure 3H-26 as sinus bradycardia with 2° AV block, Mobitz type I, *your answer would be entirely appropriate!* Nevertheless, we feel working through the above deductive process for explaining possible reasons for the short PR interval preceding beat #3 may prove insightful and help in better understanding the mechanism of certain arrhythmias.

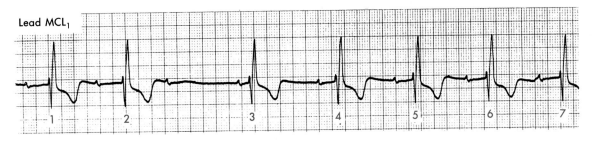

Figure 3H-26

ANSWER TO FIGURE 3H-16

Rhythm—Fairly regular
Rate—95 to 100 beats/min
P waves—?
QRS complex—Normal duration
Impression: Probable sinus rhythm, although the presence of *artifact* makes it difficult to be sure
Comment: At first glance, one might be tempted to say atrial flutter was present. However, more careful inspection suggests that the baseline deflections do not represent atrial activity at all. In adults, atrial activity with atrial flutter is almost always regular at a rate of between 250 to 350 beats/min. Typically it manifests a "sawtooth" pattern in lead II. The deflections in question for this example are more geometric in configuration (i.e., vertical), irregular, and far exceed the expected rate range for atrial flutter in an adult because they occur at a rate of between 400 to 500 times/min. A look at the patient confirmed that these small amplitude vertical deflections were the result of *tremor artifact.*

It is hard to determine what the true rhythm in Figure 3H-16 really is. The rate (95 to 100 beats/min), apparently normal QRS duration, and near regularity of the rhythm suggest a sinus etiology, but from this tracing alone one could not rule out the possibility of either accelerated junctional rhythm (since no definite P waves are seen) or atrial fibrillation (since there is a slight irregularity to the rhythm). If there was a need to know clinically, one could either attempt to repeat the rhythm strip or obtain a 12-lead ECG in the hope that other leads might be less distorted by artifact.

Although it is admittedly devious on our part to include so many examples of artifact in these exercises, we have intentionally done so because:

1. *Artifact is an extremely common finding in the real world.*
2. Patients have been medicated, and even cardioverted or defibrillated when artifact has not been recognized or has been misinterpreted.
3. Familiarity with the common types of artifact encountered, and attention to a few basic points usually makes recognition easy.
4. Failure to actively include the possibility of artifact into your differential greatly increases the chance of it being overlooked.

Suspect artifact whenever physical or electrocardiographic findings do not "fit" with the arrhythmia diagnosis being contemplated. Thus, a chaotic pattern without any or-

---

ganized activity *cannot* be ventricular fibrillation if the patient remains awake and alert. Similarly, deflections occurring at a rate of 400 to 500 times/min (as shown in Fig. 3H-16) are far too rapid to be atrial flutter, especially in view of the morphology, irregularity, and clinical history (of tremor) in this case.

ANSWER TO FIGURE 3H-17

Rhythm—Fairly regular
Rate—Less than 30 beats/min (since the R-R interval is more than 10 large boxes in duration)
P waves—Precede each QRS complex with a fixed PR interval that is not prolonged (i.e., the PR interval does not *exceed* 0.20 to 0.21 second). The atrial rhythm is almost regular at a rate of about 80 beats/min. There are three P waves for every QRS complex (i.e., there is 3:1 AV conduction).
QRS complex—Normal duration
Impression: Sinus rhythm with 2° AV block and 3:1 AV conduction, which probably represents Mobitz II
Comment: It is once again impossible from this short rhythm strip alone to diagnose the true nature of this arrhythmia with certainty. What can be said is that some type of 2° AV block is present. The fact that each QRS complex is preceded by a P wave with a *fixed* (and normal) PR interval rules out 1° and 3° AV block. What can also be said is that, because many of the P waves are not conducted, the block is "high grade." Although the constant PR interval is suggestive of Mobitz II 2° AV block, this diagnosis can *not* be made with certainty because one never sees *consecutively* conducted complexes.

On rare occasions, Mobitz I 2° AV block may manifest 3:1 AV conduction. The fact that the QRS complex is not widened is another feature in favor of Mobitz I. Thus, although the *high-grade* 2° AV block shown in Figure 3H-17 is more likely to be Mobitz II, it could also be Mobitz I. It should be emphasized that differentiation between Mobitz I and Mobitz II in Figure 3H-17 is less important clinically than the marked bradycardia. Regardless of what the conduction disturbance happens to be, stabilization of the patient and normalization of hemodynamic status have to assume first priority. If the patient was hypotensive and did not respond to atropine, pacemaker therapy would be indicated whether the block was Mobitz I or Mobitz II.

ANSWER TO FIGURE 3H-18

Rhythm—Irregular
PR interval—Normal for the sinus conducted beats
QRS complex—Normal duration except for beat #5

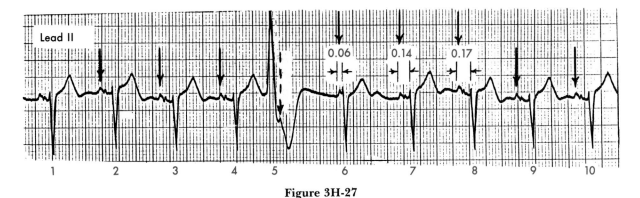

Figure 3H-27

Impression: Sinus rhythm with a PVC (beat #5)

Comment: There are three subtle points about this tracing. See if you can pick them out with the help of the following questions:

QUESTIONS:

1. Is there evidence of atrial activity within the pause that contains the PVC (i.e., between beats #4 and #6)?

2. Is the P wave that precedes beat #6 conducted? (i.e., *What kind of beat is beat #6?*)

3. Is the PR interval preceding beat #7 the same as the PR interval of other sinus conducted beats (i.e., beats #1 to #4, and #8 to #10)—or is it a *little* shorter? If so, why might this be so?

ANSWERS: Regular atrial activity continues throughout this tracing at a rate of 85 beats/min (arrows in *Figure 3H-27* above).

The notch in the downslope of the ST segment of the PVC (the dotted arrow in Fig. 3H-27) therefore represents a regularly occurring sinus P wave. This P wave is unable to conduct because it occurs at a time when the conduction system is refractory. The next sinus P wave occurs on time and just precedes beat #6. This P wave *can't* be conducting because its PR interval is far too short (i.e., only 0.06 second). Thus, beat #6 is an *escape* beat. Because its morphology is identical to that of normally conducted sinus beats, it must be a *junctional* escape beat. *The same is probably true for beat #7.* Close inspection of the PR interval preceding this beat reveals that it is ever so slightly shorter than the PR interval of *all* other sinus conducted beats (0.14 compared to 0.17 second). This makes it unlikely that the P wave preceding beat #7 is conducting, and beat #7 is probably also a junctional beat. Normal sinus rhythm resumes with beat #8.

ANSWER TO FIGURE 3H-19

Rhythm—Regular

Rate—100 beats/min

P waves—Are of small amplitude, but appear to be present and precede QRS complexes with a fixed PR interval

PR interval—Normal (i.e., *not greater* than 0.20 to 0.21 second in duration)

QRS complex—Normal duration

Impression: Sinus tachycardia at a rate of 100 beats/min. Artifact.

Comment: The most remarkable findings on this tracing are the widened, large-amplitude, upright deflections (labeled #1, #4, #8, #11, and #15) that occur approximately every 1.5 seconds. At first glance, one might be tempted to call these deflections PVCs. Closer inspection indicates that this is not the case. Instead, these deflections are artifactual. Observation of the patient reveals the source: hiccoughs!

The reason that deflections #1, #4, #8, #11, and #15 can't be PVCs is that they exert absolutely no effect on the underlying rhythm. PVCs should either delay or prevent the occurrence of the next sinus conducted beat. Furthermore, it is physiologically impossible for any impulse (sinus beat, PAC, or PVC) to be conducted during the absolute refractory period which is probably occurring at the time deflections #1, #8, and #15 are recorded. Thus, the electrocardiographic picture produced by these large amplitude, bizarre-appearing deflections is not consistent with what one would expect if they were PVCs.

ANSWER TO FIGURE 3H-20

Rhythm—Irregular

P waves—Only occasionally seen (preceding beats #2, #4, #7, #10, and #12).

PR interval—Fixed and of normal duration for each of the above noted beats.

QRS complex—Normal duration (i.e., not wider than half a large box).

Impression: Sinus rhythm with frequent PACs

Comment: The irregular irregularity of this rhythm initially suggests the possibility of atrial fibrillation. However, *definite* P waves *are* present—so that this rhythm can't be atrial fibrillation. When P waves are scarce, it is often easiest to identify atrial activity by first scanning those R-R intervals that are longest. This is the case in Figure 3H-20. Each sinus conducted beat is followed by one or more early-occurring (premature) supraventricular beats (PACs or PJCs). It is likely that distortion of the ST segments of beats #3, #5, #8, and #13 is the result of superimposed premature P waves.

> Admittedly, it is impossible to determine if the premature supraventricular beats in *Figure 3H-20* are PACs or PJCs. Statistically, the former are much more common. Practically speaking, however, differentiation is not important because the clinical significance of PACs and PJCs is virtually identical.

ANSWER TO FIGURE 3H-21

Rhythm—Irregularly irregular
P waves—Absent (although admittedly this monitoring lead is often not the best for detecting atrial activity)
QRS complex—Definitely wide
Impression: Atrial fibrillation with a rapid ventricular response
Comment: This degree of irregular irregularity in the absence of atrial activity strongly suggests atrial fibrillation as the diagnosis. QRS widening is most likely the result of preexisting bundle branch block.

Although ventricular tachycardia is not always a regular rhythm, it should *not* be this irregular. Confirmation of the diagnosis would be forthcoming if prior ECGs supported the presence of preexisting bundle branch block and a 12-lead tracing also failed to reveal P waves.

ANSWER TO FIGURE 3H-22

Rhythm—Regular
Rate—Just over 150 beats/min
P waves—Although there is evidence of atrial activity, normal (i.e., upright) P waves are not seen in this lead II monitoring lead.
QRS complex—Normal duration
Impression: Regular SVT (supraventricular tachycardia) at a rate of approximately 150 beats/min without normal P waves. Possibilities include sinus tachycardia, PSVT, and atrial flutter.
Comment: We have repeatedly emphasized how easy it is to overlook atrial flutter unless one continually maintains a high index of suspicion for this arrhythmia. *Whenever there is a regular SVT at a rate of approximately 150 beats/min and normal atrial activity is absent,* **atrial flutter** *should be assumed until proved otherwise.* This is the case in Figure 3H-22. Closer inspection (and use of calipers) confirms the presence of a regularly occurring negative *sawtooth* deflection at a rate of about 300 times/min. These negative deflections are *flutter waves.* There is 2:1 AV conduction.

ANSWER TO FIGURE 3H-23

Rhythm—Regular
Rate—65 beats/min
P waves—Appear to be present *following* each QRS complex
QRS complex—Normal duration
Impression: AV nodal (junctional) rhythm
Comment: P waves in this example are the small amplitude, upright deflections that occur *after* each QRS complex. These P waves are the result of *retrograde* conduction from the junctional rhythm. They have an R-P interval (i.e., distance from the QRS complex until the retrograde P wave) of 0.12 second. Most of the time with junctional rhythm atrial activity is either absent (i.e., hidden within the QRS complex), or P waves precede the QRS with a short PR interval. Occasionally, however, they may follow the QRS complex as they do here.

The usual rate of an AV nodal escape pacemaker in adults is between 40 to 60 beats/min. The rate in this example is slightly faster, so that technically this junctional rhythm is slightly "accelerated."

ANSWER TO FIGURE 3H-24

Rhythm—Irregular
P waves—Regular at a rate of 80 beats/min
QRS complex—Only one QRS complex is seen (at the very beginning of the tracing)
Impression: *Ventricular standstill*
Comment: Perhaps the most interesting aspect of this tracing is discussion of the semantics related to the terminology of its classification. The rhythm is not asystole. Asystole implies a total absence of electrical activity. Regular atrial activity is present here at a rate of 80 beats/min. Although none of the atrial impulses appear (are able ?) to conduct (with the possible exception of the first P wave), the rhythm should not simply be classified as 3° AV block. With "uncomplicated" 3° (complete) AV block, a lower pacemaker (junctional or ventricular) typically emerges and provides an escape rhythm that may sustain perfusion (at least to some degree). The problem in Figure 3H-24 is more profound. After the initial QRS complex, the escape focus stops . . . which is why the rhythm is probably best described as *ventricular standstill*.

Some clinicians may favor the term *"agonal"* to describe the rhythm shown in Figure 3H-24. Our conception of an agonal rhythm is a "dying heart," in which exceedingly wide, amorphous complexes are sporadically seen on the tracing. Meaningful perfusion (i.e., organized ventricular contraction) could not possibly result from such complexes. Although the rhythm shown in Figure 3H-24 may admittedly reflect a "dying heart," the ventricular complex that does appear is *not* amorphous (i.e., it is of normal duration), and organized atrial activity is present.

Semantics aside, recommended treatment for all of the entities discussed above is the same: atropine, high-dose epinephrine, pacemaker therapy, and *prayer*. Prognosis is dismal regardless of what the most appropriate terminology happens to be.

ANSWER TO FIGURE 3H-25

Rhythm—Irregular

P waves—Absent. Although there are undulations in the baseline, there are no regularly occurring deflections that would be consistent with P waves.

QRS complex—Initially narrow (for beats #1 to #4), and then wide (for beats #6 to #11)

Impression: Initially atrial fibrillation with a controlled ventricular response—then AIVR

Comment: The easiest way to approach interpretation of more complex arrhythmias is to try to determine if there is an *underlying rhythm*. The first four beats in this tracing are irregularly irregular and manifest a narrow, normal-appearing QRS complex. There are no definite P waves. This suggests that the underlying rhythm is atrial fibrillation. The QRS complex then widens (with beat #6) and becomes more regular (at a rate of 85 to 90 beats/min). This regular rhythm (represented by beats #6 to #11) appears to be ventricular in etiology (QRS widening, absent P waves) and accelerated in rate (since the usual rate of an idioventricular escape rhythm is between 30 to 40 beats/min)—which explains the impression we proposed above.

QUESTION #1: *What is beat #5?*

HINT: If beats #4 and #6 in Figure 3H-25 were "parent beats," what would you expect the QRS to look like if they "had children"?

QUESTION #2: Does the presence of beat #5 support our interpretation of this arrhythmia?

HINT: Is it likely that beats #6 to #11 are junctional? Is there any reason for beats #6 to #11 to be conducted with aberration?

ANSWERS: Beat #5 is a **fusion beat.** It is *intermediate* in morphology between the predominantly negative QRS complex of supraventricular beat #4 and the entirely positive QRS complex of ventricular beat #6.

Although it would be impossible to predict where the next supraventricular impulse after beat #4 should occur (because of the irregularity and unpredictability of the rhythm with atrial fibrillation), we would expect the ventricular complex preceding beat #6 to occur at about the time we see beat #5 (i.e., the R-R interval between beats #5 and #6 is approximately the same as the R-R interval between QRS complexes during the AIVR). Note also that the QRS complex of beat #5 appears to be even *narrower* than the QRS complex of the other supraventricular beats. *The only way this could happen is by* **fusion** *of a supraventricular complex with a* **simultaneously** *occurring ventricular beat (so as to cancel out a portion of the electrical forces).*

Identification of fusion beats in Figure 3H-25 essentially proves a ventricular etiology for beats #6 to #11. The reason these beats are unlikely to be of junctional etiology is that QRS morphology of junctional beats should generally be similar (if not identical) to that of other supraventricular complexes. There is no reason for beats #6 to #11 to conduct with aberration because beat #6 occurs late in the cycle (well after the refractory period), and the rate of the AIVR does not appear to be rapid enough to produce a rate-related bundle branch block (considering that beat #4 conducts normally).

Finally, note that beat #8 during the run of AIVR is somewhat thinner than the other ventricular beats. It is possible that there may be some degree of fusion occurring between this beat and a supraventricular impulse.

References

Berger PB, Ryan TJ: Inferior myocardial infarction: High-risk subgroups, *Circulation* 81:401-411, 1990.

Clemmensen P, Bates ER, Califf RM, Hlatky MA, Aronson L, George BS, Lee KL, Kereiakes DJ, Gacioch G, Berrios E, and the TAMI Study Group: Complete atrioventricular block complicating inferior wall acute myocardial infarction treated with reperfusion therapy, *Am J Cardiol* 67:225-230, 1991.

Constant J: Solving nomenclature problems in cardiology, *JAMA* 240:868-871, 1978.

Grauer K, Kravitz L, Curry RW, Ariel M: Computerized electrocardiogram interpretations: Are they useful for the family physician? *J Fam Pract* 24:39-43, 1987.

Grauer K, Kravitz L, Ariel M, Curry RW, Nelson WP, Marriott HJL: Potential benefits of a computerized ECG interpretation system for primary care physicians in a community hospital, *JABFP* 2:17-24, 1989.

Grauer K, Cavallaro D: *ACLS teach kit: An instructor's resource*, St. Louis, 1990, Mosby–Year Book.

Grauer K: *A practical guide to ECG interpretation*, St. Louis, 1992, Mosby–Year Book.

Henson JR: Descartes and the ECG lettering series, *J Hist Med* 26:181-186, 1971.

Julian DG: Nomenclature in cardiology: More on "extrasystole," *Heart Lung* 16:121, 1987.

Marriott HJL: Arrhythmia versus dysrhythmia, *Am J Cardiol* 54:628, 1984.

Marriott HJL: More comments on proper terminology for the VPC, *Am J Cardiol* 57:191-192, 1986 (letter).

Marriott HJL: Depolarization, contraction, systole, complex, or beat? Take your choice, but may my sinus node go on *beating! Heart Lung* 16:117-119, 1987.

Schamroth L: North American malady: Usage and meaning of "extrasystole," *Heart Lung* 16:119-121, 1987.

Spodick DH: Cardiolocution: The cardiologist's assault on English, *Am J Cardiol* 48:973-974, 1981.

Surawicz B, Uhley H, Borun R, Laks M, Crevasse L, Rosen K, Nelson W, Mandel W, Lawrence P, Jackson L, Flowers N, Clifton J, Greenfield J, Robles de Medine EO: Task force I: Standardization of terminology and interpretation, *Am J Cardiol* 41:130-145, 1978.

CHAPTER 4

PUTTING IT ALL TOGETHER: PRACTICE FOR MEGA CODE

The essentials of running a code are contained within the algorithms presented in Chapter 1. The problem is that memorization of material presented in "algorithmic" form is often difficult unless one is able to practice applying it. Unfortunately being able to recite the exact sequence of an algorithm in the peace and quiet of one's own study facility does not necessarily correlate with the ability to command instant recall of the same material in an emergency situation *(or when you are being tested at the MEGA CODE station!)*.

The exercises in this chapter have been selected to provide you with an opportunity to *"put it all together"* and apply the information covered up to this point. Four basic scenarios of cardiac arrest are presented. The rationale for the treatment given in each of these scenarios closely follows the protocols laid out in the algorithms and commentary presented in Chapter 1. *The material is probably very similar to what you will be tested on at the MEGA CODE station.* It also comprises the KEY core content of what you need to know to successfully manage most real code situations.

To obtain maximum benefit from these exercises, *mentally transport YOURSELF to the bedside for each case.* Imagine the events transpiring before you as they might actually occur. Then assume the position of the code director—*and take over the management of each case!*

CASE STUDY A

You are working in the emergency department where a middle-aged man suddenly collapses. A *code blue* is called. Within seconds, a full complement of qualified assistants have assembled around *YOU,* waiting for *your* next command. *How would you proceed?*

Plan

1. Confirm unresponsiveness.
2. Open the airway.
3. Verify apnea. Then administer two *slow,* full breaths.
4. Verify pulselessness. Then begin CPR.
5. Call for help—*although there is no need to do so in this case since you are already surrounded by qualified assistants ready to assume your every command.*
6. Bring over the crash cart, turn on the defibrillator, and apply the quick-look paddles.

All of these steps are accomplished within 40 seconds. Application of quick-look paddles reveals the rhythm shown in *Figure 4A-1* on the monitor. What is this rhythm? *How would you treat it?*

Analysis of Figure 4A-1 and Plan

There is a total lack of organized electrical activity. The rhythm is *ventricular fibrillation.*

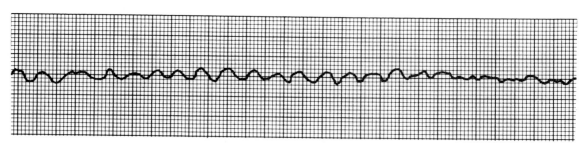

Figure 4A-1. Initial rhythm of the patient in Case Study A (as demonstrated by application of quick-look paddles).

7. <u>Defibrillate</u> the patient *as soon as this is possible.* In preparing to do this, apply conductive medium to the paddles (or put on defibrillator pads), ensure that no one is in contact with the patient, apply firm pressure to the paddles (pressing down with approximately 25 lb of force), and discharge. Use <u>200 joules</u> of delivered energy for this initial countershock attempt.

Two points are deserving of special mention about the initial steps followed in this protocol. They regard use of the *precordial thump* and application of *mouth-to-mouth ventilation.*

Application of a **precordial thump** is indicated at the onset of pulseless rhythms (such as pulseless ventricular tachycardia, ventricular fibrillation, and/or asystole). Practically speaking, the chance that the thump will work in this situation is small. However, *there is little to lose* by trying the thump (since the patient is pulseless)—and occasionally the 2 to 5 joules of energy it delivers will be enough to convert the patient to sinus rhythm. In contrast, use of the precordial thump is no longer recommended for treatment of rhythms associated with a pulse (as may be the case for some patients with sustained ventricular tachycardia). This is because delivery of mechanical energy at a random point in the cardiac cycle (as occurs with the thump) may precipitate deterioration of ventricular tachycardia to ventricular fibrillation or asystole (if the impulse happens to be delivered during the vulnerable period). In this particular case study, *one could have delivered a precordial thump immediately after Step #4* (i.e., immediately after confirming pulselessness). Alternatively—since it was known that a defibrillator would be available momentarily—it was reasonable (and perhaps even preferable) to withhold the thump and await arrival of the defibrillator.

The setting described by this case scenario is one in which an emergency care provider is present at the scene of a cardiopulmonary arrest and confronted with an apneic victim *WITHOUT* the benefit of any ventilatory adjuncts. In recent years, emergency care providers have become increasingly reluctant to perform **mouth-to-mouth ventilation** in this situation (see *Section D of Chapter 10*). Practically speaking, it may be helpful to realize that there are *four* ways to approach this problem:

1. Deliver mouth-to-mouth ventilation YOURSELF if it is needed *until* the arrival of suitable equipment (i.e., a ventilatory adjunct). If you select this course of action, take comfort in the fact that the statistical likelihood of AIDS transmission by performance of mouth-to-mouth ventilation is *exceedingly* small (if not negligible)—especially if mucous membranes in the mouth are intact.

2. Let *someone else* be the one to deliver mouth-to-mouth ventilation. . . .

3. Intentionally STALL—*especially* if help (in the form of an Ambu bag) is expected *momentarily.* If you select this course of action, *be sure to initiate chest compressions.* Take comfort in the fact that performance of several cycles of chest compressions (even *without* accompanying ventilation!) may effectively circulate a small (but nevertheless important) amount of partially oxygenated blood (that had been present in the victim's blood vessels at the time of the arrest). *Then hope that the Ambu bag arrives shortly. . . .*

4. Prevention/anticipation—*clearly the BEST course of action!* Ready availability of a disposable pocket mask (with an exhalation valve) at the bedside—or in areas where cardiopulmonary arrest is likely to occur—would go a long way to alleviating the reluctance of health care providers to perform rescue breathing.

The patient has been defibrillated with 200 joules of delivered energy. He remains pulseless and unresponsive. Quick-look paddles now reveal the rhythm shown in *Figure 4A-2. What would you do at this point?*

Analysis of Figure 4A-2 and Plan

The patient is still in *ventricular fibrillation.*

8. Repeat <u>defibrillation</u> *as soon as this is possible* (i.e., as soon as the defibrillator is recharged). Use <u>300 joules</u> for this second countershock attempt.

Minimizing the time between countershock attempts reduces transthoracic resistance. This allows a greater amount of *current* to pass through the chest wall (and therefore through the heart) with each defibrillation. Increasing the energy selected (to 300 joules in this case) further ensures that a greater amount of current will pass through the chest wall with this second defibrillation attempt.

The patient fails to respond. He remains pulseless and in ventricular fibrillation. *What should be done next?*

Plan

9. <u>Defibrillate</u> a *third* time—again, *as soon as this is possible.* Use full energy (i.e., <u>360 joules</u>) for this third countershock attempt.

The rationale for adding the third countershock attempt is that some patients will only respond to defibrillation with maximal energy.

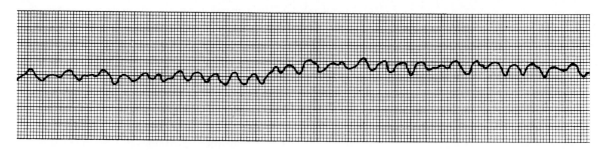

Figure 4A-2.   Rhythm of the patient in Case Study A after receiving an initial countershock of 200 joules. He is still pulseless and unresponsive. *What would you do at this point?*

Despite delivery of the third countershock, the patient remains pulseless and in ventricular fibrillation. *What next?*

Plan

10. Resume CPR.
11. Establish an airway. *Ventilate* the patient—and then *intubate* (if possible).
12. Establish *intravenous access.*

> *Success at defibrillation is inversely proportional to the amount of time between the onset of ventricular fibrillation and the application of electrical countershock.* As a result, any intervention that might delay defibrillation at all (such as intubation, achieving IV access, and administration of drugs) is best deferred until *after* the initial series of countershocks has been completed. Intubation may not even be needed if defibrillation is successful in restoring an effective cardiac rhythm. Achieving IV access may also be far simpler to accomplish if a spontaneous rhythm can be restored (since the caliber of venous vessels will be naturally greater with spontaneous perfusion than in the arrested heart).

The patient is intubated, and *IV* access is secured with a large-bore catheter inserted into the antecubital fossa.

> It is essential to secure *effective* IV access as soon as possible after the initial series of countershocks. Although ideally this entails establishment of an *upper torso* central line (subclavian or internal jugular), a large-bore IV catheter in a proximal upper extremity site (such as the antecubital fossa) may be almost as good if medications are "flushed" after administration (by a 50- to 100-cc bolus of fluid) and the extremity is elevated (to favor venous return). Alternatively, certain drugs (recalled by the mnemonic **A-L-E** = **A**tropine, **L**idocaine, and **E**pinephrine) can be given by the *endotracheal* (ET) route if IV access has not yet been established.
>
> It should be emphasized that the femoral line is no longer recommended as a site for IV access during cardiac arrest (since blood flow below the diaphragm is minimal in an arrest situation). Establishment of a "butterfly" in a distal IV site (i.e., dorsum of the wrist) is also unlikely to provide adequate access to the central circulation in a code situation.

The patient is *still* in ventricular fibrillation. As noted above, there has been no response to three defibrillation attempts (with 200, 300, and 360 joules). *What should you do at this point?*

13. Administer epinephrine. Begin with SDE (i.e., 1 mg), given *either* intravenously (IV) or down the endotracheal (ET) tube–*depending on whichever route was established first.* Be ready to increase the dose of epinephrine (i.e., to HDE) if there is no response.

> Administration of epinephrine by the ET route is a suitable alternative when a large-bore IV site is not yet available. Absorption of endotracheally administered drug is rapid and complete for epinephrine, although somewhat higher doses may be needed to achieve the same effect as from IV administration. As a result, *at least* 10 ml (= 1 ampule) of the 1:10,000 solution (= 1 mg of epinephrine) should be injected down the ET tube. This should be immediately followed by several forceful insufflations of the Ambu bag to ensure good distal distribution of drug. More epinephrine may be needed if the patient fails to respond to this SDE dose.

An initial 1-mg dose of epinephrine is given IV—and is immediately followed by a bolus of fluid and elevation of the arm.

> Note that mention of **sodium bicarbonate** has been *intentionally omitted* up to this point. This is because the acidosis that occurs during the *initial* minutes of cardiac arrest is primarily respiratory in nature (due to hyp**o**ventilation). Recommended treatment for this respiratory acidosis is to improve ventilation–*NOT to give sodium bicarbonate!* On the contrary, early administration of sodium bicarbonate may actually worsen the situation by producing a *paradoxical* intracellular acidosis (that may lead to further depression of myocardial function). *Use of sodium bicarbonate in the usual code situation is to be strongly discouraged for AT LEAST the first 5 to 10 minutes of the arrest!*
>
> A possible exception to this general rule may be when a severe preexisting metabolic acidosis was known to be present at the time of the arrest (as may be the case for a patient with diabetic ketoacidosis

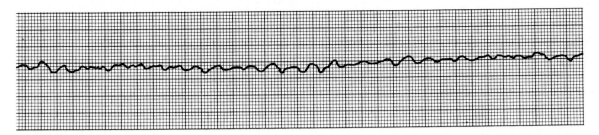

Figure 4A-3.   Rhythm demonstrated on ECG monitoring leads. The patient is still unresponsive. *What should be done at this point?*

or lactic acidosis)—especially if the metabolic acidosis was thought to have contributed to causing the arrest. However, *recent data now question whether sodium bicarbonate should even be given under these circumstances (because of its potentially deleterious effects).*

CPR is continued (to circulate the epinephrine given above). A respiratory therapist at the bedside draws blood for a set of ABGs from the femoral pulse that is palpated with each external chest compression. *What should you do at this point?*

14. Have your assistants hook the patient up to *monitoring leads* (or preferably an ECG machine) to provide *continuous* ECG monitoring.
15. Reassess the patient.

The patient remains unresponsive. Monitoring leads demonstrate the rhythm shown in *Figure 4A-3*. *What should be done at this point?*

Analysis of Figure 4A-3 and Plan
Once again the rhythm is ventricular fibrillation.

16. *Recheck the pulse!*

It is imperative to *ALWAYS* check for a pulse after EVERY **intervention—and/or *WHENEVER* the rhythm changes on the monitor.** Even though the electrocardiographic appearance of the rhythm shown in Figure 4A-3 is still that of ventricular fibrillation, a monitor lead may have fallen off . . . *in which case another rhythm may actually be present* (and the patient might *not* necessarily need defibrillation!).

There is no pulse—which means that the rhythm shown in Figure 4A-3 is truly *ventricular fibrillation.*

17. Defibrillate the patient again (since he is still in ventricular fibrillation). Use maximum delivered energy (i.e., 360 joules) for this *fourth* defibrillation attempt.

There is no response to countershock. The patient remains pulseless, unresponsive, and in persistent (i.e., *refractory*) ventricular fibrillation. Interventions attempted up to this point include:

* *Defibrillation × 3* (with 200, 300, and 360 joules)
* Intubation/establishment of IV access
* Administration of *epinephrine*
* *Defibrillation* with 360 joules

What should be done next?

Plan
18. Try antifibrillatory therapy. Although a number of agents might be listed under this therapeutic heading, lidocaine is generally accepted as the drug of choice for *initial* medical treatment of *refractory* ventricular fibrillation. Administer an IV-loading bolus of between 50 and 100 mg ($\approx$ 1 mg/kg).

Other *antifibrillatory measures* to consider include bretylium tosylate, amiodarone, and magnesium sulfate. Despite much enthusiasm in the past for the use of **bretylium** as an antifibrillatory agent, studies to date have failed to demonstrate any clear advantage for this drug compared to lidocaine. Because lidocaine may be a safer agent, and most emergency care providers are more familiar and comfortable with its use, it is currently favored for *initial* medical treatment of refractory ventricular fibrillation.

Amiodarone holds promise of becoming a drug of choice for antifibrillatory therapy. Future years may see emergency IV loading regimens of the drug (i.e., administration of between 150 and 500 mg over a 5- to 10-minute period) become reality. At the present time, however, controlled studies on the use of amiodarone in the setting of cardiac arrest are extremely limited, and the drug is not yet available for general use.

Use of **magnesium sulfate** in the setting of cardiac arrest is *purely empiric*. Although one might expect this agent to be most effective in the treatment of patients with low *prearrest* serum magnesium levels, advocates of its use maintain that magnesium may also be effective when serum levels are normal. Clinically, serum magnesium levels do *not* always correlate well with body (i.e., intracellular) stores of this cation. Moreover, the emergency care provider will often (usually) *not* *know* the victim's serum magnesium level at the time the arrest occurs–nor will he/she usually have access to STAT serum magnesium determinations in a timely enough fashion to be able to act accordingly. Thus, many questions about the use of this drug in the setting of cardiac arrest remain *unanswered* at this time. *Whether to EMPIRICALLY administer magnesium sulfate to a patient in refractory ventricular fibrillation—and if so, at what point during the resuscitation effort to try this therapy—are issues* that must therefore be left to the judgment of the resuscitation team. Practically speaking, however, *there may be little to lose by empiric administration (of 1 to 2 gm IV) of magnesium sulfate to a patient in refractory ventricular fibrillation who has not responded to other measures. . .*

19. *Consider* beginning an <u>IV maintenance infusion</u> of lidocaine (at <u>2 mg/min</u>).

Pharmacokinetically, it is *not* essential to begin an IV maintenance infusion of lidocaine *until* the spontaneous circulation is restored. This is because lidocaine metabolism is markedly reduced in the arrested heart. As a result, the duration of action of each lidocaine bolus that is given will be significantly prolonged, and no more than one (or *at most* two) lidocaine boluses need be given for as long as the patient remains in ventricular fibrillation.

Practically speaking, we find it easiest to routinely initiate an IV maintenance infusion of lidocaine *whenever* we initiate IV loading of the drug. However, the point to emphasize is that if you choose not to begin a continuous IV infusion at the time you administer antifibrillatory therapy, *it is IMPERATIVE to remember to do so AS SOON AS the heart is restarted.*

A lidocaine bolus of 75 mg is administered IV. *What should you do next?*

20. *Circulate the bolus of drug* (by performing CPR for a period of time). Then <u>defibrillate</u> again. Use maximal energy <u>(360 joules)</u>.

At least 1 to 2 minutes of CPR appear to be needed for the lidocaine to "circulate" (i.e., reach the central circulation).

Despite administration of lidocaine and subsequent defibrillation, the patient remains pulseless, unresponsive, and in ventricular fibrillation. *What next?*

Plan

21. *Look for some other factor that might explain the patient's refractory condition.* Thus, you might mentally run down the following checklist in search of a *potentially correctable* cause of ventricular fibrillation (beginning with the **ABCs**):

- *Is the **A**irway secure?*
- *Is mechanical **B**reathing effective?* (Are good bilateral breath sounds present? (Is the PaO_2 adequate?)
- *Is **C**irculation adequate?* (Does CPR produce a pulse?)

Other items to consider might include the following:

- Could some *preexisting* metabolic condition (i.e., diabetic ketoacidosis, hyperkalemia) have precipitated the arrest (and need correction)?
- Was the patient hypovolemic? (Is there evidence of blood loss? marked dehydration?)
- Could the patient be hypothermic? *(Do you know the patient's temperature?)*
- Could the patient have overdosed on any medications? (cocaine? tricyclics? narcotics?)
- Might a complication from CPR have developed during resuscitation? (tension pneumothorax? pericardial tamponade?)

Although the above checklist is by no means complete, it does include some of the more common/most important *potentially reversible* causes of refractory ventricular fibrillation. Alternatively, the patient could have suffered a massive myocardial infarction or ruptured an aortic aneurysm—*causes of refractory ventricular fibrillation that would be extremely unlikely to respond to any treatment at this point in the process.*

No potentially reversible cause of ventricular fibrillation is found. It is not known why the patient collapsed in the emergency department. Interventions attempted up to this point include:

- *Defibrillation × 3* (with 200, 300, and 360 joules)
- Intubation/establishment of IV access
- Administration of *epinephrine*
- *Defibrillation* with 360 joules
- *Antifibrillatory therapy* (with a *lidocaine* bolus of 75 mg and initiation of an IV infusion of 2 mg/min)
- *Defibrillation* with 360 joules
- A search for a potentially correctable, underlying cause of the arrest

Despite these actions, the patient remains in ventricular fibrillation. *What would you do now?*

Plan

22. Repeat <u>epinephrine</u> administration (using <u>HDE</u>— *if you have not already done so*).
23. *Possibly reconsider* whether you want to use <u>sodium bicarbonate.</u>

It is likely that *at least* 10 minutes will have passed by this time (which may be long enough for a metabolic component to the acidosis to develop)–*although there is NO evidence that giving sodium bicarbonate at any time during resuscitation will improve prognosis—and doing so could be harmful.*

24. Consider a trial of *additional* antifibrillatory measures. This might include one (or more) of the following:

- A *second* (50 to 75 mg) IV bolus of lidocaine
- Magnesium sulfate (1 to 2 g IV)—*if you have not already tried this*
- Bretylium tosylate (1 ampule = 500 mg) as an initial IV bolus—followed by a *second* bolus (of 10 mg/kg—or approximately 1 to 2 ampules)—and additional (10 mg/kg) boluses as needed (up to a total dose of 30 mg/kg).

Bretylium is an effective antifibrillatory agent, and an *empiric* trial of this drug would be completely appropriate at this point. Although administration of bretylium rarely results in spontaneous conversion of ventricular fibrillation to sinus rhythm, it may *facilitate* conversion to sinus rhythm with subsequent countershocks. The antifibrillatory effect of the drug usually begins to work within a few minutes, but occasionally may be delayed for *as long* as 10 to 15 minutes. As a result, once the decision is made to try bretylium, it is important *not* to terminate resuscitation efforts until adequate time has been allowed for the drug to work.

25. Circulation of drug(s) by resumption of CPR (for 1 to 2 minutes) before *repeat* defibrillation (with 360 joules).
26. Repeat Steps #22, #24, and #25 (i.e., epinephrine, *additional* antifibrillatory measures, CPR, and defibrillation)—*as often as needed* (i.e., until *either* the patient responds to treatment, or the decision is made to terminate resuscitation efforts).

An initial IV bolus (of 500 mg) of bretylium is given and "circulated" with CPR for approximately 2 minutes. Another countershock (with 360 joules) is then delivered, but the patient remains in ventricular fibrillation. However, immediately following a second bolus of bretylium (and the accompanying countershock), the rhythm shown in *Figure 4A-4* is noted. What has happened? *What should you do next?*

Analysis of Figure 4A-4 and Plan

Sinus rhythm is noted on the monitor.

27. *Check for a pulse!*

    If no pulse were present, the rhythm would be EMD! In this case, CPR would need to be resumed immediately.

A bounding pulse is associated with the rhythm shown in Figure 4A-4. The patient's blood pressure is 120/80 mm Hg, and he is beginning to open his eyes. *What should be done BEFORE transfer to the coronary care unit?*

Plan

28. Rebolus the patient with (50 to 75 mg of) lidocaine, and begin a maintenance infusion (at a rate of 2 mg/minute)—*if you have not already done so.*

    Alternatively—since the patient only responded to defibrillation after antifibrillatory therapy with bretylium, you might initiate an IV maintenance infusion of this drug *instead* of lidocaine.

Discussion

This case illustrates the steps in the algorithm for resuscitation of a patient in ventricular fibrillation *(see Fig. 1-2).* Several points are deserving of special mention.

It is important to emphasize that the likelihood of successfully resuscitating a patient in cardiac arrest is inversely proportional to the interval between the onset of ventricular fibrillation and the application of countershock. *This is why ALL patients should be defibrillated as soon as the diagnosis of ventricular fibrillation is established.* Delay for the purpose of intubation and/or starting an IV line (i.e., to administer epinephrine) is unwarranted, and may adversely affect the patient's chance for survival. To assist in making the most rapid diagnosis of ventricular fibrillation possible, *quick-look paddles* should be applied as soon as the defibrillator arrives. This pertains *both* to arrests that occur within the hospital, as well as to those that occur outside of the hospital. *Application of quick-look paddles should only take a few seconds.* If the patient is in ventricular fibrillation—*immediately countershock* before you do anything else.

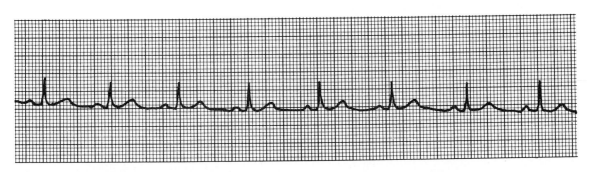

Figure 4A-4. Rhythm resulting from countershock after the second bolus of bretylium. *What should you do next?*

The final point is that *there is no limit to the number of times that the patient may be defibrillated!* As long as the rhythm is ventricular fibrillation—the rhythm is *potentially treatable.* A potentially correctable underlying cause of the refractory ventricular fibrillation should be sought. This was done—but *none was to be found* in this particular case. Instead, the patient remained refractory to all of the usual treatment measures until after the second dose of bretylium was given. If he had remained in ventricular fibrillation beyond this point, repetition of Steps #22, #24, and #25 in the above sequence would be in order. This would entail the use of more epinephrine, *additional* antifibrillatory measures (such as a second dose of lidocaine, a third dose of bretylium, and/or magnesium sulfate), and further attempts at defibrillation until the patient was either converted out of ventricular fibrillation, or cardiovascular unresponsiveness could be conclusively established.

One antifibrillatory measure that was not included in this case scenario is the use of an IV β-blocker (i.e., **IV propranolol** in a dose of 0.5 to 1 mg administered *slowly* up to a total dose of 5 mg). The most difficult part about making recommendations for the use of IV β-blockers in the setting of cardiopulmonary arrest is knowing when to administer these drugs. Clearly there are times when all other treatment measures will fail, and *only* IV β-blockers may save the patient. Situations in which this is most likely to occur are those in which excessive sympathetic tone is implicated as an important etiologic factor (i.e., in the setting of acute ischemia and/or *anterior* infarction—especially when cardiac arrest is preceded by a period of tachycardia or hypertension—or in the setting of cocaine overdose or severe stress during the prearrest period). If any of these factors were known to be present, an empiric trial of an IV blocker would have been reasonable (in Step #18—or at any point thereafter).

CASE STUDY B

You are on call making your rounds when a *code blue* is called. You run to the room of the code and find numerous hopsital personnel standing around the bed of an elderly woman. The patient is awake and alert, but a little bit short of breath. She is not having any chest pain. The ECG monitor reflects the rhythm shown in *Figure 4B-1.*

What is the rhythm? *What should you do?*

Analysis of Figure 4B-1 and Plan

The first thing to do is to take your own pulse! Although the rhythm on the monitor is clearly worrisome, the patient (at least for the moment) is awake, alert, and appears to be *hemodynamically stable!* Therefore, you DO have a moment to compose yourself—catch your breath—and formulate a plan. Your approach might be to:

1. Check the patient's blood pressure, and provide supplemental oxygen.

2. Remember the four questions, and systematically apply them to analyze the arrhythmia.

The patient's blood pressure is 90/60 mm Hg.

The rhythm in Figure 4B-1 is a *wide-complex tachycardia* at a heart rate of about 150 beats/min. No P waves are evident. The differential should include **five** entities:

   i) VENTRICULAR TACHYCARDIA
   ii) VENTRICULAR TACHYCARDIA
   iii) VENTRICULAR TACHYCARDIA
   iv) Supraventricular tachycardia with a preexisting bundle branch block
   v) Supraventricular tachycardia with aberrant conduction

Although there is some irregularity to the rhythm and the patient is awake and alert, *VENTRICULAR TACHYCARDIA must be assumed until proved otherwise!*

The following point cannot be emphasized too strongly:

Lead II

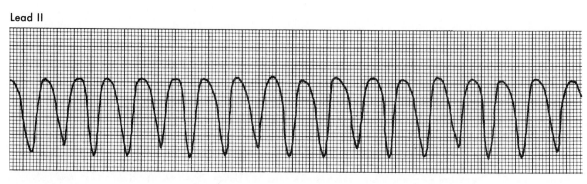

Figure 4B-1.   Initial rhythm of patient in Case Study B. Despite the rhythm, the patient is awake and alert.

> *Not every patient with ventricular tachycardia will immediately decompensate.* On the contrary, patients may sometimes remain in sustained VT for minutes— and even *hours* at a time.

The chance that a particular patient in sustained VT will remain hemodynamically stable is greatest when the rate of the ventricular response is not excessively rapid. This is the case here, since the heart rate in this example is not much over 150 beats/min. Rapid hemodynamic decompensation is much more likely to occur with heart rates in excess of 180 to 200 beats/min.

There are several things one could do to help determine whether the rhythm shown in Figure 4B-1 could possibly be supraventricular. Perhaps the simplest measure would be to look for a previous ECG recording from the patient to see what the QRS complex normally looked like when sinus (or some other supraventricular) rhythm was present. Obtaining a 12-lead ECG may prove equally valuable by confirming QRS widening, demonstrating the appearance of the QRS complex in other leads, and/or by identifying occult atrial activity. Other points to consider are discussed in detail in Chapters 15 and 16 (and include assessment of QRS morphology and physical examination signs). However, for now, *one HAS to assume that the regular (or at least fairly regular) wide-complex tachycardia shown in Figure 4B-1 is VENTRICULAR TACHYCARDIA until proved otherwise.* More important, *one should treat the patient accordingly* (i.e., as if the rhythm was ventricular tachycardia— until proved otherwise).

3. Consider <u>cough version</u>.

Although the mechanism of action is not exactly clear, instructing a patient who is still conscious to forcefully cough at the onset of ventricular tachycardia may maintain coronary and cerebral perfusion, and will occasionally convert the tachyarrhythmia to sinus rhythm. There is little to lose from a trial of cough version, and the maneuver may sometimes provide definitive therapy.

4. Administer a 50- to 100-mg IV bolus of <u>lidocaine</u>. Begin an infusion at 2 mg/min.

Given the extremely high likelihood that the rhythm shown in Figure 4B-1 is ventricular tachycardia—and the fact that the patient is still hemodynamically stable—a presumptive trial of medical therapy (with lidocaine) is the preferred course of action at this point.

5. *Think ahead.* Anticipate the *worst* thing that could happen to the patient—*and what you would do if this were to occur.*

Anticipating "the worst possible case scenario" can be helpful in two ways. First, it allows you to prepare the next line of medications and/or therapeutic modalities that you are likely to turn to if your present therapy does not work. Second

(and equally important), is that *thinking ahead* (and being able to formulate your next plan of attack) often has a *calming* effect—and increases your confidence in being able to successfully manage whatever future problems you might encounter.

> In this particular case, the "worst case scenarios" that could develop include *sudden decompensation* of the patient (i.e., loss of the pulse and/or blood pressure)—and/or development of ventricular fibrillation.

The lidocaine administered in Step #4 above has not had any effect. The patient's rhythm remains unchanged. Clinically she is still alert, fairly comfortable, and is maintaining a blood pressure of 90/60 mm Hg. *What to do now?*

Plan

6. Repeat the lidocaine bolus in several minutes. (A dose of between 50 and 75 mg IV is usually selected for the second bolus.)

QUESTION

If the patient did not respond to this second bolus of lidocaine, what would be your therapeutic options at this point? In other words, *how would you manage* **sustained ventricular tachycardia** *in a patient who remains hemodynamically stable?*

ANSWER

Therapeutic options to be considered *at this point* for treatment *of hemodynamically stable* sustained ventricular tachycardia might include:

1. Completing the protocol for lidocaine loading (by administration of a *third* bolus [of 50 to 75 mg] of IV lidocaine within 5 to 10 minutes after the second bolus was given).
2. A trial of *procainamide*
3. A trial of *bretylium*
4. *Synchronized cardioversion*
5. Alternative therapy.....

Although there is little likelihood that a third bolus of lidocaine will convert the patient if the first two boluses have not worked, this is still a reasonable therapeutic option at this point.

Procainamide is generally recommended as the *second* drug of choice (after lidocaine) for medical treatment of hemodynamically stable ventricular tachycardia. The drug is usually given in the form of 100 mg IV increments—each administered over a 5-minute period (at a rate of about 20 mg/min) until one of the following *end points* is achieved:

1. The patient has received a total loading dose of 500 to 1,000 mg
2. The arrhythmia is suppressed

3. Hypotension develops
4. QRS widening occurs

Alternatively, 500 to 1,000 mg of procainamide may be diluted in 100 ml of D5W and infused over 30 to 60 minutes. If successful, either loading regimen may be followed by a maintenance infusion of procainamide (beginning at an initial rate of 2 mg/min).

Use of **bretylium** has been deemphasized for treatment of ventricular tachycardia. In general, the drug is usually reserved for those cases of ventricular tachycardia that have not responded to other measures (i.e., neither lidocaine nor procainamide has been effective).

When bretylium is used to treat sustained ventricular tachycardia, it is probably best administered as a *slow* IV loading infusion. This may be prepared by mixing 500 mg (1 ampule) in 50 ml of D5W, and infusing this amount over a 10-minute period. If successful, bretylium loading may be followed by a maintenance infusion of the drug at a rate of 1 to 2 mg/min. Special attention should be directed at monitoring blood pressure during bretylium infusion (in view of the fact that hypotension is the most common adverse effect associated with use of the drug).

If there is no response to a trial of medical therapy (i.e., administration of lidocaine, and perhaps procainamide and/or alternative therapy), consideration might be given at this point to the use of **synchronized cardioversion.** As long as the patient remains hemodynamically stable, the procedure may be carried out under "semielective" circumstances. Ideally this will entail:

1. Sedation (with diazepam or another agent)
2. Calling anesthesia to the bedside (to assist with intubation if needed)—so as to leave you FREE to concentrate on managing the arrhythmia
3. A trial at a lower energy level (i.e., 50 joules initially, increasing to 100 to 200 joules as needed).

It should be emphasized that if the patient decompensates *at any time* during the treatment process, synchronized cardioversion is *immediately* indicated. Use of a higher initial energy level (of at least 100 to 200 joules) may be preferable in this situation.

Finally, consideration should be given to **alternative measures** that may be useful in the treatment of sustained ventricular tachycardia, especially if standard therapy has not been effective. Alternative measures might include one or more of the following:

1. Ruling out an underlying metabolic/acid-base abnormality (by STAT laboratory analysis of ABGs or serum electrolytes)
2. A trial of an *IV β-blocker* (i.e., **IV propranolol** in a dose of 0.5 to 1 mg IV, administered *slowly* up to a total dose of 5 mg)
3. A trial of IV magnesium.

Situations in which an IV **β-blocker** is most likely to be effective are those in which excessive sympathetic tone is implicated as an important etiologic factor (i.e., in the setting of acute ischemia and/or *anterior* infarction, particularly when cardiac arrest is preceded by a period of tachycardia or hypertension).

IV magnesium is clearly a drug of choice for treatment of torsade de pointes and for ventricular arrhythmias that occur in association with hypomagnesemia. In addition, it should be emphasized that IV magnesium may sometimes also be useful for treatment of ventricular arrhythmias *even when serum magnesium levels are normal.* As a result, administration of IV magnesium (in a dose of 1 to 2 g IV) on a purely *empiric basis* would not be unreasonable at this point in the therapeutic process.

The second bolus of lidocaine you have given has not been effective. You are about to administer a third (and final) bolus *when the patient suddenly loses consciousness.* The pulse has weakened, yet the rhythm on the monitor remains unchanged (i.e., sustained ventricular tachycardia is still present). *What should you do now?*

Plan

7. Think back to the "worst possible case scenarios" you had anticipated earlier. The patient has suddenly decompensated, and you are now dealing with a sustained ventricular tachycardia that has become *hemodynamically unstable.* As a result, *immediate* cardioversion is now in order. There is no time (or need in an unconscious patient) for sedation. Use *at least* 100 joules for this *emergency* cardioversion.

Immediately following synchronized cardioversion with 200 joules, the rhythm shown in *Figure 4B-2* develops. The

Lead II

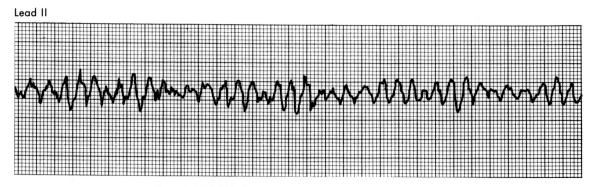

Figure 4B-2. Rhythm resulting from emergency cardioversion of hemodynamically significant ventricular tachycardia. There is no longer any pulse.

Lead II

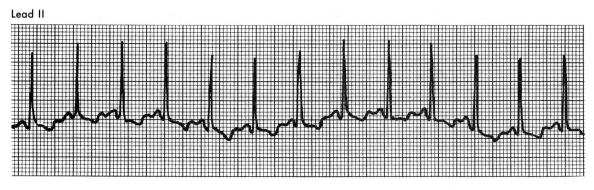

Figure 4B-3. Rhythm resulting from defibrillation of Figure 4B-2.

patient is unresponsive, and there is no pulse. What is the rhythm? *What to do now?*

Analysis of Figure 4B-2 and Plan

The patient has gone into *ventricular fibrillation*.

8. Shut off the synchronized mode and *immediately* <u>defibrillate</u> the patient with 200 joules.

 In view of the fact that the likelihood of successfully resuscitating a patient in ventricular fibrillation is *inversely proportional* to the interval between the onset of this rhythm and the application of countershock, this is probably the best chance you will *ever* have of converting a patient out of ventricular fibrillation. *You are right on the scene with a defibrillator, and should be able to apply countershock immediately.*

Your immediate defibrillation results in the rhythm shown in *Figure 4B-3. What should you do now?*

Analysis of Figure 4B-3 and Plan

Sinus tachycardia at a heart rate of 125 beats/min is seen on the monitor.

9. *Check for a pulse!* If a pulse is present, check for a blood pressure.

The pulse is strong and the blood pressure is 140/80 mm Hg. The patient is regaining consciousness.

 Note that morphology of the QRS complex in this lead is very different from what it was during the wide-complex tachycardia (Fig. 4B-1). This rules out a preexisting bundle branch block as the etiology for the rhythm that was shown in Figure 4B-1 and adds credence to our previous assumption that ventricular tachycardia was present.

10. Maintain the patient on a lidocaine infusion (at 2 mg/min).

Discussion

 This case illustrates the steps in the algorithm for treatment of sustained ventricular tachycardia *(see Fig. 1C-1).* The KEY factor resides in the first step: *identification of VT **and** assessment of hemodynamic status.* If a patient is hemodynamically compromised, it no longer matters whether the tachyarrhythmia is supraventricular or not since the treatment is the same—*emergency cardioversion to stabilize the patient!*

 On the other hand, if the patient is stable one has the luxury of trying antiarrhythmic agents and/or synchronized cardioversion on a relatively "semielective" basis. As emphasized earlier, if decompensation develops *at any time* during the treatment process, emergency synchronized cardioversion (with at least 100 joules) should then be *immediately* performed.

CASE STUDY C

You are obtaining a history from a middle-aged man who has just been admitted to the coronary care unit for evaluation and treatment of new-onset chest pain. He is still wearing a *nitroglycerin patch* on his chest which he had put on at home that morning. He has received 2 sublingual nitroglycerin tablets since arriving in the hospital. A peripheral IV of D5W at KVO has been inserted. Blood pressure is 100/70 mm Hg, the monitor shows sinus rhythm, and the patient is complaining of only mild chest discomfort—*when he suddenly loses consciousness.* You note the

rhythm shown in *Figure 4C-1* on the monitor. *What do you do?*

Analysis of Figure 4C-1 and Plan

The rhythm appears to be *ventricular fibrillation*.

1. Confirm unresponsiveness. Verify pulselessness. Deliver a <u>precordial thump</u>. Then yell for help and begin CPR.

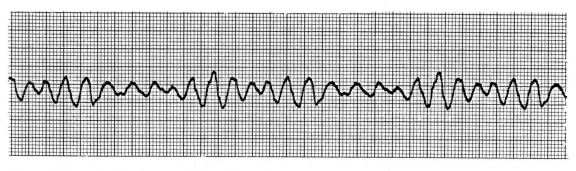

Figure 4C-1.   Initial rhythm of the patient in Case Study C. The patient has just been admitted to the hospital for new-onset chest pain. He suddenly loses consciousness as this rhythm strip is recorded.

This situation is one of the few indications for the precordial thump—*presence at the onset of ventricular fibrillation (witnessed by an ACLS provider)*. There is little to lose (the patient is pulseless), and definitive backup in the form of a defibrillator will soon be on hand.

There is no response to the precordial thump you deliver. Several CCU nurses with a crash cart and defibrillator have already joined you in the room. *What do you do next?*

    2. <u>Defibrillate</u> the patient with <u>200 joules</u> of delivered energy.

       As always before defibrillating, it is essential for the *code director* (= YOU!) to be sure that no one is in contact with the patient. Add conductive medium to the paddles, and apply firm pressure as you hold the paddles to the chest wall when discharging.

In this particular case, *what else should have been done BEFORE defibrillating?* (HINT: Refer back to the *second sentence* of the opening paragraph of this case study.)

Answer

    The patient's chest should have been wiped clean (and the nitroglycerin patch removed!) *before* defibrillating. If a patch (or nitroglycerin paste) is left on the chest of a patient who is defibrillated, sparks may fly (and/or much worse could happen).

    Defibrillation is successful in producing the rhythm shown in *Figure 4C-2. What is the rhythm?* How would you proceed? (i.e., *What would you do first?*)

Plan

    3. Check for a pulse!

       Even before attempting to interpret the rhythm, *it is essential to determine if a pulse is present*. If not, the rhythm is EMD (by definition!)—and this would mandate an entirely different therapeutic approach (e.g., immediate resumption of CPR, treatment with epinephrine, looking for an underlying cause of EMD).

    Despite the fact that the patient is still unresponsive, he is being adequately ventilated (with a bag-valve-mask and supplemental oxygen), and a pulse IS present. The pulse is associated with a palpable pressure of 60 mm Hg. In view of this, how would you interpret the rhythm shown in Figure 4C-2? *How would you proceed with treatment?*

Analysis of Figure 4C-2

    A bradyarrhythmia is seen in which the QRS complex is wide and the ventricular rate regular at 35 to 40 beats/min. The atrial rate is also fairly regular at about 90 beats/min. However, P waves are seen to "march through the QRS complex", and are totally unrelated to it (i.e., the PR interval constantly changes). This is *complete (3°) AV block*.

    4. Administer <u>atropine</u>.

       The suggested protocol for administration of atropine has been to give 0.5 mg IV every 5 minutes until a total dose of 2 mg is given. However, at the slow heart rate seen in Figure 4C-2 (and with this low a blood pressure), it would be quite reasonable to administer a larger initial dose of atropine (i.e., 1 mg). Alternatively, if one still preferred to begin with the

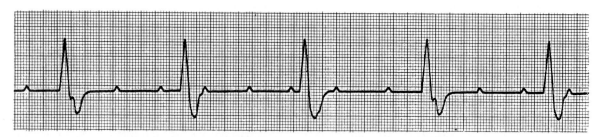

Figure 4C-2.   Rhythm resulting from defibrillation of Figure 4C-1.

lower dose of (0.5 mg) of atropine, a second dose (of 0.5 to 1 mg) of the drug can be given sooner (i.e., within 2 to 3 minutes, instead of waiting for a full 5 minutes) if the desired clinical response is not achieved.

5. Insert a <u>transvenous pacemaker.</u> Practically speaking, *pacemaker therapy* is the intervention of choice for treatment of hemodynamically significant 3° AV block that develops in the setting of cardiac arrest.

The patient fails to respond to 1 mg of atropine. You request assistance from cardiology for pacemaker insertion, but are told that it will be *at least* 10 minutes before the person on call will be able to get there. *What to do in the meantime?*

Plan

6. Intubate (since the patient is still unresponsive).
7. Repeat the atropine (by giving another 1 mg IV to complete the 2 mg "atropinization" dose.)
8a. While doing this, have your assistant prepare the <u>pressor agent of your choice</u> (in the event that the additional atropine is not effective).

                    and/or

8b. Set up an <u>external pacemaker.</u>

Isoproterenol and dopamine have both been commonly used as pressor agents in the setting of cardiac arrest. Recent years have seen a trend favoring much greater use of the latter. At low-to-moderate infusion rates (i.e., 2 to 10 μg/kg/min), **dopamine** primarily exerts a β-adrenergic effect. This leads to an increase in heart rate and stroke volume without necessarily increasing blood pressure. The α-adrenergic (vasoconstrictor) effect of the drug becomes more prominent at higher infusion rates (i.e., >10 μg/kg/min). Clinically, one usually begins a dopamine infusion at a rate of between 2 and 5 μg/kg/min. The drip is then titrated upward as needed according to the clinical response.

In contrast, **isoproterenol** works primarily by providing *chronotropic* support (as a result of its potent pure β-adrenergic effect). Overall, cardiac output usually increases with the use of this drug, but it may do so at the expense of excessive peripheral vasodilation and an increase in myocardial oxygen consumption.

A third alternative that may be used as a pressor agent is **epinephrine**—*when the drug is given as an **IV infusion.*** Bolus therapy with epinephrine is generally *not* recommended for treatment of bradyarrhythmias that are associated with a pulse and blood pressure because there is simply no way to titrate

the dose once the drug has been injected. Use of an IV infusion allows fine tuning of the dose with gradual adjustment of the amount administered as needed according to the clinical response. However, because of the potent α-adrenergic activity of epinephrine (which acts to vasoconstrict and increase afterload) as well as its potential arrhythmogenic effect, use of this drug is probably best reserved for treatment of slower bradyarrhythmias that cause a more significant degree of hemodynamic compromise than is the case here.

It should be emphasized that *regardless* of which drug is chosen, use of a pressor agent for treatment of atropine-resistant, hemodynamically significant bradycardia is *ONLY* a stopgap (i.e., temporizing) measure until pacemaker therapy is available.

Use of the **external pacemaker** has rapidly expanded in recent years. Obvious advantages of this device are that it is easy to apply (both in a hospital and prehospital setting), effective, and completely noninvasive. In a hospital setting, use of an external pacemaker may provide adequate hemodynamic support during the critical period while awaiting more definitive therapy (i.e., insertion of a transvenous pacemaker). Occasionally, use of the device as a temporizing measure may even obviate the need for subsequent transvenous pacing (i.e., if the bradyarrhythmia resolves). Finally, external pacing may be preferable to pharmacologic therapy because it does not produce adverse effects such as uncontrolled tachycardia, exacerbation of ventricular arrhythmias, or increased oxygen consumption that are sometimes seen with the use of atropine or a pressor agent.

If a *reliable* unit is readily available, **external pacing** is probably the ideal *initial* approach to management of *hemodynamically significant* bradyarrhythmias associated with cardiac arrest.

The second (1 mg) dose of atropine has no effect. The external pacemaker has been sent for. While awaiting its arrival, a dopamine infusion is begun. Moments later, the

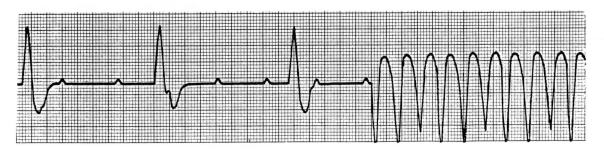

Figure 4C-3.   Rhythm that develops shortly after starting the dopamine infusion.

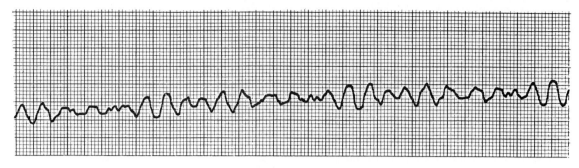

Figure 4C-4.   Rhythm resulting from delivery of a precordial thump.

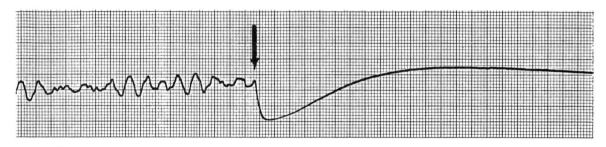

Figure 4C-5.   The patient is defibrillated with 200 joules at the point indicated by the arrow. What follows? *What to do?*

rhythm shown in *Figure 4C-3* is seen on the monitor. The patient is still unresponsive. A pulse is present, but it is hard to obtain a blood pressure. What has happened? *What should you do?*

Analysis of Figure 4C-3 and Plan

Midway through the rhythm strip shown above, the patient develops *ventricular tachycardia*.

> 9. *Stop the dopamine!* Reassess the patient.
>
>   It is all too easy to lose track of which medications have been given during a code (and in what dose), as well as which IV infusions are still ongoing. Clearly, if initiation of an IV infusion of a particular pressor agent results in an adverse hemodynamic effect, *the infusion must be stopped immediately.*

Despite stopping the dopamine, ventricular tachycardia persists. The patient remains unresponsive. The tachy-arrhythmia is associated with a weak pulse and a barely palpable systolic blood pressure of 60 mm Hg. A decision is made to deliver a *precordial thump*. The result is the rhythm shown in *Figure 4C-4*.

The pulse has been lost. What has happened? *What should you do now?*

Analysis of Figure 4C-4 and Plan

The precordial thump has precipitated *ventricular fibrillation*.

> 10. *Immediately* <u>defibrillate</u> the patient. Use 200 joules.
>
>   Since 200 joules were effective in converting the patient out of ventricular fibrillation at the onset of the code, it is reasonable to try this energy level again at this point.

The arrow in *Figure 4C-5* indicates the moment at which the electrical discharge is delivered. What follows? *What to do?*

Analysis of Figure 4C-5 and Plan

Defibrillation has resulted in *asystole*.

> 11. Since the rhythm on the monitor has changed again, reassess the patient (one more time) to verify continued unresponsiveness and pulselessness.
> 12. If no pulse is present—*immediately* resume CPR!
> 13. Verify that the rhythm is truly asystole (and *not* fine ventricular fibrillation) by quickly checking for a flat-line recording in several other leads.
> 14. Administer <u>epinephrine</u> (by either the IV or the ET route). Begin with <u>SDE</u>—and *rapidly increase* to <u>HDE</u> if there is no response.
>
>   Epinephrine (in as high of a dose as is needed) is the medical treatment of choice for asystole. Other potential therapeutic options for this disorder include atropine, sodium bicarbonate, and/or pacemaker therapy. The patient has already received the usual "full atropinzation dose" (of 2 mg), and an external pacemaker has already been sent for.
>
>   Use of sodium bicarbonate has been deemphasized for treatment of cardiac arrest. The drug is probably *not* indicated in this particular case (at least at this point), since the duration of the arrest is still relatively short, CPR was promptly initiated, and the patient is being adequately ventilated. One might want to obtain ABGs and perhaps consider bicarb administration *IF* the pH was excessively low (i.e., *less* than 7.15)—and/or if it were known that the patient had a severe *preexisting* metabolic acidosis. Even if these indications were present, many would still argue against using sodium bicarbonate because: (1) this therapy has *never* been shown to improve sur-

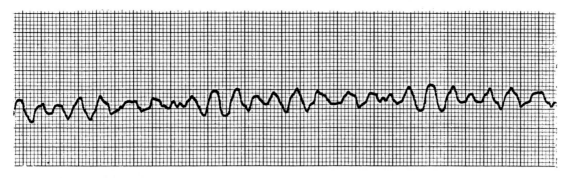

Figure 4C-6.   Rhythm resulting from treatment of asystole with HDE. Would you say that the epinephrine was effective? *How would you proceed?*

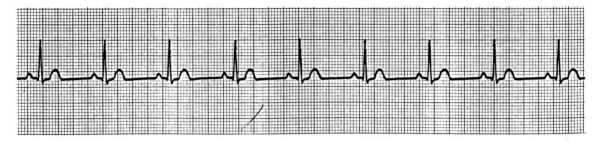

Figure 4C-7.   Rhythm resulting from defibrillation of ventricular fibrillation. *What is the first thing to do after seeing this rhythm?*

vival; (2) bicarb administration could be harmful (i.e., it may produce a paradoxical *intracellular* acidosis); and (3) adequate ventilation is the treatment of choice for the initial minutes of cardiac arrest (since it appears to take *at least* 5 to 15 minutes for a metabolic component of the acidosis to develop).

The presence of a true flat-line recording (i.e., definite asystole) is confirmed in several other leads. The decision is made not to give sodium bicarbonate. Instead, HDE is administered. A moment later the rhythm shown in *Figure 4C-6* is seen on the monitor. There is still no pulse.

Would you say that the epinephrine was effective? *How would you proceed?*

Analysis of Figure 4C-6 and Plan

Ventricular fibrillation is again evident on the monitor. Considering that the patient was in asystole, generation of ventricular fibrillation IS a beneficial response to administration of epinephrine *(since ventricular fibrillation is a rhythm you can treat!)*.

15. <u>Defibrillate</u> the patient with 200 joules.

   Since the last defibrillation attempt produced asystole, it may be advisable to remain at the lower energy level of 200 joules for this attempt.

Defibrillation results in the rhythm shown in *Figure 4C-7. What is the first thing to do after seeing this rhythm?*

Analysis of Figure 4C-7 and Plan

The monitor shows *normal sinus rhythm.* Practically speaking however, the *electrical* rhythm means *nothing* unless you . . . . . .

16. *Check for a pulse!*
17. If a pulse is present, *check for a blood pressure.* Reassess the patient clinically.

A strong pulse is present. Clinically, the rhythm shown in Figure 4C-7 is associated with a blood pressure of 130/85 mm Hg, but the patient has not regained consciousness.

   Despite the fact that the patient has not regained consciousness, he appears to be stabilizing (at least *hemodynamically!*). The time may be right to reassess selected clinical and laboratory parameters.

18. Verify again that ventilation is adequate and that equal (or appropriate) breath sounds are present bilaterally. It may also be a good idea to verify that the dopamine infusion you had previously asked to be discontinued (in Step #9) was in fact stopped at that time.
19. Consider obtaining the following laboratory tests: ABGs (if these have not yet been ordered), a chest x-ray (for endotracheal tube placement), a 12-lead ECG, and blood chemistries (as indicated).

   As emphasized earlier, it is extremely important to keep track of ALL medications that are given during the resuscitation effort, and to be aware of ALL *ongoing* IV infusions. It is not unusual for some patients to require temporary infusion of a pressor agent for hemodynamic support during the early postresuscitation period. However, it IS essential to know which drugs are being given, and to try to limit the amount infused to the lowest level needed to achieve (and maintain) the desired hemodynamic effect.

Considering that the patient has just been converted out of ventricular fibrillation (and is now hemodynamically stable), one more drug should be started (if you have not already done so). *Which drug?*

> 20. <u>Lidocaine.</u> Load the patient (with a 50- to 100-mg IV bolus), and start an IV infusion of lidocaine at a rate of 2 mg/min.
>
> > Administration of lidocaine is routinely recommended as a *prophylactic* measure to be started at the *earliest* opportunity in the resuscitation process (i.e., as soon as a patient is converted out of ventricular fibrillation and into a stable rhythm) in an attempt to minimize the chance that ventricular fibrillation will recur.

Discussion

In addition to reviewing the KEY steps in the algorithm for management of bradyarrhythmias **(Figure 1D-1),** a number of important issues are raised by this case study. Thus, one might ask:

1. Should a *precordial thump* have been given at the onset of ventricular tachycardia (in Fig. 4C-3)? Or, in view of the fact that the rhythm was associated with a pulse, *would you have managed this arrhythmia in a different manner?*
2. *How much energy should be used for defibrillation when ventricular fibrillation recurs during a code?* In this particular case study, an energy level of 200 joules was selected on two occasions for defibrillation when ventricular fibrillation recurred (i.e., in Steps #10 and #15). Although successful in the latter instance, defibrillation precipitated asystole in Step #10. *Was this complication avoidable?*
3. Defibrillation of the rhythm shown in Figure 4C-6 resulted in restoration of sinus rhythm (Fig. 4C-7) with a strong pulse and a blood pressure of 130/85 mm Hg. *But how would you have managed the patient if restoration of sinus rhythm was associated with hypotension?*

Perhaps the most difficult thing to do *after* participating in a code is to *review the process.* Although "hindsight is 100% accurate"–and success can *never* be guaranteed *(even if the optimal management approach is followed perfectly!)*–thoughtful review of the sequence of events of a code *immediately after* the acute situation has passed will often provide invaluable insight into the process, and help to improve the quality of care delivered with future resuscitation efforts.

> In this particular case, despite reasonable treatment and a favorable final outcome, *things did not go quite as well as they might have.* Thus, initial defibrillation was carried out with a nitroglycerin patch still on the patient's chest (Step #2); the external pacemaker was nowhere to be found in its greatest "moment of need" (Step #8b); administration of dopamine precipitated ventricular tachycardia (Step #8a)–delivery of the precordial thump caused this rhythm to deteriorate into ventricular fibrillation–and countershock resulted in further deterioration to asystole (Step #10). *Thoughtful reflection of these events may help improve future care.*

Use of the *precordial thump* has been deemphasized. The problem with this procedure is that there is no way to control the point in the cardiac cycle at which the energy will be delivered. As a result, use of *synchronized cardioversion* would seem to be far preferable to random delivery of the small amount of energy that the thump provides. Because of the unstable nature of this particular patient (the ventricular tachycardia was associated with a barely palpable systolic blood pressure of 60 mm Hg), a relatively high energy level (i.e., 100 to 200 joules) would seem preferable for the initial attempt at cardioversion.

Defibrillation is not benign. Use of excessive energy levels in the application of electrical countershock may produce additional damage to the conduction system. As a result, we generally favor using the lowest possible energy level for defibrillation during cardiopulmonary resuscitation *(and therefore routinely tend to drop back to an energy level of 200 joules when ventricular fibrillation recurs during cardiac arrest).* Despite this precaution, defibrillation precipitated development of asystole in Step #10 of this case study. Until further refinement of current-based defibrillation *(see Section D of Chapter 2),* the occasional occurrence of this complication would seem to be unavoidable. Use of the lowest energy level possible for defibrillation might limit its incidence.

> As discussed in Case Study B of this chapter, **anticipation** (of the "worst possible case scenario") may help in planning ahead and increasing your comfort in dealing with whatever situation you happen to encounter. In this case, anticipating "the worst that could happen" after Step #8a (and contemplating how you would approach management of the patient if "the worst" did occur) would have helped prepare you for the series of events that followed—including development of hemodynamically unstable ventricular tachycardia (Fig. 4C-3), ventricular fibrillation (Fig. 4C-4), and asystole (Fig. 4C-5).

A final issue raised by this case study relates to the question of how you would manage the patient if restoration of sinus rhythm at the end of the code (in Fig. 4C-7) would have been associated with hypotension. The answer would have to depend on the reason for the hypotension. Fluid resuscitation would be indicated if the patient was hypovolemic. Invasive hemodynamic monitoring might be needed if the diagnosis was unclear (and/or to guide therapy) in the postresuscitation period *(see Section D of Chapter 12).* Practically speaking, however, empiric treatment with a *dopamine* infusion is often tried initially in an attempt to resolve the problem.

CASE STUDY D

You are called to the emergency department where a *code in progress* has just been brought in. The patient is an elderly woman who had been found at home in an unresponsive state. The time from collapse until arrival of the EMS unit is unknown. CPR is being performed, the patient is intubated, and a large-bore peripheral IV is in place. One ampule of sodium bicarbonate and two ampules of epinephrine have already been given. Nothing else has been done. The patient is unresponsive. There is no spontaneous pulse, and monitor leads reveal the rhythm shown in *Figure 4D-1*. What do you do?

Analysis of Figure 4D-1 and Plan

The patient is in *ventricular fibrillation*.

1. <u>Defibrillate</u> with <u>200 joules</u> of delivered energy.

What should have been done before your arrival?

Answer

The patient should have been defibrillated!

Electrical defibrillation is by far the most important therapeutic intervention available for treatment of ventricular fibrillation. Consequently, as soon as one documents the presence of this rhythm, the patient should be defibrillated. Delay for the purpose of intubating the patient and/or insertion of an IV line is unacceptable. Use of quick-look paddles facilitates the process of documentation, and may save precious seconds that are wasted if time is taken to put monitor leads on.

There is no response. The rhythm shown in Figure 4D-1 persists. What next?

Plan

2. Verify pulselessness, immediately recharge the defibrillator paddles, and <u>defibrillate</u> again—this time with <u>300 joules</u>.

Once again there is no response. What next?

Plan

3. Verify pulselessness, immediately recharge the defibrillator paddles, and <u>defibrillate</u> a third time—this time with <u>360 joules</u>.

The patient is converted to the rhythm shown in *Figure 4D-2*. What now?

Plan

4. Check for a pulse.

There is *no pulse!!!!*
What does this mean? What treatment is indicated?

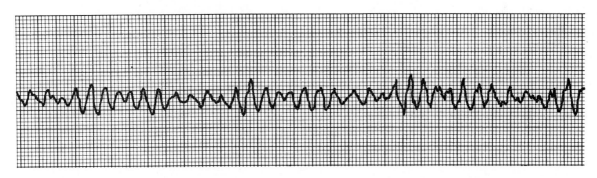

Figure 4D-1.   Initial rhythm of the patient in Case Study D. The patient is unresponsive and there is no pulse.

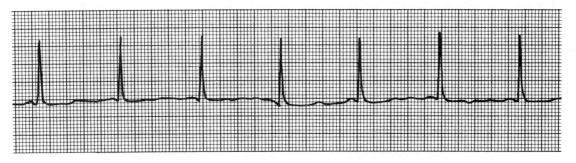

Figure 4D-2.   Rhythm resulting after the third countershock. *What now?*

Analysis and Plan

By definition the patient is in EMD, since there is organized electrical activity (i.e., the rhythm shown in Fig. 4D-2) but no effective mechanical contraction (i.e., there is no pulse!).

  5. Resume CPR.
  6. Repeat the epinephrine.
  7. Assess the patient clinically, and look for a *potentially reversible* cause of the EMD.

An ampule of epinephrine is given. Lung auscultation reveals no breath sounds on the left. After withdrawal of the endotracheal tube "a tad," bilateral breath sounds can be heard. Shortly thereafter, a weak pulse is felt. Blood pressure is 70 mm Hg systolic. *What to do?*

Plan

  8a. Begin dopamine.

  Prepare the drip by mixing 1 ampule of drug (200 mg) in 250 cc of D5W, and begin the infusion at 15 to 30 drops/min (≈2 to 5 μg/kg/min). Gradually increase the rate of infusion until the desired pressor response is seen.

or

  8b. Consider a trial of volume infusion.

Dopamine is begun and the blood pressure increases to 100/70 mm Hg. What should be done at this point? Sinus rhythm is still present on the monitor.

Plan

  9. Load the patient with a 50- to 100-mg IV bolus of lidocaine, and begin an infusion at 2 mg/min.

  Once again, administration of lidocaine after a patient is converted out of ventricular fibrillation into a stable rhythm is strongly recommended as a prophylactic measure in the hope of preventing recurrence of the event.

The patient is transferred to the coronary care unit.

QUESTION

  What would you have done if the pulse did not return after slight withdrawal of the endotracheal tube? That is, *how would you have managed persistent EMD?*

ANSWER

  The three KEY therapeutic measures for treatment of EMD are:

  1. Continue CPR.
  2. Administer epinephrine.
  3. Determine the underlying cause, and correct it if at all possible.

  If the patient in this case had failed to respond to initial therapeutic measures, one would therefore continue CPR, increase the dose of epinephrine (i.e., use HDE), and intensify

efforts to find the underlying cause. *Empiric therapy* (i.e., with fluid infusion and/or other interventions) would be indicated at this point *(see Discussion below.)*.

  Atropine may sometimes be effective for treatment of EMD associated with persistent bradycardia (Vanags et al, 1989). However, it is unlikely to be successful in this case because the heart rate of the rhythm shown in Figure 4D-2 is not excessively slow.

Discussion of Case D

  This case underscores the importance of *always* checking for a pulse after every therapeutic intervention (and/or change in the patient's status or cardiac rhythm). The appearance of sinus rhythm on the monitor means little when there is no accompanying pulse. *Without a pulse, EMD is the diagnosis.*

  In most cases, EMD is *secondary* to some other underlying disorder. Success with treatment will almost always depend on identifying and correcting this underlying cause. The most important etiologies to consider are shown in *Table 4D-1.*

Table 4D-1

Underlying Etiologies of Electromechanical Dissociation

Inadequate ventilation

- Intubation of right mainstem bronchus
- Tension pneumothorax (trauma, asthma, patient on ventilator)
- Bilateral pneumothorax (trauma)

Inadequate circulation

- Pericardial effusion with tamponade (trauma, pericarditis, uremia, too vigorous CPR)
- Myocardial rupture or rupture of aortic aneurysm
- Massive pulmonary embolism
- Hypovolemia due to:
  • Acute blood loss (trauma, GI bleeding)
  • Dehydration
  • Septic shock
  • Cardiogenic shock (acute myocardial infarction, myocardial contusion)
  • Anaphylactic shock
  • Neurogenic shock (cervical spine fracture)

Metabolic disorders

- Persistent acidosis (diabetic ketoacidosis, lactic acidosis)
- Electrolyte disturbance (severe hyperkalemia, hypokalemia, hypomagnesemia)
- Overdose of cardiac depressant drugs

Adapted from Grauer K: *Am Fam Physician* 29:223, 1984.

Therapeutically, the first thing to do when confronted with a patient in EMD is to resume CPR (since by definition EMD is a *nonperfusing* rhythm). Following this epinephrine should be given.

> The reason for using epinephrine in the treatment of EMD is that it favors blood flow to the heart and brain. This is important because some cases of EMD are *"primary"*—that is, the result of *diffuse myocardial ischemia* rather than the result of some other underlying cause (Ewy, 1984). Clinically, this situation is most likely to occur as the end point of a prolonged and unsuccessful resuscitation effort, although inadequate coronary perfusion per se may occasionally be a direct precipitant of EMD. In either case, treatment directed at optimizing myocardial blood flow may be effective in restoring mechanical function, and epinephrine would seem to be the ideal agent for accomplishing this (Nieman et al, 1986).

If a patient with EMD doesn't rapidly respond to epinephrine, a vigorous search for an underlying *secondary* etiology must be undertaken (Table 4D-1). Practically speaking, if EMD is due to rupture of an aortic aneurysm or massive pulmonary embolism, there is little one can do to save the patient. On the other hand, there are a number of *potentially reversible* causes of EMD that *CAN* be effectively treated if they are identified in time.

> Clinically, attention should focus on aspects of the history and physical examination that may suggest one of the causes of EMD listed in Table 4D-1. Use of selected laboratory tests (either obtained from review of the patient's chart and/or ordered STAT) may provide additional clues to the underlying cause.
>
> The most common potentially reversible cause of EMD is a *respiratory* disorder (Stueven et al., 1989). As a result, the first thing to check for on physical examination is the **adequacy of ventilation.** Absence of breath sounds on the left suggests intubation of the right mainstem bronchus. Simply withdrawing the endotracheal tube a small distance should restore bilateral breath sounds (as it did in this particular case study). If this maneuver is not successful—and/or breath sounds are absent on the right and tracheal deviation is present, the possibility of tension pneumothorax should be considered. One's index of suspicion for tension pneumothorax might be further increased in certain clinical settings (i.e., if there was a history of significant trauma, or in patients with asthma or chronic obstructive pulmonary disease—especially if they have been on a ventilator). In such cases, if time does not allow for the luxury of radiographic confirmation, a *diagnostic* (and *potentially therapeutic!*) tap with a large-bore needle (or Heimlich valve) may be indicated.

> The point of insertion for **emergency decompression** of *suspected tension pneumothorax* is in the second or third intercostal space. Pass the large-bore (16- or 18-gauge) needle *over the top of the rib* (to avoid the intercostal vessels that run along the lower border of each rib)—and insert the needle in the *midclavicular line* (to avoid the internal mammary artery that lies medially). Air under tension produces a hissing sound—*and dramatic improvement of the patient's hemodynamic condition should immediately follow.*

If inadequate ventilation is not the problem, attention should next be directed at **assessing volume status.**

> Clinically, the questions to address are:
>
> 1. Is the patient dehydrated?
> 2. Has the patient gone into cardiogenic shock (i.e., from a massive myocardial infarction)?
> 3. Was the patient at risk for throwing a pulmonary embolus?
> 4. Was there a known aortic aneurysm?
> 5. Could the patient have been in septic shock?

> Practically speaking, **hypovolemia** is one of the more easily potentially correctable causes of EMD. With this in mind, *even without an obvious reason for hypovolemia, empiric administration of a fluid challenge should be strongly considered at this point.*

A number of other potentially reversible causes of EMD should be considered including **persistent acidosis** (i.e., diabetic ketoacidosis, lactic acidosis), a severe **electrolyte disturbance** (i.e., hyperkalemia, hypokalemia, hypomagnesemia), and pericardial effusion with **tamponade.**

> Laboratory evaluation (i.e., with ABGs and STAT serum electrolytes) will assess some of these possibilities.
>
> *If cardiac tamponade is at all suggested* either by history (i.e., known uremia or pericarditis)—by the course of resuscitation (i.e., suspicion of fractured ribs from too vigorous CPR)—and/or by physical examination (presence of jugular venous distention or muffled heart sounds)—*pericardiocentesis* should be attempted. *Withdrawing as little as 50 ml of fluid under these circumstances may be lifesaving.*

> **Emergency pericardiocentesis** is best performed through a subxiphoid approach with insertion of the needle at a 20- to 30-degree angle with respect to the frontal plane. The needle should be directed toward the tip of the left shoulder. Aspiration is continuously applied. Entry into the pericardium usually produces a distinct "giving" sensation that should be followed by the appearance of *nonclotting* blood in the syringe. If the blood clots, it most likely has been removed from the right ventricle.

Finally, special consideration should be given to EMD that occurs in association with **trauma.** This situation should prompt the emergency care provider to actively consider an alternative set of causes.

> The mechanism of injury may be enlightening. For example, learning that a victim's automobile was demolished in a high-speed freeway accident in which the patient's chest deformed

the steering wheel before his head crashed through the windshield should suggest *at least* four possible etiologies for EMD including:

1. Acute blood loss (internal hemorrhage from abdominal injury, pelvic fracture, etc.)
2. Cardiogenic shock from myocardial contusion (the result of the steering wheel injury)
3. Neurogenic shock from cervical spine injury
4. Pericardial tamponade, bilateral pneumothorax, or tension pneumothorax from trauma to the chest wall

RECENT DEVELOPMENTS IN OUR UNDERSTANDING OF EMD

EMD has always been defined as the presence of *organized electrical activity* (in the form of a rhythm on the ECG monitor) *in the absence of meaningful cardiac contraction* (Ewy, 1984). Clinically this means that the patient is pulseless, and that there is no detectable blood pressure. However, recent evidence suggests this working definition may not be completely accurate. Rather than an "all-or-none" phenomenon, it now appears that the clinical entity of EMD really encompasses a *spectrum* of disorders in which some mechanical function is actually present in many (if not most!) patients.

> Support for this theory was provided in an echocardiographic study by Bocka et al (1988) in which an overwhelming majority of patients diagnosed as having EMD demonstrated at least some degree of meaningful (i.e., organized) mechanical activity—albeit insufficient to generate a palpable pulse. In another study by Berryman (1986), almost half of a group of patients initially "thought to be in EMD" were found to have detectable systolic blood pressure readings of between 40 to 100 mm Hg when arterial pressure was measured directly.

It therefore appears that EMD is really a *relative* finding, and that many patients diagnosed with this disorder actually have "undetected perfusion" (Callaham and Barton, 1990). These results may have a number of potentially important clinical implications:

1. *The prognosis of patients diagnosed as having EMD may not be as uniformly dismal as was once thought.* On the contrary, certain subsets of patients may have a surprisingly good chance for recovery. Some degree of organized myocardial contractility is likely to be preserved in such individuals, and intensive medical therapy stands a reasonable chance of restoring a pulse. At the other end of the spectrum is the subset of patients for whom EMD is a preterminal rhythm. Meaningful cardiac function is unlikely to be present, and medical therapy is usually futile.

2. Attention to certain clinical features may help determine where in this spectrum of EMD a particular patient lies. Awareness of this information may prove useful *prognostically* (when deciding how far to pursue the resuscitation effort), as well as *therapeutically* (in

determining the most appropriate dose of epinephrine to use).

Rhythm analysis and use of ET CO_2 monitoring may both provide insight in this regard. Thus, survival from EMD appears to be most likely if there is *organized atrial activity*—either on the initial ECG—or if organized atrial activity develops in response to treatment (Aufderheide et al, 1989; Stueven et al, 1989). In contrast, ultimate survival from EMD is much less likely when organized atrial activity is absent, the QRS complex is wide, and/or bradycardia persists despite medical treatment. Prognosis is poorest when the initial rhythm associated with EMD manifests QRS widening with a monophasic complex and no atrial activity at all (Stueven et al, 1989). These adverse rhythm prognostic indicators probably reflect a prolonged period of anoxia, and correlate clinically with a poor prognosis *irrespective* of whatever additional therapeutic interventions are tried (Aufderheide et al., 1989; Stueven et al, 1989).

ET CO_2 monitoring may also be helpful in predicting the potential viability of patients with EMD. Thus, a relatively high initial ET CO_2 reading (i.e., ≥15 torr) suggests that at least some meaningful myocardial contraction may exist. Restoration of a spontaneous pulse appears to be much more likely in such individuals (Callaham and Barton, 1990). In contrast, low ET CO_2 readings (either initially, or after therapy) augur for a much poorer prognosis.

3. Consideration might also be given to *doppler determination* of blood pressure to explore (rule out) the possibility of subclinical contractile activity (in the form of a measurable, but nonpalpable systolic blood pressure). If present, this may indicate a group of patients at the less severe end of the spectrum. Such patients would seem to be the group most likely to respond to treatment with epinephrine, since this drug is the ideal agent for stimulating contractile function in the setting of cardiac arrest (Bocka et al, 1988). Lower doses of drug (i.e., SDE) may suffice in some cases, and *could* be tried first. If unsuccessful, *rapid titration* to HDE is indicated. On the other hand, it would seem much less likely that SDE will work when there is no contractile activity at all—especially when the initial rhythm associated with EMD is one of the adverse prognostic indicators described above (and/or initial ET CO_2 readings are extremely low). Maximal doses of epinephrine should be tried much sooner in such individuals—and even then, the chances for long-term survival are dismal.

References

Aufderheide TP, Thakur RK, Stueven HA, Aprahamian C, Zhu YR, Fark D, Hargarten K, Olson N: Electrocardiographic characteristics in EMD, *Resuscitation* 17:183-193, 1989.

Berryman CR: Electromechanical dissociation with directly measurable arterial blood pressures, *Ann Emerg Med* 15:625, 1986 (abstract).

Bocka JJ, Overton DT, Hauser A: Electromechanical dissociation in human beings: An echocardiographic evaluation, *Ann Emerg Med* 17:450-452, 1988.

Callaham M, Barton C: Prediction of outcome of cardiopulmonary resuscitation from end-tidal carbon-dioxide concentration, *Crit Care Med* 18:358-362, 1990.

Charlap S, Kahlam S, Lichstein E, Frishman W: Electromechanical dissociation: Diagnosis, pathophysiology, and management, *Am Heart J* 118:355-360, 1989.

Ewy GA: Defining electromechanical dissociation, *Ann Emerg Med* 13:830-832, 1984.

Nieman JT, Haynes KS, Garner D, Rennie CJ, Jagels G, Stormo O: Postcountershock pulseless rhythms: Response to CPR, artificial cardiac pacing, and adrenergic agonists, *Ann Emerg Med* 15:112-120, 1986.

Stueven HA, Aufderheide TP, Waite EM, Mateer JR: Electromechanical dissociation: Six years prehospital experience, *Resuscitation* 17:173-182, 1989.

Stueven HA, Aufderheide TP, Thakur RK, Hargarten K, Vanags B: Defining electromechanical dissociation: Morphologic presentation, *Resuscitation* 17:195-203, 1989.

Vanags B, Thakur RK, Stueven HA, Aufderheide TP, Tresch DD: Interventions in the therapy of electromechanical dissociation, *Resuscitation* 17:163-171, 1989.

CHAPTER 5

FINDING THE ERROR: MORE PRACTICE FOR MEGA CODE

This chapter has been added to provide a final practice for MEGA CODE. Six *code vignettes* are presented. For each, the patient's rhythm is shown, and information regarding clinical appearance and hemodynamic status is provided. *One or more flagrant errors in treatment have been made.* You are asked to review the sequence of events and the treatment that was given for the present scenario—*and then to "Find the Error(s)."*

The points brought out by these code scenarios should once again reinforce the principles that are essential to master in order to effectively run a cardiac arrest. Recognition of these errors—and understanding why a particular treatment given is not the most appropriate course of action—are important preparatory exercises for the MEGA CODE station.

EXERCISE A

Preceding Scenario

A middle-aged man of average (≈70 kg) size is admitted to the coronary care unit (CCU) with chest pain to rule out acute myocardial infarction. He is on oxygen and has received some morphine, but no other medications. Shortly thereafter, the rhythm shown in *Figure 5A-1* is noted on telemetry.

Present Scenario

Clinical Appearance: The patient is alert and complaining of chest discomfort at the time the rhythm shown in Figure 5A-1 is recorded.

Hemodynamic Status: BP = 90 palpable.

Sequential Treatment Given for the Present Scenario:

1. <u>Lidocaine</u>—75 mg by IV bolus.
2. <u>Bretylium</u>—infusion of 500 mg (mixed in 50 ml of <u>D5W</u>) over a 10-minute period–and followed by a continuous infusion at a rate of 2 mg/min.
3. <u>Epinephrine</u>—1 mg by IV bolus (i.e., SDE).
4. <u>Defibrillation</u>—with 200 joules.

Find the Error(s)

- **How would you interpret the rhythm shown in Figure 5A-1?**
- **Do you agree with the treatment given?** *What might you have done differently?*

Analysis

Rhythm Interpretation: A regular, wide QRS complex tachycardia is present at a rate of about 115 beats/min. There is no sign of atrial activity. One must therefore assume this to be *ventricular tachycardia* until proven otherwise.

Treatment Analysis: Although the rate of the VT shown in Figure 5A-1 is not extremely rapid, a number of other factors about this case scenario are definite cause for concern. These include the fact that the patient has been admitted to the hospital for suspected acute infarction, that he is still having chest discomfort, and that the arrhythmia is associated with a barely adequate systolic blood pressure (of 90 palpable). Treatment is clearly indicated.

Because the patient is conscious, alert, not in acute dis-

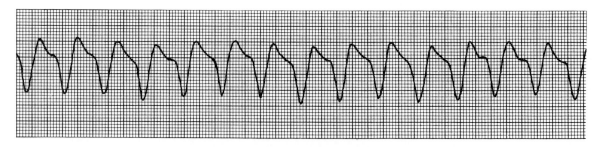

Figure 5A-1. Rhythm obtained from a middle-aged man with new-onset chest pain.

tress, and still maintaining a blood pressure of 90 mm Hg, a *brief* trial of medical therapy is reasonable. Were hemodynamic decompensation to occur at any time during such therapy, immediate *synchronized* cardioversion would be indicated.

> Alternatively, some emergency care providers might argue that cardioversion should be performed initially, given the patient's somewhat precarious hemodynamic status. This approach would also be reasonable. If this course of action was chosen, there would be time to sedate the patient, call anesthesia to the bedside, and select a relatively low energy level (50 joules) for the initial cardioversion attempt.

If you chose to begin with medical therapy, lidocaine would be the drug of choice. The initial bolus prescribed in Step #1 above (75 mg) is an appropriate amount, considering the size of the patient (who we are told weighs ≈70 kg). However, in addition to a bolus, a continuous infusion of the drug should have also been started (to prevent the effect of the bolus from wearing off).

Administration of bretylium is *not* the next step. Although bretylium is an effective *antifibrillatory* agent, its use has been de-emphasized for treatment of ventricular tachycardia. In general, lidocaine *and* procainamide should both be tried (in therapeutic doses) *before* turning to bretylium. Thus in this particular case, if the initial 75-mg IV bolus of lidocaine didn't work, the next step would be to rebolus with one or more additional 50- to 75-mg doses of lidocaine before moving on to procainamide.

Administration of epinephrine (Step #3) is obviously wrong, since the potent chronotropic and inotropic action of this agent can only make the arrhythmia worse. Epinephrine is the drug of choice for medical treatment of *ventricular fibrillation*, but it is contraindicated with ventricular tachycardia.

Finally, the patient should *not* have been defibrillated with an *unsynchronized* countershock (Step #4). If the need for electrical therapy arose (i.e., if hemodynamic decompensation developed and/or medical therapy failed to convert the arrhythmia), energy delivery should have been *synchronized* to minimize the chance that the electrical impulse will occur on the T wave (the vulnerable period) and precipitate ventricular fibrillation.

EXERCISE B
Preceding Scenario

An EMS unit is called to the scene of a cardiac arrest. The victim is an elderly woman who has been "down" for an estimated "5 minutes" before arrival. CPR was performed by a witness at the scene. The paramedics immediately intubated the patient, and have just secured a peripheral IV line. The rhythm observed on quick-look paddles is shown in *Figure 5B-1*.

Present Scenario

Clinical Appearance: The patient is unresponsive.
Hemodynamic Status: No pulse. No blood pressure.
Sequential Treatment Given for the Present Scenario:

1. Epinephrine—1 mg by ET administration.
2. Sodium bicarbonate—2 ampules IV.
3. Defibrillation—with 300 joules.
4. Defibrillation—with 360 joules.
5. Bretylium—500 mg by IV bolus.
6. Epinephrine—1 mg (this time by IV bolus). Repetition of this dose every 5 minutes thereafter.

Find the Error(s)

- **How would you interpret the rhythm shown in Figure 5B-1?**
- **Do you agree with the treatment given?** *What might you have done differently?*

Analysis

Rhythm Interpretation: The patient is in *ventricular fibrillation*.

Treatment Analysis: The KEY to treating ventricular fibrillation is to defibrillate the patient *as soon as possible*. Although quick-look paddles were used on the scene to identify the initial rhythm of the arrest, *defibrillation was unnecessarily delayed!* Clearly the patient should have been defibrillated *BEFORE* being intubated, having an IV started, and receiving epinephrine and sodium bicarbonate.

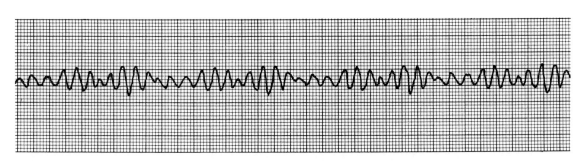

Figure 5B-1.   Rhythm observed on quick-look paddles applied to an elderly woman who has been "down" for an estimated "5 minutes."

The recommended energy level for the *initial* counter-shock attempt is 200 joules—*not* the 300 joules that were administered in Step #3 of this scenario.

> The lower energy level of 200 joules appears to be equally effective for this first countershock, yet less likely to produce asystole or other conduction system disturbance than if a higher initial energy level was used. If initial defibrillation is unsuccessful, a second countershock attempt with increased energy (300 joules) should be tried, to be followed in rapid succession by a *third* attempt with maximal energy (360 joules). *Only two attempts at defibrillation were made in this case.*

If defibrillation is unsuccessful in converting ventricular fibrillation, administration of epinephrine becomes the intervention of choice. The drug should be given *as soon as possible* after the initial series of countershocks via the *first* medication access route established. Thus, ET administration of 1 mg of epinephrine (as was given in Step #1 of this scenario) was completely appropriate. However, this should probably have been followed by IV administration of the drug at a sooner point in the process than Step #6. More important, in view of the substantial "down time" *before* arrival of the EMS unit (estimated to be "5 minutes"), *much larger* doses of epinephrine (i.e., HDE) should have been tried *much sooner* in the process (if not *immediately* after establishing IV access).

> Layperson estimation of "down time" is an exceedingly difficult phenomenon to interpret—especially when such estimation is purely subjective (i.e., untimed), and made by an individual who has just seen a loved one suddenly collapse in front of them. *Minutes may seem like hours* . . . . (or the other way around). Although realistically, the chance for long-term recovery (with intact neurologic function) is practically nil if a patient with out-of-hospital cardiac arrest is initially found in asystole, this is *not* necessarily the case for a patient who is initially found in ventricular fibrillation. Moreover—even if the patient has been truly "down" for an *extended* period of time—there is no way to know if they had been in cardiac arrest for this entire period, or if perhaps they were in a perfusing rhythm (i.e., sustained ventricular tachycardia with a pulse) that only later deteriorated to ventricular fibrillation. Practically speaking then, one *ALWAYS* has to err on the side of the patient—which means: *initiate (and continue) intense resuscitation efforts UNTIL there is conclusive evidence of cardiovascular unresponsiveness.*

Regarding other interventions in this particular code scenario, the advisability of administering sodium bicar-bonate in Step #2 is questionable. Unless there was clear evidence of a severe, preexisting metabolic acidosis, it would seem preferable to try other measures (i.e., defibrillation, HDE, optimizing ventilation) *prior* to administering sodium bicarbonate—especially since sufficient time (i.e., *more than* 5 to 10 minutes) may not yet have passed for a metabolic component of the acidosis to develop.

> Hyperventilation (rather than sodium bicarbonate) is the treatment of choice for the acidosis that develops during the *initial* minutes of cardiac arrest. The value of sodium bicarbonate has never been proved, and the drug may be counterproductive (i.e., it may exacerbate the degree of intracellular acidosis).

Bretylium is not the drug of choice for medical treatment of refractory ventricular fibrillation. Thus instead of administering 500 mg of IV bretylium in Step #5, it would have been preferable to try lidocaine first.

> Because of the markedly decreased clearance of lidocaine in the arrested heart, it is not essential to start an infusion of this drug as long as ventricular fibrillation persists. Once converted out of ventricular fibrillation, however, the patient should be rebolused with lidocaine, and an infusion begun.

If one (or two) bolus of lidocaine was unsuccessful, it would then be appropriate to try either bretylium and/or other antifibrillatory measures (i.e., empiric use of magnesium sulfate or perhaps an IV β-blocker).

> The final point to emphasize about antifibrillatory therapy is that administration of a drug by itself rarely results in spontaneous conversion of ventricular fibrillation. Instead, CPR must be performed for 1 to 2 minutes following administration in order to circulate the drug. Repeating defibrillation after that period of time may then be effective.

EXERCISE C
Preceding Scenario

An elderly man is admitted to the CCU for evaluation and treatment of new-onset chest pain. His symptoms are relieved by small doses of morphine and nitroglycerin. A 12-lead ECG initially shows a regular sinus rhythm with evidence of acute *inferior* myocardial infarction. Shortly thereafter, the rhythm changes *(Figure 5C-1)*.

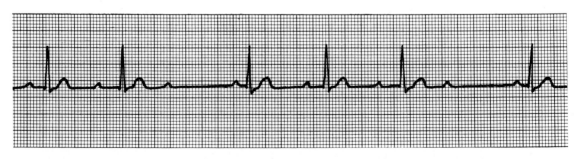

Figure 5C-1.   Rhythm obtained from an elderly man admitted to the CCU for acute *inferior* infarction. He is asymptomatic at the time of this recording.

Present Scenario

Clinical Appearance: The patient is comfortable and is not having any more chest pain at the time the rhythm shown in Figure 5C-1 is recorded.

Hemodynamic Status: Blood pressure is 110/70 mm Hg.

Sequential Treatment Given for the Present Scenario

1. Atropine—1 mg by IV bolus.
2. Cardiology consultation (for transvenous pacemaker insertion).
3. Repetition of the 1-mg dose of atropine while waiting for cardiology to come.
4. Preparation to begin an isoproterenol infusion if the patient fails to respond to atropine.

Find the Error(s)

- **How would you interpret the rhythm shown in Figure 5C-1?**
- **Do you agree with the treatment given?** *What might you have done differently?*

Analysis

Rhythm Interpretation: Despite the obvious irregularity of the ventricular response, the atrial rate is regular for the most part. Each QRS complex is preceded by a P wave, and the PR interval gradually prolongs until a beat is dropped. The rhythm is 2° *AV block, Mobitz type I (Wenckebach)*.

Treatment Analysis: Mobitz type I 2° AV block occurs *much more* commonly than does the Mobitz type II form of 2° AV block. This is fortunate because the overall prognosis for Mobitz I is much better than it is for Mobitz II.

> Mobitz I 2° AV block is most commonly seen in the setting of acute *inferior* myocardial infarction. Patients are usually hemodynamically stable, and do *not* require treatment in most cases. Thus, the conduction disturbance generally resolves spontaneously, and pacemaker insertion is only *rarely* needed.
>
> In contrast, Mobitz II more often occurs in association with acute anterior myocardial infarction. The level of the block is usually lower in the conduction system (i.e., *below* the AV node). As a result, the QRS complex will almost always be wide (whereas it is most often narrow with Mobitz I), and the ventricular response slower and less reliable. Pacemaker insertion is essential.

In this particular case scenario, the patient does not require any treatment at this time because:

1. He is asymptomatic.
2. He is hemodynamically stable.
3. AV block is of the Mobitz I type in the setting of acute *inferior* infarction.

Instead, the preferred course of action is close observation (and perhaps standby availability of an external pacemaker in the unlikely event it is needed). If the patient

was symptomatic *from the bradycardia*, treatment with atropine would be indicated. However, it should be emphasized that atropine is *not* a benign medication, and that this drug should be used *only* if there is evidence of *hemodynamic compromise* (i.e., hypotension, mental confusion, chest pain). Because this is clearly not the case here, no atropine at all should have been given in Steps #1 and #3.

> Activity of *both* sympathetic and parasympathetic components of the autonomic nervous system is often increased with acute myocardial infarction. With inferior infarction, parasympathetic tone usually predominates (which is why one commonly sees associated bradycardia and hypotension). Administration of vagolytic doses of atropine blocks this parasympathetic tone. However, if underlying sympathetic hyperactivity is also present, it may now be unopposed. This explains how giving atropine could result in tachycardia, increased oxygen consumption, and/or potentially serious ventricular tachyarrhythmias. It is therefore important to administer the drug with caution to patients with acute myocardial infarction, limiting the dose to 0.5 mg at a time (especially if the patient shows signs of only "mild" hemodynamic compromise). In contrast, when heart rate is markedly decreased (i.e., 40 beats/min or less) and/or blood pressure is extremely low (60 mm Hg systolic or less), administration of 1-mg increments of atropine is reasonable.

Even greater caution is advised for administration of isoproterenol (Step #4) than with atropine. Potential adverse effects that may result from use of this pressor agent include precipitation/aggravation of ventricular arrhythmias and/or increased myocardial oxygen consumption. As a result, use of a pressor agent (be it isoproterenol, dopamine, or epinephrine by infusion) is indicated *only* as a stopgap measure for treatment of atropine-resistant, hemodynamically significant bradyarrhythmias while awaiting pacemaker therapy.

Obvious advantages of external pacing are that it is effective, rapidly applied, and entirely noninvasive. Thus, standby availability of this modality will often be all that is needed in the management of relatively benign conduction system disorders (such as hemodynamically stable Mobitz I 2° AV block) that usually resolve on their own.

EXERCISE D

Preceding Scenario

An elderly woman arrests in the outpatient clinic. She is immediately attended to by the staff, who utilize the clinic crash cart at the scene. An initial rhythm of ventricular fibrillation responds to the first 200-joule countershock attempt and converts to the rhythm shown in *Figure 5D-1*. An IV of D5W has been started.

Present Scenario

Clinical Appearance: The patient is unresponsive and is not spontaneously breathing.

Hemodynamic Status: There is no pulse and no

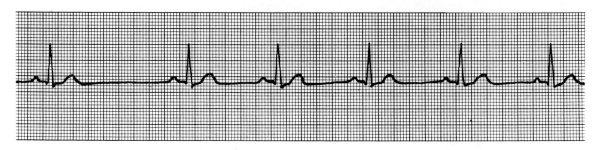

Figure 5D-1.   Rhythm resulting from defibrillation of an elderly woman who had just arrested in the outpatient clinic.

blood pressure at the time the rhythm shown in Figure 5D-1 is recorded.

Sequential Treatment Given for the Present Scenario:

1. Intubation.
2. Atropine—1 mg by IV bolus. Repetition of this dose (i.e., 1 mg) 5 minutes later.
3. Sodium bicarbonate—2 ampules.
4. Isoproterenol—infusion at an initial rate of 2 μg/min, with upward dose titration as needed.
5. Calcium chloride—500 mg by IV bolus.

Find the Error(s)

- **How would you interpret the rhythm shown in Figure 5D-1?**
- **Do you agree with the treatment given? *What might you have done differently?***

Analysis

Rhythm Interpretation: The mechanism of the rhythm is sinus, as each QRS complex is preceded by a P wave with a fixed PR interval. A pause follows the first beat, after which the rhythm becomes regular at 52 beats/min. It is hard to be sure of the reason for the pause with only this short rhythm strip available. However, this becomes academic when one considers that the patient is pulseless and unresponsive. She is therefore in *electrical-mechanical dissociation (EMD)*.

Treatment Analysis: Three KEY measures are essential to the management of EMD:

1. *Continuous* performance of CPR (since by definition EMD is a *nonperfusing* rhythm).
2. Administration of epinephrine (in a dose of 1 mg initially—*rapidly increasing* to HDE if there is no response).
3. Search for an underlying cause of the EMD.

Practically speaking, *the chance for meaningful* (i.e., neurologically intact) *survival depends on identifying AND correcting the underlying cause of the disorder.* Epinephrine (in as high a dose as is needed) is indicated because it is the drug of choice for optimizing coronary and cerebral perfusion in the arrested heart. Administration of atropine (in a dose of 1 mg IV, and repeated 5 min later) may occasionally

be helpful in cases of EMD associated with bradycardia—which justifies its use in this case (Step #2). However, *epinephrine should have been tried first.* Intubation is appropriate because the patient was unresponsive and not spontaneously breathing (Step #1). But *NONE of the other medications given were indicated at this point in the resuscitation process.* Thus, it is unlikely that sufficient time (i.e., *more than* 5 to 10 minutes) had yet passed to justify the use of sodium bicarbonate (Step #3); the vasodilatory effect of isoproterenol *lowers* aortic diastolic pressure, and is therefore couterproductive in the setting of cardiac arrest (Step #4); and calcium chloride, if anything, appears to adversely affect survival of patients with EMD who are not hyperkalemic (Step #5).

EXERCISE E

Preceding Scenario

A middle-aged man complaining of chest pain presents to the emergency department. An IV is started, and he is hooked up to a monitor. As the rhythm shown in *Figure 5E-1* is recorded, the patient becomes unresponsive.

Present Scenario

Clinical Appearance: Unresponsive. Not breathing spontaneously.

Hemodynamic Status: No pulse can be palpated in association with the rhythm strip shown in Figure 5E-1.

Sequential Treatment Given for the Present Scenario:

1. Lidocaine—100 mg by IV bolus, followed by continuous IV infusion of the drug at a rate of 2 mg/min.
2. Rebolus (with 75 mg) of lidocaine, with increase in the rate of the IV infusion to 3 mg/min.
3. *Synchronized* cardioversion with 200 joules.

Find the Error(s)

- **How would you interpret the rhythm shown in Figure 5E-1?**
- **Do you agree with the treatment given? *What might you have done differently?***

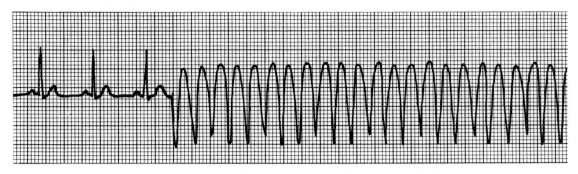

Figure 5E-1. Rhythm obtained from a middle-aged man who becomes unresponsive as this strip is recorded.

Analysis

Rhythm Interpretation: Sinus rhythm is present for the first three beats of this strip. This is interrupted by a run of sustained *ventricular tachycardia* with an extremely rapid ventricular response.

Treatment Analysis: The treatment approach for ventricular tachycardia depends on the patient's hemodynamic status during the tachyarrhythmia. If hemodynamic compromise develops at any time, restoring perfusion MUST assume highest priority. In the case of *pulseless* ventricular tachycardia (as occurs here), this should be accomplished by *immediate* delivery of *unsynchronized* countershock (with 200 joules). A precordial thump could be tried first (while someone is getting the defibrillator and charging it), but *there is NO justification for delaying therapy to administer lidocaine when the patient is pulseless* (Steps #1 and #2). Similarly, time should not be wasted attempting synchronization (Step #3) in the setting of a nonperfusing rhythm.

In contrast, if a pulse and acceptable blood pressure were present in association with sustained ventricular tachycardia (as was the case in Exercise A), a trial of medical therapy with lidocaine would be completely appropriate.

> The reason *unsynchronized countershock* is generally preferred (over synchronized cardioversion) for treatment of pulseless ventricular tachycardia is simply that it can be applied faster with *at least* equal success. The extremely rapid rates of ventricular tachycardia that usually accompany the pulseless state frequently preclude accurate synchronization by the defibrillator. Distinction between the QRS complex and the T wave becomes difficult (and/or *the T wave itself* may be sensed *instead of* the QRS—especially if the T wave is relatively tall in amplitude). Routine use of *unsynchronized countershock* for treatment of pulseless ventricular tachycardia obviates this problem.

Thus, the easiest way to conceptualize the treatment approach of sustained ventricular tachycardia is to categorize the arrhythmia according to the patient's hemodynamic status. One of three situations will be present:

1. *The patient will be pulseless.* In this case, the rhythm is treated *exactly* the same as ventricular fibrillation—with application of *unsynchronized countershock* as soon

as this is possible. Lidocaine is begun immediately *after* defibrillation.

2. *A pulse will be present and the patient is hemodynamically stable.* In this case there is at least some time for a trial of medical therapy (with lidocaine and/or other measures). Immediate *synchronized* cardioversion is indicated if hemodynamic decompensation occurs at any point during the treatment process.

3. *A pulse will be present, but the patient shows signs of hemodynamic compromise* (i.e., hypotension, chest pain, mental confusion). Immediate *synchronized* cardioversion is indicated. Lidocaine is begun immediately *after* cardioversion.

EXERCISE F
Preceding Scenario

A cardiac arrest has been in progress. The patient was initially in ventricular fibrillation which converted to a supraventricular tachycardia after a third countershock with maximal energy. Lidocaine was administered, but despite this, ventricular fibrillation recurred. Repeat countershock produced the rhythm shown in *Figure 5F-1*. The patient has been intubated, a large-bore peripheral IV has been started, and CPR is being performed. An estimated 5 minutes have passed since the code began.

Present Scenario

Clinical Appearance: The patient is unresponsive. No spontaneous respirations.

Hemodynamic Status: There is no pulse and no blood pressure at the time the rhythm shown in Figure 5F-1 is recorded.

Sequential Treatment Given for the Present Scenario:

1. Sodium bicarbonate—2 ampules IV.
2. Atropine—0.5 mg by IV bolus. Repetition of this dose (0.5 mg) 5 minutes later.
3. Dopamine—infusion at an initial rate of 30 drops/min (having mixed 200 mg in 250 ml of D5W)—

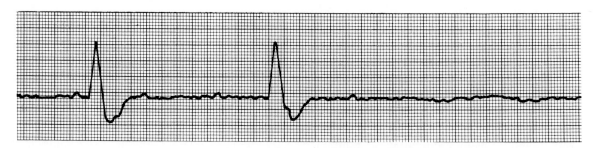

Figure 5F-1.   Rhythm obtained from a patient in cardiac arrest after 5 minutes of resuscitation. The recording is the result of the last defibrillation attempt.

with upward titration of the rate of infusion as needed.
4. Transvenous pacemaker insertion.
5. Calcium chloride—500 mg by IV bolus.
6. Epinephrine—0.5 mg by IV bolus. Repetition of this dose (0.5 mg) every 5 minutes thereafter.

Find the Error(s)

- **How would you interpret the rhythm shown in Figure 5F-1?**
- **Do you agree with the treatment given?** *What might you have done differently?*

Analysis

Rhythm Interpretation:. Two wide (idioventricular) complexes are seen, and then asystole results. This is an *agonal rhythm.*

Treatment Analysis: The sequential treatment administered in this case scenario is far from ideal. Sodium bicarbonate should *not* be routinely given during the early minutes of cardiac arrest (Step #1). Atropine may occasionally be effective in the treatment of asystole, and its administration is reasonable in this particular case. However, the optimal dose of atropine for this indication is probably 1 mg (and *not* 0.5 mg that was given here). Furthermore, considering the seriousness of the situation, this 1-mg dose should probably have been repeated in very

short order (i.e., in *less* than 5 min) if there was no response (Step #2). Low-dose dopamine (as was ordered in Step #3) would be unlikely to exert a potent enough α-adrenergic (vasoconstrictor) effect to adequately favor myocardial blood flow. Pacemaker insertion is indicated, but its effectiveness with asystole tends to be inversely proportional to the amount of time that has passed until such therapy is instituted. Application of an external pacer would therefore be preferred in this situation, since it is much more likely to be accomplished in a timely fashion than is insertion of a transvenous pacemaker (as was tried in Step #4). Finally, calcium chloride, if anything, appears to adversely affect survival of patients with asystole (or agonal rhythm) who are not hyperkalemic (Step #5).

The treatment of choice for asystole (and/or agonal rhythm) is to resume CPR and administer epinephrine. In this particular case, it seems as if this drug was given almost as an afterthought (in Step #6) at a point when all other medications and modalities had been tried and failed. Instead, *early administration of epinephrine in much larger amounts is essential.* If the decision is made to begin with SDE (i.e., use of a 1-mg dose of epinephrine), the amount of drug should be *rapidly* increased (i.e., to HDE) if there is no response.

Use of a 12-lead ECG machine would help to verify that the rhythm shown in Figure 5F-1 was truly asystole (and not fine ventricular fibrillation that is "masquerading" as asystole in the one lead being monitored).

CHAPTER 6

SELF-ASSESSMENT: PRACTICE FOR THE WRITTEN TEST

This chapter provides an opportunity for *self-assessment* and preparation for the written test in the ACLS course. Select the best answer(s) to the following questions. *(Many questions have more than one answer.)*

1. Steps in the assessment and management of the unconscious victim include:
   i)   Calling for help.
   ii) Establishing unresponsiveness.
   iii) Positioning the victim.
   iv) Applying the ABCs of CPR.

   Which of the following indicates the correct order in which these steps should be performed?
   a. i, ii, iii, iv
   b. i, iii, ii, iv
   c. ii, i, iii, iv
   d. ii, iii, iv, i
   e. iv, i, ii, iii

2. Treatment for asystole includes which of the following?
   a. Epinephrine
   b. Atropine
   c. Calcium chloride
   d. Pacemaker insertion
   e. Isoproterenol

3. The *single* most common cause of airway obstruction in the unconscious victim is:
   a. A foreign body
   b. Food
   c. Dentures
   d. The tongue
   e. Edema from epiglottitis or tracheobronchitis.

4. Regarding the diagnosis of acute myocardial infarction, which one of the following is the *most* important factor to consider in deciding whether to admit a patient with chest pain?
   a. Initial ECG
   b. Chest x-ray film
   c. Cardiac enzymes
   d. Technetium pyrophosphate scan
   e. History

5. Which of the following measures may be useful in the treatment of paroxysmal supraventricular tachycardia?
   a. Sedation
   b. Verapamil
   c. Carotid sinus massage
   d. Infusion of isoproterenol
   e. Adenosine

6. Pulse oximetry provides information on:
   a. End-tidal carbon dioxide level.
   b. Arterial carbon dioxide content.
   c. Arterial carbon dioxide saturation.
   d. Arterial oxygen saturation.
   e. End-tidal oxygen level.

7. For optimal effectiveness of external chest compression in an adult, it is recommended that the sternum be depressed:
   a. 0.5 to 0.75 inch.
   b. 1 inch.
   c. 1.5 to 2 inches.
   d. 2.5 inches.
   e. 3 to 4 inches.

8. Which of the following statements is (are) true regarding supraventricular bradyarrhythmias with acute myocardial infarction?
   a. They are particularly common during the first hour following the onset of symptoms.
   b. They are most often associated with anterior infarction.

   c. They usually reflect increased parasympathetic tone.
   d. They should be routinely treated with atropine.
   e. All of the above.

9. Which of the following statements is (are) true regarding recommendations for the performance of two-rescuer CPR in the unintubated patient?
   a. At least 80 compressions should be performed each minute.
   b. There should be a 15:2 ventilation to compression ratio.
   c. Each compression should be sustained for 40% of the cycle.
   d. CPR may be stopped for up to 45 seconds at a time when needed for endotracheal intubation or moving a patient.
   e. The cardiac output produced by properly performed external chest compression may be 60% of normal output.

10. Pulselessness in an infant is established by checking for the presence of:
    a. A carotid pulse.
    b. A brachial pulse.
    c. A radial pulse.
    d. Precordial activity.
    e. A femoral pulse.

11. The most common mechanism of sudden cardiac death is:
    a. Ventricular tachycardia/fibrillation.
    b. Asystole.
    c. Electromechanical dissociation.
    d. Long QT syndrome.
    e. Idioventricular rhythm.

12. In an unmonitored arrest situation, which of the following should be done first after the diagnosis of ventricular fibrillation has been established?
    a. Apply countershock with 200 joules of delivered energy.
    b. Apply countershock with 360 joules of delivered energy.
    c. Administer epinephrine IV or by intratracheal instillation.
    d. Administer sodium bicarbonate.
    e. Administer lidocaine.

13. Which of the following statements about sodium bicarbonate is (are) true?
    a. The drug should be routinely given as soon as possible in cardiac arrest.
    b. The initial dose for a patient in cardiac arrest is 0.5 mEq/kg.

   c. Indiscriminate use may result in a paradoxical intracellular acidosis.
   d. The drug is probably unnecessary if the period of cardiac arrest is only a few minutes in duration.
   e. Each ampule of sodium bicarbonate contains 25 mEq of drug.

14. The appropriate amount of drug for IV administration of SDE (standard-dose epinephrine) is:
    a. 0.1 mg of a 1:10,000 solution.
    b. 1 mg of a 1:10,000 solution.
    c. 10 mg of a 1:10,000 solution.
    d. 1 mg of a 1:1000 solution.
    e. 10 mg of a 1:1000 solution.

15. Relative or absolute contraindications to thrombolytic therapy include which of the following?
    a. Age over 65
    b. Recent history of peptic ulcer disease
    c. Severe hypertension
    d. Recent history of a TIA (transient ischemic attack)
    e. Atrial fibrillation

16. The most important priority in the management of cardiopulmonary resuscitation of children is to:
    a. Establish an intravenous line.
    b. Defibrillate the patient.
    c. Manage the airway.
    d. Administer epinephrine.
    e. Suction the patient.

17. Which of the following statements about procainamide is (are) true?
    a. The drug may be administered in 100-mg increments IV every minute until a loading dose of 1 g has been given.
    b. Its use is indicated for ventricular arrhythmias that are resistant to lidocaine.
    c. Its use may result in widening of the QRS complex.
    d. It rarely causes hypotension when given IV.
    e. The drug may lengthen the QT interval.

18. Which of the following statements about dopamine is (are) true?
    a. The drug is a chemical precursor of norepinephrine.
    b. At doses above 20 µg/kg/min it dilates renal and mesenteric blood vessels.
    c. It primarily exerts an α-receptor stimulating action at low doses.
    d. It is indicated for treatment of cardiogenic shock and hemodynamically significant hypotension.
    e. It comes in 1-ml ampules that contain 500 mg of drug.

19. Cannulation of the internal jugular vein by the central approach is performed by introducing the needle:
    a. 1 cm below the junction of the middle and medial thirds of the clavicle.
    b. At the midpoint of the anterior border of the sternomastoid muscle.
    c. At the junction of the lower and middle thirds of the anterior border of the sternomastoid muscle.
    d. At the apex of the triangle formed by the two heads of the sternomastoid muscle and the clavicle.
    e. Under the sternomastoid muscle near the junction of the middle and lower thirds of the lateral border of this muscle.

20. Which of the following statements about airway obstruction is (are) true?
    a. Dentures and an elevated blood alcohol level are frequently associated with choking on food.
    b. Foreign body obstruction of the airway accounts for nearly as many cases of cardiopulmonary arrest as does coronary heart disease.
    c. Back blows and manual thrusts should be applied in the management of both partial and total airway obstruction.
    d. Foreign body obstruction of the airway rarely occurs during eating.
    e. The abdominal thrust to relieve airway obstruction cannot be applied by the victim on himself/herself.

21. Which of the following statements is (are) true regarding the performance of basic life support in infants and children?
    a. Adequate external chest compression in the infant may be performed with only two fingers.
    b. The proper area of compression in the infant is the midsternum.
    c. The sternum should be depressed 0.25 to 0.5 inch with external chest compression in the infant.
    d. The compression to ventilation ratio is 5:1 for both one and two rescuers.
    e. The compression rate in infants is at least 80/min.

22. What is the recommended initial energy dose for the defibrillation of a 20-kg child?
    a. 10 joules
    b. 20 joules
    c. 40 joules
    d. 60 joules
    e. 80 joules

23. A BVM device should consist of which of the following characteristics?
    a. A clear mask

b. An easy-to-grip bag
    c. A system to deliver supplemental O_2
    d. An oxygen reservoir
    e. No pop-off valve

24. The most common cause of sudden cardiac death in adults is:
    a. Mitral valve prolapse.
    b. Coronary artery disease.
    c. Acute myocardial infarction.
    d. Hypertrophic cardiomyopathy.
    e. Massive pulmonary thromboembolism.

25. Which of the following statements about Mobitz I 2° AV block is (are) true?
    a. The level of this block usually originates below the AV node.
    b. The conduction defect is usually transient.
    c. The block may be the result of the increased parasympathetic tone that is commonly associated with acute inferior infarction.
    d. Group beating is commonly seen.
    e. The block may be caused by digitalis toxicity.

26. Which of the following statements about atrial flutter in adults is (are) true?
    a. The atrial rate is usually between 200 and 240 beats/min.
    b. The ventricular response is usually between 100 and 120 beats/min.
    c. The rhythm is a common manifestation of digitalis toxicity.
    d. It can usually be converted to sinus rhythm with low-energy cardioversion.
    e. Application of carotid sinus massage may be helpful in confirming the diagnosis.

27. Which of the following factors would suggest that an abnormal QRS complex is an aberrantly conducted PAC rather than a PVC?
    a. The finding of a premature P wave in front of the abnormal complex
    b. The presence of a full compensatory pause
    c. A QRS complex width of greater than 0.14 second for the abnormal complex
    d. A typical right bundle branch block pattern of the abnormal complex in a right-sided monitoring lead
    e. The presence of atrial fibrillation

28. Treatment of ventricular tachycardia may include which of the following?
    a. Cardioversion
    b. Lidocaine
    c. Procainamide

d. Verapamil
e. Bretylium

29. Treatment for 3° AV block may include which of the following?
a. Verapamil
b. Isoproterenol or dopamine
c. Insertion of a pacemaker
d. Calcium chloride
e. Atropine

30. Insertion of a subclavian or internal jugular line is preferable on the right side because of which of the following reasons?
a. The dome of the right lung and pleura is lower than that of the left side.
b. Both veins are larger on the right side.
c. There is more or less a straight line to the atrium.
d. The landmarks are easier to recognize on the right side.
e. The large thoracic duct is not endangered.

31. The esophageal obturator airway (EOA):
a. Requires visualization of the airway for insertion.
b. When removed is frequently followed by immediate regurgitation.
c. Should be removed before endotracheal intubation is performed.
d. Presents some potential for damage to the esophagus.
e. Is a superior technique to endotracheal intubation.

32. Endotracheal intubation:
a. Should be performed as the first step in CPR.
b. Should be preceded by oxygenation of the lungs by other methods of ventilation.
c. Allows adequate lung inflation without causing gastric distention.
d. Is always necessary for adequate lung ventilation.
e. Provides an alternative route for administration of medication.

33. Oxygen-powered mechanical breathing devices for use during CPR:
a. Are satisfactory only if pressure cycled.
b. Are satisfactory only if manually triggered.
c. Are safest when the flow rate is set at below 60 L/min.
d. Are not capable of delivering high concentrations of oxygen to the patient
e. Can be used in patients of all ages and sizes.

34. Epinephrine:
a. Increases peripheral vascular resistance.
b. Can restore electrical activity in asystole.

c. Can facilitate defibrillation of ventricular fibrillation
d. Increases myocardial contractility.
e. Is contraindicated in electromechanical dissociation.

35. Atropine sulfate:
a. Is of no value in ventricular tachycardia.
b. Is always required if the heart rate is less than 50 beats/min.
c. Is usually given in 0.1 mg boluses up to a total of 0.5 mg.
d. May be of value in symptomatic bradyarrhythmias.
e. Is a benign treatment.

36. Lidocaine:
a. May facilitate defibrillation of ventricular fibrillation.
b. Usually has no significant effect on myocardial contractility.
c. May be useful in treating multiform PVCs.
d. May cause asystole.
e. May cause seizures.

37. Which of the following ECG rhythms may mimic ventricular tachycardia?
a. Paroxysmal supraventricular tachycardia (PSVT) with aberration.
b. PSVT with left bundle branch block (LBBB)
c. Atrial tachycardia with block
d. Very rapid atrial fibrillation with LBBB
e. PSVT with right bundle branch block (RBBB)

38. Which of the following drugs may be useful in preparing the heart for electrical conversion from ventricular fibrillation to an effective rhythm?
a. Oxygen
b. Calcium chloride
c. Epinephrine
d. Morphine
e. Verapamil

39. Isoproterenol:
a. Increases myocardial irritability.
b. Results in α-adrenergic stimulation.
c. Lowers peripheral vascular resistance.
d. Speeds the heart rate.
e. Increases myocardial oxygen consumption.

40. Which of the following drugs when used in therapeutic doses will usually not directly depress cardiac contractility?
a. Atropine
b. Lidocaine
c. Propranolol

d. Isoproterenol
e. Verapamil

41. Arterial blood gas values of pH = 7.3, P_{CO_2} = 60 mm Hg, and HCO_3 = 30 mEq/L suggest which of the following:
    a. Metabolic acidosis
    b. Metabolic alkalosis
    c. Respiratory acidosis
    d. Respiratory alkalosis
    e. A mixed acid-base disorder

42. Risk factors of coronary artery disease include:
    a. Hypertension.
    b. Smoking.
    c. Level of fitness.
    d. Male sex.
    e. Type A personality.

43. Which of the following drugs/therapeutic measures may be useful for treating asystole after an unwitnessed cardiac arrest?
    a. Lidocaine, epinephrine, and sodium bicarbonate
    b. Epinephrine, atropine, pacemaker therapy
    c. Verapamil, atropine, and calcium chloride
    d. Isoproterenol, dopamine, and atropine
    e. Epinephrine, bretylium, calcium chloride

44. Which of the following statements regarding IV lines in the setting of cardiac arrest is (are) true?
    a. A large-bore IV is preferable.
    b. A femoral line is undesirable for administrating drugs.
    c. Sterile technique must be used.
    d. The first thing to do in an arrest is to start an IV.
    e. Drug delivery may be improved by following drug administration with a bolus of fluid.

45. Cardiac arrest in children is usually preceded by/the result of:
    a. Myocardial infarction.
    b. Cardiac arrhythmias.
    c. Hypoxia secondary to respiratory arrest.
    d. SIDS (sudden infant death syndrome).
    e. Valvular heart disease.

46. Nitroglycerin:
    a. May be effective in treating angina pectoris.
    b. Reduces preload in patients with congestive heart failure.
    c. Relieves bronchospasm.
    d. Is useful in treating the chest pain of acute myocardial infarction.
    e. May lower blood pressure in patients with acute myocardial infarction.

47. How much pressure should be exerted on each electrode paddle during adult defibrillation?
    a. 5 lb
    b. 10 lb
    c. 15 lb
    d. 20 lb
    e. 25 lb

48. Which of the following are considered end points during the administration of IV procainamide?
    a. QRS widening of 100% of its pretreatment width
    b. Hypotension
    c. A loading dose of 2 g
    d. Control of the arrhythmia
    e. Hypertension

49. During the course of synchronized cardioversion, a patient suddenly develops ventricular fibrillation. Which of the following steps should be taken?
    a. Begin external chest compression immediately.
    b. Administer 50 to 100 mg lidocaine IV.
    c. Immediately repeat synchronized cardioversion with the same energy.
    d. Immediately turn off the synchronizer switch and proceed with unsynchronized countershock.
    e. Administer epinephrine.

50. Reasons sodium bicarbonate has been de-emphasized in the treatment of cardiac arrest are that:
    a. It may shift the oxyhemoglobin dissociation curve to the right (thus resulting in easier release of oxygen to the tissues).
    b. It may cause a paradoxical intracellular acidosis.
    c. It may cause hypoosmolality.
    d. Its use may result in production of iatrogenic metabolic alkalosis.
    e. Hyperventilation is the preferred way to correct the acidosis that occurs during the initial minutes of the arrest.

51. Clinical indications of lidocaine toxicity include which of the following?
    a. Disorientation
    b. Paresthesias
    c. Diarrhea
    d. Agitation
    e. Seizures

52. Clinical factors that suggest a patient with acute myocardial infarction is likely to benefit greatly from thrombolytic therapy include which of the following?
    a. Recent onset of symptoms (i.e., symptom duration of *less* than 4 hours)
    b. Marked ST segment elevation on the initial ECG
    c. Marked reciprocal ST segment depression on the initial ECG

d. Anterior location of infarction
e. Absence of Q waves on the initial ECG

53. Adenosine:
    a. Is much more effective than verapamil in the treatment of PSVT.
    b. Is usually effective in the treatment of atrial fibrillation.
    c. Has a half-life of only 60 seconds.
    d. May cause transient bradycardia.
    e. May need to be repeated in the acute treatment of PSVT.

54. The recommended technique for opening the airway in a patient with suspected neck injury is:
    a. Head tilt–chin lift.
    b. Jaw thrust.
    c. Chin lift.
    d. Head tilt–jaw thrust.
    e. Head tilt–neck lift.

55. Parameters that are helpful in assessing the work of breathing include:
    a. Tachycardia.
    b. Use of accessory chest muscles.
    c. Use of abdominal muscles.
    d. Suprasternal and substernal retractions.
    e. Nasal flaring.

56. Which of the following factors are important in determining survival from out-of-hospital ventricular fibrillation?
    a. Prompt recognition of cardiac arrest by the lay public (and early activation of emergency medical services)
    b. Initiation of CPR by a bystander within 4 minutes
    c. Initiation of ACLS within 8 minutes
    d. The mechanism of the arrest
    e. All of the above

57. Which of the following ventilatory assist measures/devices is (are) *not* recommended for use in children?
    a. Endotracheal intubation
    b. Pocket mask
    c. Esophageal obturator airway
    d. BVM device
    e. Oxygen-powered breathing device

58. What would you expect the pH to be for a patient with a *pure* respiratory acidosis if the $PaCO_2$ is 55 mm Hg?
    a. 7.36
    b. 7.32
    c. 7.28
    d. 7.24
    e. 7.20

59. Inspiratory stridor suggests:
    a. Lower airway obstruction.
    b. Upper airway obstruction.
    c. Bronchial obstruction.
    d. Chronic obstructive pulmonary disease.
    e. Pneumonia.

60. Potential indications for synchronized cardioversion include:
    a. Ventricular fibrillation.
    b. Rapid atrial fibrillation in a hypotensive patient.
    c. Sinus tachycardia in a hypotensive patient.
    d. Ventricular tachycardia in a hypotensive patient.
    e. Asystole.

TRUE/FALSE QUESTIONS

61. In the "sniffing" position, the neck is extended backward as the head is flexed forward.

62. To intubate a patient with a curved blade, the tip is inserted into the vallecula, and traction is exerted upward and forward to displace the epiglottis anteriorly and expose the glottis.

63. The tidal volumes generated with a bag-valve mask device are much greater than those delivered by the mouth-to-mouth technique.

64. A Venturi mask is advantageous for use in patients with chronic obstructive pulmonary disease because of its ability to deliver a controlled oxygen concentration.

65. The femoral vein lies medial to the artery in the femoral sheath.

66. In adults, ventricular tachycardia is a much more common cause of a regular wide complex tachycardia than SVT with aberration.

67. Nitroglycerin is contraindicated in the management of acute myocardial infarction, since there is the risk of its causing hypotension.

68. Ventricular fibrillation is at least 10 times more common during the first 2 hours after the onset of symptoms of an acute myocardial infarction than during the subsequent 24 hours.

69. The Killip classification for patients with acute myocardial infarction can reliably predict which patients will have elevated pulmonary capillary wedge pressures with hemodynamic monitoring.

70. Induction of diuresis is the treatment of choice for right-sided heart failure associated with pure right ventricular infarction.

71. Insertion of a pacemaker significantly reduces mortality in patients who develop complete right bundle branch block with acute myocardial infarction.

72. Isoproterenol may be useful in the treatment of cardiac arrest because of its pure β-adrenergic effect, which favors coronary perfusion.

73. The dose of lidocaine should be reduced in the presence of congestive heart failure.

74. For a malpractice claim to be successful, the plaintiff must establish only that a patient-physician relationship existed and that the physician was negligent in the care rendered to the patient.

75. A "do not resuscitate" (DNR) order cannot be written unless the patient and the family are both competent and willing.

76. The AED (automatic external defibrillator) is intended primarily for use by the lay public (i.e., spouse or family of the victim of a cardiac arrest).

77. Acute epiglottitis is most commonly seen in patients who are older than 2 years of age.

78. The usual pediatric response to hypoxemia is tachycardia.

79. A 3° AV block that occurs in the setting of acute *inferior* infarction will almost always require pacemaker insertion.

80. The esophageal obturator airway (EOA) is inserted with the patient's head in the sniffing position.

81. The presence of *"warning arrhythmias"* reliably predicts those patients who are most likely to develop ventricular fibrillation in the setting of acute myocardial infarction.

82. Lidocaine is the treatment of choice for sustained ventricular tachycardia associated with hypotension.

83. Initial evaluation of a patient with new-onset chest pain (to rule out acute myocardial infarction) is primarily based on the initial ECG and cardiac enzymes.

84. The cause of acute myocardial infarction is almost always acute occluding thrombus formation in a major coronary vessel.

85. It is unsafe to perform cardiac catheterization and/or angioplasty in the setting of acute myocardial infarction.

86. An important factor to consider in the selection of respiratory assist devices for administration of supplemental oxygen is whether the patient is breathing through their nose or mouth.

87. Tidal volumes attainable by ventilation with a pocket mask are significantly less than those achieved from ventilation with a BVM device.

88. End-tidal carbon dioxide monitoring can be used to help confirm endotracheal tube placement.

89. In patients with acute myocardial infarction, the initial ECG may provide important prognostic information even when it is normal.

90. When suctioning an unconscious patient, the suction catheter should be inserted through the lumen of the oral pharyngeal airway.

91. When performing external cardiac compressions on infants, finger placement should be parallel to the nipple line.

92. In an intubated patient, ventilation need not be synchronized to external chest compressions.

93. The most common terminal event in pediatric cardiopulmonary arrest is asystole.

94. When using an AED (automatic external defibrillator) for resuscitation of a victim of out-of-hospital cardiac arrest, it is important to first perform rescue breathing before defibrillating.

95. The dose of atropine for a 15-kg infant is 0.75 mg IV.

96. It is likely that the use of HDE (high-dose epinephrine) will significantly increase long-term survival rates for patients with out-of-hospital ventricular fibrillation that has not responded to defibrillation.

97. Mobitz I 2° AV block is slightly more common than Mobitz II with acute myocardial infarction.

98. The most common potentially reversible cause of EMD is hypovolemia.

99. The most common adverse reaction to a bretylium infusion is hypertension.

100. A patient in ventricular tachycardia may remain conscious for several hours without sign of hemodynamic compromise.

Answers to Self-Assessment: Practice for the Written Test

1. The correct order of steps in assessment and management of the unconscious victim is **establishing unresponsiveness (ii), calling for help (i), positioning the victim (iii), and applying the ABCs of CPR (iv). (Choice C)**

   (See Section A of Chapter 10.)

2. Treatment for asystole includes **epinephrine (A), atropine (B), and pacemaker insertion (D).**

   Calcium chloride is no longer recommended for treatment of asystole. Data proving its efficacy are lacking, and some studies suggest mortality to be increased with the use of this agent. Similarly, isoproterenol is no longer recommended for treatment of asystole. The vasodilatory effect of this agent *lowers* aortic diastolic blood pressure, resulting in reduced myocardial blood flow. (See Chapters 1 and 2.)

3. The *single* most common cause of airway obstruction in the unconscious victim is **the tongue (D).**

   The tongue has been affectionately named as "the enemy of the airway." This is because in the unconscious victim the musculature that normally supports the tongue relaxes, allowing this structure to fall back and obstruct the airway. (See Chapter 7.)

4. The *most* important factor to consider in deciding whether to admit a patient with chest pain to the hospital is **the history (E).**

   Despite the tremendous diagnostic and prognostic importance of the initial ECG, it is often not the deciding factor that determines whether or not to admit the patient to the hospital. Moreover, the initial ECG may remain normal for the first few hours of acute infarction. Occasionally it *never* shows changes. Cardiac enzymes should *not* be used to decide whether to admit the patient, and neither the chest x-ray nor the technetium pyrophosphate scan is of much help in the acute decision-making process. In contrast, if the history is at all suggestive, the patient should be admitted. (See Section A of Chapter 12.)

5. Measures that may be useful in the treatment of paroxysmal supraventricular tachycardia include **sedation (A), verapamil (B), carotid sinus massage (C), and adenosine (E).**

   Verapamil and adenosine are equally effective for the acute treatment of PSVT in adults. Vagal maneuvers (such as carotid sinus massage) may occasionally be effective even without medication. Not generally appreciated is the fact that sedation may also be helpful. In addition to relieving the anxiety that so often accompanies this tachyarrhythmia, sedation reduces sympathetic tone. This is important because enhanced sympathetic tone may help perpetuate PSVT by shortening the refractory period of AV nodal tissue and speeding up conduction through the area. (See Chapter 1 and Section B of Chapter 16.)

6. Pulse oximetry provides information on **arterial oxygen saturation (D).**

   Oximetry is a noninvasive way to provide continuous measurement of the *arterial oxygen saturation* (SaO_2) of the blood. When oxygen saturation values are high (i.e., in the range 95-100%), the emergency care provider can feel comfortable that PaO_2 concentrations will also be quite good. However, it is important to realize that a relatively small decrease in the oxygen saturation value (i.e., to the 90-95% range) may correspond to a surprisingly large drop in the PaO_2 reading. When in doubt (i.e., whenever oxygen saturation values drop into the low range), strong consideration should be given to obtaining an ABG study to determine the true oxygen content of the blood. (See Chapter 7).

7. For optimal effectiveness of external chest compression in an adult, it is recommended that the sternum be depressed **1.5 to 2 inches (C).**

   For optimal effectiveness of chest compression, the sternum should be depressed between 0.5 to 1 inch for infants, 1 to 1.5 inches for children (i.e., between 1 to 8 years old), and 1.5 to 2 inches for older children and adults. (See Section C of Chapter 17.)

8. Supraventricular bradyarrhythmias with acute myocardial infarction **are particularly common during the first hour following the onset of symptoms (A), and usually reflect increased parasympathetic tone (C).**

   Supraventricular bradyarrhythmias are most commonly associated with acute *inferior* infarctions. Treatment with atropine should be administered only if the patient is symptomatic (hypotensive, or having chest pain, dyspnea, mental status changes, or ventricular ectopy) as a result of the bradycardia. (See Chapter 3, Section D of Chapter 12, and Chapter 16.)

9. Recommendations for performance of two-rescuer CPR in the unintubated patient are that **at least 80 compressions should be performed each minute (A).**

   Recommendations for performance of two-rescuer CPR are to maintain a 5:1 compression:ventilation ratio in which compressions are delivered at a rate of 80 to 100/min, with a 1 to 1.5-second pause for slow ventilation to be inserted after each five compressions. The 15:2 compression:ventilation ratio is still recommended for performance of one-rescuer CPR, whereas ventilations and compressions in the intubated patient may be asynchronous. (See Section A in Chapter 10.)

10. Pulselessness in an infant is established by checking for the presence of a **brachial pulse (B).**

    Because of the short, chubby neck of infants, determination of the location of the carotid pulse is extremely difficult in this age group (i.e., infants simply "don't have necks."). After 1 year of age, either the carotid or brachial pulse may be used.

In the past, the femoral pulse had been selected as an alternative site for palpating the pulse during CPR. Unfortunately, the femoral *vein* (rather than the artery) will sometimes be palpated when this method is used! (See Chapter 17.)

11. **Ventricular tachycardia/fibrillation (A)** is the most common mechanism of sudden cardiac death.

    In the past, ventricular fibrillation had always been cited as the most common mechanism of sudden cardiac death. Recently it has become evident that a period of ventricular tachycardia probably precedes development of ventricular fibrillation in most cases of cardiac arrest. (See Section A of Chapter 11.)

12. In an unmonitored arrest situation, as soon as the diagnosis of ventricular fibrillation has been established, one should **apply countershock with 200 joules of delivered energy (A).**

    Prior to countershock, a precordial thump may be delivered. (See Chapters 1 and 2.)

13. Regarding sodium bicarbonate, **indiscriminate use may result in a paradoxical intracellular acidosis (C), and the drug is probably unnecessary if the period of cardiac arrest is only a few minutes in duration (D).**

    Each ampule of sodium bicarbonate contains 50 mEq of drug. More important than a patient's weight in determining the dose to administer is the clinical circumstance of the arrest. In the absence of a severe, preexisting metabolic acidosis, sodium bicarbonate is definitely not indicated if the period of arrest is brief. (See Chapter 2.)

14. The appropriate amount of drug for IV administration of SDE (standard-dose epinephrine) is **1 mg of a 1:10,000 solution (B).**

    If SDE is ineffective, higher doses (i.e., HDE or high-dose epinephrine) should probably be tried. The optimal amount of drug for IV administration of HDE remains controversial. (See Section B of Chapter 2.)

15. Relative or absolute contraindications to thrombolytic therapy include **recent history of peptic ulcer disease (B), severe hypertension (C), and recent history of a TIA (D).**

    Traditionally, most centers have used 75 years of age as the cutoff for the use of thrombolytic agents, although age per se should not be thought of as an absolute contraindication—and it appears that many patients *over* 75 years of age may also benefit from this treatment. Atrial fibrillation is not a contraindication to thrombolytic therapy. (See Section C of Chapter 12.)

16. The most important priority in the management of cardiopulmonary resuscitation of children is to **manage the airway (C).**

    The KEYs to pediatric resuscitation are achieving and maintaining a patent airway, and ensuring adequate venti-

lation. Administration of drugs and defibrillation are much less important priorities. (See Chapter 17.)

17. Procainamide **is indicated for ventricular arrhythmias that are resistant to lidocaine (B), may widen the QRS complex (C), and may lengthen the QT interval (E).**

    Procainamide should not be given more rapidly than 20 mg/min, or hypotension is likely to occur. (See Chapter 14.)

18. Dopamine is **a chemical precursor of norepinephrine (A), and is indicated for treatment of cardiogenic shock and hemodynamically significant hypotension (D).**

    The drug is usually dispensed in ampules of 200 mg. The dopaminergic effect (dilatation of renal and mesenteric blood vessels) prevails at low infusion rates (1-2 μg/kg/min), while α-receptor stimulating effects predominate at high infusion rates (>10 μg/kg/min). At intermediate infusion rates (2-10 μg/kg/min), β-receptor stimulating effects predominate. (See Section B of Chapter 2.)

19. Cannulation of the internal jugular vein by the central approach is performed by introducing the needle **at the apex of the triangle formed by the two heads of the sternomastoid muscle and the clavicle (D).**

    (See Section A of Chapter 8.)

20. Regarding airway obstruction, **dentures and an elevated blood alcohol level are frequently associated with choking on food (A).**

    Foreign body airway obstruction frequently occurs during eating, especially in patients with dentures who have consumed too much alcohol. Although back blows are no longer recommended by the AHA for relief of complete airway obstruction in the adult, there are still some advocates of its use. However, *neither* back blows nor abdominal thrusts should be delivered to the patient manifesting only *partial* airway obstruction! (See Chapter 7 and Fig. 7-50)

21. Regarding the performance of basic life support in infants and children, **adequate external chest compression in the infant may be performed with only two fingers (A), and the compression to ventilation ratio is 5:1 for both one and two rescuers (D).**

    The sternum must be depressed at least 0.5 to 1 inch for infants, and the compression rate should be at least 100 times/min. The recommended hand position for infants is no longer over the midsternum (parallel to the nipple line), but instead should be one fingerbreadth *below* the nipple line. (See Section C of Chapter 17.)

22. The recommended initial energy dose for the defibrillation of a 20-kg child is **40 joules (C).**

    The energy recommended for the initial countershock attempt in children is 2 joules/kg. If unsuccessful, this energy level should be doubled (to 4 joules/kg) for repeat defibrillation. (See Chapter 17.)

23. A BVM device should consist of **a clear mask (A), an easy-to-grip bag (B), a system to deliver supplemental O_2 (C), an oxygen reservoir (D), and no pop-off valve (E).**

> The reason for the clear mask is that it allows the emergency care provider to see if regurgitation has occurred. An easy-to-grip bag facilitates handling the unit when ventilating the patient. A system to deliver supplemental O_2 which includes an oxygen reservoir is needed to provide high concentrations of oxygen. However, pop-off valves are not desirable because of the dramatic decrease in lung compliance that may occur in the setting of cardiac arrest. (See Chapter 7.)

24. The most common cause of sudden cardiac death in adults is **coronary artery disease (B).**

> The overwhelming majority of victims of out-of-hospital cardiac arrest have underlying coronary artery disease. Surprisingly, only about one third of such individuals have an acute myocardial infarction at the time of their episode. (See Section E of Chapter 11.)

25. Regarding Mobitz I 2° AV block, **the conduction defect is usually transient (B), the block may be the result of the increased parasympathetic tone that is commonly associated with acute inferior infarction (C), group beating is commonly seen (D), and the block may be caused by digitalis toxicity (E).**

> Mobitz I 2° AV block usually originates at the level of the AV node. In contrast, the level of Mobitz II 2° AV block usually originates *below* the AV node (which is why this form of block is usually associated with a less reliable escape focus and QRS widening). (See Chapter 3.)

26. Regarding atrial flutter in adults, **it can usually be converted to sinus rhythm with low-energy cardioversion (D), and application of carotid sinus massage may be helpful in confirming the diagnosis (E).**

> The usual atrial rate of flutter in adults is approximately 300 beats/min (250-350 beats/min range)—provided that the patient is not being treated with a medication (such as quinidine or procainamide) that might slow the atrial response. Most commonly there is 2:1 AV conduction, so that the usual ventricular response will be about 150 beats/min. Although digitalis toxicity may produce almost any arrhythmia, it rarely produces atrial flutter. (See Section B of Chapter 3.)

27. Factors suggesting that an abnormal QRS complex is an aberrantly conducted PAC include **the finding of a *premature* P wave in front of the abnormal complex (A), and a typical right bundle branch block pattern in a right-sided monitoring lead (D).**

> The finding of a full compensatory pause and a QRS complex width of greater than 0.14 second are factors in favor of ventricular ectopy. The finding of atrial fibrillation by itself is of little help. (See Chapter 15.)

28. Treatment of ventricular tachycardia may include **cardioversion (A), lidocaine (B), procainamide (C), and bretylium (E).**

> Verapamil is *contraindicated* for the treatment of ventricular tachycardia because its cardiac depressant and vasodilatory effects frequently result in deterioration of the rhythm to ventricular fibrillation. For this reason, verapamil should *not* be given as a therapeutic trial to patients with a regular wide complex tachycardia when the possibility exists that the rhythm may be ventricular tachycardia. (See Chapters 1 and 2.)

29. Treatment for 3° AV block may include **isoproterenol or dopamine (B), insertion of a pacemaker (C), and atropine (E).**

> Initial treatment of hemodynamically significant AV block consists of atropine or pacemaker therapy. Pressor therapy (with dopamine, epinephrine infusion, or isoproterenol) is sometimes used as a stopgap measure until pacemaker therapy is available. Neither verapamil nor calcium has any role in the treatment of this disorder. (See Chapter 1.)

30. Insertion of a subclavian or internal jugular line is preferable on the right side because **the dome of the right lung and pleura is lower than the dome on the left side (A), there is more or less a straight line to the atrium (C), and the large thoracic duct is not endangered (E).**

> (See Section A of Chapter 8.)

31. The esophageal obturator airway (EOA) **when removed is frequently followed by immediate regurgitation (B), and presents some potential for damage to the esophagus (D).**

> An EOA provides a means of controlling the airway when operators skilled in endotracheal intubation are not available. An advantage of the EOA is that it can be inserted without the need for visualization of the airway. To minimize the chance of regurgitation, the EOA should *not* be removed until after endotracheal intubation has been performed. (See Chapter 7.)

32. Endotracheal intubation **should be preceded by oxygenation of the lungs by other methods of ventilation (B), allows adequate lung inflation without causing gastric distention (C), and provides an alternative route for administration of medication (E).**

> Endotracheal intubation need *not* be performed as the first step in CPR. Instead, it should be at least briefly preceded by ventilation and oxygenation by other methods. Adequate ventilation can often be maintained by proper use of respiratory adjuncts. (See Chapter 7.)

33. Oxygen-powered mechanical breathing devices for use during CPR **are satisfactory only if manually triggered (B).**

Oxygen-powered mechanical breathing devices have come under increasing scrutiny in recent years. Although capable of delivering high concentrations of oxygen, they are especially prone to producing gastric insufflation when used in the patient with an unprotected airway. Newer devices are safer because they have reduced the flow rate to 40 L/min. The device should not be used in children. (See Chapter 7.)

34. Epinephrine **increases peripheral vascular resistance (A), can restore electrical activity in asystole (B), can facilitate defibrillation of ventricular fibrillation (C), and increases myocardial contractility (D).**

    All of the selections except (E) are true. Epinephrine is a treatment of choice for EMD. (See Section B of Chapter 2.)

35. Atropine sulfate **is of no value in ventricular tachycardia (A), and may be of value in symptomatic bradyarrhythmias (D).**

    Atropine is usually administered in 0.5 to 1 mg boluses given as needed up to a total of 2 mg. Because of its potential to produce supraventricular or ventricular tachyarrhythmias, the drug should *not* be used to treat bradycardia unless the patient is symptomatic. (See Section B of Chapter 2.)

36. Lidocaine **may facilitate defibrillation of ventricular fibrillation (A), usually has no significant effect on myocardial contractility (B), may be useful in treating multiform PVCs (C), may cause asystole (D), and may cause seizures (E).**

    (See Section B of Chapter 2 and Sections B and E of Chapter 12.)

37. ECG rhythms that may mimic ventricular tachycardia include **paroxysmal supraventricular tachycardia (PSVT) with aberration (A), PSVT with LBBB (B), very rapid atrial fibrillation with LBBB (D), and PSVT with RBBB (E).**

    Although one should always assume that a wide complex tachycardia is ventricular tachycardia until proved otherwise, the possibility of a supraventricular tachycardia with either preexisting bundle branch block or aberrancy should also be kept in mind. Because rapid atrial fibrillation often appears as a fairly regular rhythm, it may also mimic ventricular tachycardia if there is preexisting bundle branch block. (See Section B of Chapter 3 and Chapter 15.)

38. Drugs that may be useful in preparing the heart for electrical conversion from ventricular fibrillation to an effective rhythm include **oxygen (A) and epinephrine (C).**

    (See Chapter 1.)

39. Isoproterenol **increases myocardial irritability (A), lowers peripheral vascular resistance (C), speeds the heart rate (D), and increases myocardial oxygen consumption (E).**

Isoproterenol produces pure β-adrenergic stimulation. Because of the effects of this drug, its use has been de-emphasized in recent years. Isoproterenol is best reserved as a temporizing measure for treatment of hemodynamically significant bradyarrhythmias that have not responded to atropine. (See Section E of Chapter 2.)

40. Drugs that usually do not directly depress cardiac contractility when used in therapeutic doses include **atropine (A), lidocaine (B), and isoproterenol (D).**

    Propranolol and verapamil are both negative inotropic agents, so that use of these drugs must proceed with extreme caution (if at all) in patients with a history of congestive heart failure. (See Section B of Chapter 2 and Chapter 14.)

41. Arterial blood gas values of pH = 7.3, P_{CO_2} = 60 mm Hg, and HCO_3 = 30 mEq/L suggest **a mixed acid-base disorder (E).**

    The acid-base abnormality in this example is *mixed*, since both P_{CO_2} and the HCO_3 values are abnormal. The P_{CO_2} is increased by 20 mm Hg over the normal value of 40 (respiratory *acidosis*), while HCO_3 is increased by 5 mEq/L over the normal value of 25 (metabolic *alkalosis*). Since the body usually does not overcorrect the pH—and an acidosis is present, one can presume that this is probably the *primary* abnormality.

    In the acute setting, a change in Pa_{CO_2} (either up or down) of 10 mm Hg is associated with a change in pH of 0.08 units in the *opposite* direction. Thus one would have expected the pH to drop by 0.16 units (to a pH = 7.24) if one were simply dealing with an acute respiratory acidosis. The fact that the pH is higher than this (i.e., 7.3), and that HCO_3 has also been increased suggests metabolic *adaptation* by the body in an attempt to compensate for the primary acid-base disorder. Thus, this example illustrates a *primary respiratory acidosis* with partial *metabolic compensation*.

42. Risk factors of coronary artery disease include **hypertension (A), smoking (B), level of fitness (C), male sex (D), and type A personality (E).**

    The five most important risk factors for coronary artery disease are smoking, hypertension, positive family history, an abnormal lipid profile (high cholesterol/low HDL values), and level of fitness. Lesser risk factors include male sex, age, obesity, diabetes mellitus, and type A personality. Although family history, sex, and age cannot be changed, the other risk factors may all be modified to at least some extent by a motivated patient.

43. Drugs/therapeutic measures that may be useful for treating asystole after an unwitnessed cardiac arrest include **epinephrine, atropine, and pacemaker therapy (B).**

    (See Chapters 1 and 2.)

44. Regarding the use of IV lines in the setting of cardiac arrest, **a large bore IV is preferable (A), a femoral line is undesirable for administering drugs (B), and drug delivery may be improved by following drug administration with a bolus of fluid (E).**

Circulation of drugs in the arrested heart is most effectively accomplished when administered into a *central* vein such as the internal jugular or subclavian. However, achieving access at these sites requires the presence of a provider skilled in their insertion, and may still be attended by complications such as pneumothorax. The femoral vein is no longer recommended as a site for drug delivery during cardiac arrest because blood flow during CPR is significantly diminished below the diaphragm. Drug delivery from a peripheral IV line may be optimized if a proximal site (such as the antecubital fossa) is chosen, a large-bore needle is used, a 50- to 100-ml bolus of fluid "flushes" the medication in, and the arm is elevated after drug administration. (See Section A of Chapter 8.)

45. Cardiac arrest in children is usually due to **hypoxia secondary to respiratory arrest (C).**

    (See Chapter 17.)

46. Nitroglycerin **may be effective in treating angina pectoris (A), reduces preload in patients with congestive heart failure (B), is useful in treating the chest pain of acute myocardial infarction (D), and may lower blood pressure in patients with acute myocardial infarction (E).**

    (See Section B of Chapter 12 and Chapter 14.)

47. The amount of pressure that should be exerted on each electrode paddle during adult defibrillation is **25 lb (E).**

    Among the factors that decrease transthoracic resistance (TTR) during defibrillation are the pressure of the electrode paddles against the chest wall, and the phase of ventilation of the patient. Exerting firm pressure (of 25 lb) on each paddle may lower TTR by up to 25%. It also helps assure forced expiration of the victim, thus decreasing the distance between paddle electrodes and the heart, and further lowering TTR. (See Section D of Chapter 2.)

48. End points during the administration of IV procainamide include **hypotension (B), and control of the arrhythmia (D).**

    Other end points for the IV administration of procainamide include QRS widening by 50% of the pretreatment width, and infusion of the full 1-g loading dose. (See Chapter 14.)

49. If during the course of synchronized cardioversion a patient suddenly develops ventricular fibrillation, one should **immediately turn off the synchronizer switch and proceed with unsynchronized countershock (D).**

    Immediately defibrillating the patient minimizes the time that ventricular fibrillation is present and maximizes the chance for successful conversion. A precordial thump may be delivered prior to countershock. (See Chapter 1 and Section D of Chapter 2.)

50. Reasons sodium bicarbonate has been de-emphasized in the treatment of cardiac arrest are that **it may cause a paradoxical intracellular acidosis (B), its use may result in production of iatrogenic metabolic alkalosis (D), and hyperventilation is the preferred way to correct the acidosis that occurs during the initial minutes of the arrest (E).**

Significant metabolic acidosis will usually not develop in cardiopulmonary arrest for at least a period of time (5-15 min?) after patient collapse. Since the primary abnormality during the initial minutes is hypoventilation (i.e., *respiratory* acidosis), it would therefore seem far more appropriate to correct the acidosis of cardiac arrest by improving ventilation (by hyperventilating the patient) than by administering sodium bicarbonate.

Sodium bicarbonate therapy is *not* benign. Adverse effects of excessive administration of this agent include extreme alkalosis, hyperosmolality, hypokalemia, sodium overload, shifting of the oxyhemoglobin dissociation curve *leftward* (with consequent impaired oxygen release to the tissues), and precipitation of convulsions and/or arrhythmias. Moreover, unless adequate ventilation is achieved, carbon dioxide (CO_2) will tend to accumulate. Since CO_2 is freely diffusible across cellular and organ membranes, it readily enters the brain and heart where it may further depress function by producing a *paradoxical intracellular acidosis*. Giving sodium bicarbonate only aggravates this acidosis. (See Section E of Chapter 2.)

51. Clinical indications of lidocaine toxicity include **disorientation (A), paresthesias (B), agitation (D), and seizures (E).**

    (See Section E of Chapter 12.)

52. Clinical factors that suggest a patient with acute myocardial infarction is likely to benefit greatly from thrombolytic therapy include **recent onset of symptoms (A), marked ST segment elevation (B), marked reciprocal ST segment depression (C), anterior location of infarction (D), and absence of Q waves on the initial ECG (E).**

    The sooner a patient with acute myocardial infarction is treated with thrombolytic therapy, the more they are likely to benefit from this form of treatment (*especially* when they are treated within the first 4 hours after the onset of symptoms). In addition, the larger the infarct, the greater the potential benefit is likely to be. The findings of marked ST segment elevation, marked reciprocal ST segment depression, and anterior location all suggest more extensive infarction. The absence of Q waves on the initial ECG suggests a greater likelihood of potential reversibility—and therefore a greater likelihood of benefiting from acute thrombolytic therapy. (See Table 12A-2.)

53. Adenosine **may cause transient bradycardia (D), and may need to be repeated in the acute treatment of PSVT (E).**

    Verapamil appears to be equally effective as adenosine in the acute treatment of PSVT (with both drugs demonstrating 90-95% efficacy in acute conversion rates). Adenosine is *not* effective for treatment of atrial fibrillation. It may transiently slow the ventricular response, but rapid atrial fibrillation invariably resumes as soon as the effect of the drug wears off. The half-life of adenosine is on the order of 10 seconds (rather than 60 seconds).

Drawbacks to the use of adenosine are that it may cause transient bradycardia, and that the short half-life of its action makes it likely that PSVT will recur. Thus long-term antiarrythmic therapy may be needed to maintain sinus rhythm after the acute use of IV adenosine. Another reason why the drug may need to be repeated is that the initial dose (i.e., of 6 mg IV) may not be enough in some patients—and that an additional one or two 12-mg IV boluses may be required (up to a maximum total dose of 30 mg). (See Section B in Chapter 2.)

54. The recommended technique for opening the airway in a patient with suspected neck injury is the **jaw thrust (B).**

   Although slightly more difficult to perform than the head-tilt/chin-lift maneuver, the *jaw thrust* allows the rescuer to support the head and open the airway without having to flex the cervical spine. (See Chapter 7.)

55. Parameters that are helpful in assessing the work of breathing are **tachycardia (A), use of accessory chest muscles (B), use of abdominal muscles (C), suprasternal and substernal retractions (D), and nasal flaring (E).**

   In healthy individuals, airway resistance is relatively low. As a result, descent of the diaphragm and the outward expansion of the chest musculature produced by normal respiration will generally produce sufficient negative intrathoracic pressure to fill the lungs with air. However, in patients with pulmonary disease, and in the presence of respiratory distress, airway resistance is greatly increased. In this situation, all of the compensatory actions listed above are called into play to maximize air entry into the lungs and optimize oxygen delivery. (See Chapter 7 and Section A of Chapter 17.)

56. Factors important in determining survival from out-of-hospital ventricular fibrillation include **prompt recognition of cardiac arrest by the lay public (and early activation of emergency medical services), initiation of CPR by a bystander within 4 minutes, initiation of ACLS within 8 minutes, and the mechanism of the arrest (all of the above = Choice E).**

   (See Section A of Chapter 11.)

57. Ventilatory assist devices that are not recommended for use in children are **esophageal obturator airways (C) and oxygen-powered breathing devices (E).**

   An esophageal obturator airway is not indicated for use in children for two principal reasons. First, the length of a standard EOA tube is simply too long compared to the relatively short length of the pediatric esophagus. Thus, if an EOA/EGTA was inserted into a child, the distal tip and balloon would extend into the patient's stomach (rather than come to rest in its normal position in the esophagus). In addition, the large EOA balloon might cause rupture of the pediatric esophagus.
   Oxygen-powered breathing devices (O₂PBD) are also not indicated for pediatric patients because the increased airway pressures they generate are sufficiently high to produce a pneu-

mothorax. Furthermore, as a result of the high flow rate of the O₂PBD, resistance of the small pediatric airway may be increased to the point that ventilation of the patient is significantly reduced. (See Chapter 17.)

58. For a patient with a *pure* respiratory acidosis in which the PaCO₂ is 55 mm Hg, one would expect the pH to be **7.28 (C).**

   In the acute setting, a change in PaCO₂ (either up or down) of 10 mm Hg is associated with an approximate increase or decrease in pH of 0.08 units. Since the PaCO₂ in this example was increased by 15 (over the usual PaCO₂ of 40 mm Hg), one would expect the pH to decrease by 0.12 units. *(This inverse relationship between pH and PaCO₂ is the only one of the original "Golden Rules" that is still felt to be clinically relevant.)*

59. Inspiratory stridor suggests **upper airway obstruction (B).**

   During inspiration, extrathoracic airways narrow. As a result, stridor is produced. Croup and epiglottitis are examples of acute respiratory disorders that are characterized by inspiratory stridor. (See Chapter 17.)

60. Potential indications for synchronized cardioversion include **rapid atrial fibrillation in a hypotensive patient (B), and ventricular tachycardia in a hypotensive patient (D).**

   Synchronization of the electrical discharge to the upstroke of the R wave minimizes the chance of delivering the impulse during the "vulnerable period." The method is effective for treatment of supraventricular or ventricular tachyarrhythmias (sush as rapid atrial fibrillation or ventricular tachycardia) that fail to respond to medical therapy, and/or when (if) the patient becomes hemodynamically unstable. Cardioversion is ineffective for treatment of either ventricular fibrillation or asystole (because there is no QRS complex to synchronize to). Treatment of sinus tachycardia is always dependent on identifying and correcting the underlying cause. (See Section D of Chapter 2.)

TRUE/FALSE QUESTIONS

61. **False.**

   The "sniffing" position is achieved in children by sliding a small rolled washcloth (or your hand) under the patient's shoulders. This allows the head to tilt slightly *backward* on its axis until the jaw forms a 90-degree angle to the long axis of the body. (See Section A of Chapter 17.)

62. **True.**

   This differs from intubation with a straight blade in which the epiglottis is directly lifted to expose the epiglottis. (See Chapter 7.)

63. **False.**

   The most difficult part about using a bag-valve-mask device is that one rescuer must simultaneously perform *three* tasks. A patent airway and tight face seal must be maintained with one hand, while the other hand is used to ventilate the patient.

The tidal volume generated by squeezing the reservoir bag with one hand is significantly less than that delivered by the mouth-to-mouth technique. (See Chapter 7.)

64. **True.**

(See Chapter 7.)

65. **True.**

The mnemonic **VAN,** may help recall that the femoral vein lies medial to the artery, and the artery lies medial to the nerve. (See Section A of Chapter 8.)

66. **True.**

By far the most common cause of a regular, wide complex tachycardia (in which atrial activity is not apparent) is ventricular tachycardia—especially in adults who have a history of underlying heart disease. (See Section B of Chapter 3 and Chapter 15.)

67. **False.**

Although in the past nitroglycerin was not used in acute myocardial infarction for fear of causing hypotension, the drug is now commonly recommended in this setting as an agent of choice for treatment of chest pain, ischemia, or hypertension. If administered cautiously to patients with systolic blood pressure readings of at least 100 mm Hg, hypotension usually does not pose a problem. Hypotension is most likely to occur when nitroglycerin is given to patients who are hypovolemic and/or who have acute right ventricular infarction. (See Section B of Chapter 12 and Chapter 14.)

68. **True.**

The importance of this statistic lies with the fact that educating the public to seek medical assistance sooner may be the single most important intervention we can make toward reducing mortality from acute myocardial infarction. (See Chapter 11.)

69. **False.**

The Killip classification of patients with acute myocardial infarction was first proposed in 1967 and is still in use today. It consists of four classes:

Class I—uncomplicated myocardial infarction (i.e., no rales or S3)
Class II—mild ventricular failure (i.e., rales in the lower lung field and an S3)
Class III—severe ventricular failure (i.e., pulmonary edema)
Class IV—cardiogenic shock (i.e., systolic blood pressure of less than 90 mm Hg, oliguria, mental obtundation)

The problem with this classification is that it is based on bedside assessment of the patient's circulatory status. Differentiation of patients with mild-to-moderate failure from those with severe failure is sometimes quite difficult to do on clinical grounds alone. (See Chapter 12.)

70. **False.**

Diuresis is an important component of the therapy of patients with acute myocardial infarction and left ventricular failure. In contrast, *volume expansion* (rather than diuretic therapy) is the initial treatment of choice for hemodynamically significant right ventricular infarction. The goal is to increase right ventricular contractility by the Frank-Starling principle. Decreasing preload (with diuretics) would be counterproductive. (See Section A of Chapter 12.)

71. **False.**

Development of intraventricular conduction defects with acute myocardial infarction is thought to reflect extensive myocardial damage. Mortality most often results from power failure rather than from progression of the conduction disturbance to complete AV block. Consequently, prophylactic pacing usually will not increase survival, although on rare occasions it may benefit patients with bundle branch block and high-degree AV block who do not have significant heart failure. (See Chapter 12.)

72. **False.**

The pure β-adrenergic effect of isoproterenol is the reason this drug is *contraindicated* in the arrested heart. As a result of this action, vasodilatation is produced and coronary perfusion is reduced! In contrast, the α-adrenergic effect of epinephrine produces vasoconstriction (which leads to an increase in aortic diastolic pressure and improved coronary perfusion). (See Section E of Chapter 2.)

73. **True.**

Lidocaine is eliminated from the body by hepatic metabolism. The half-life of this elimination phase is proportional to hepatic blood flow, and under normal circumstances takes between 1 and 2 hours. Patients in shock or congestive heart failure in whom hepatic blood flow may be greatly diminished would be expected to have a prolonged elimination phase half-life and be more susceptible to accumulation of drug and lidocaine toxicity. Other groups at high risk of developing lidocaine toxicity include patients with liver disease, those taking drugs such as propranolol or cimetidine (that decrease hepatic clearance of lidocaine), the elderly (in whom cardiac output is less), and patients with low body weight. (See Sections B and E of Chapter 12.)

74. **False.**

For a malpractice claim to be successful, four conditions must be satisfied:

1. A relationship must have been established between the patient and health care provider.
2. Negligence on the part of the health care provider must have occurred.
3. The patient must have suffered an injury.
4. A direct *cause-and-effect* relationship must be *proved* to exist between the negligence and the injury that results. (See Section A of Chapter 18.)

75. **False.**

"Do not resuscitate" (DNR) orders may be written if the patient is competent and willing. If the patient was competent in the past and made out a valid advance directive, or if the legal guardian and/or proxy decision-maker of an incompetent patient agrees with the physician that a DNR order is in the best interests of the patient, the order may also be written. Finally, the physician may write a DNR order in cases where cardiopulmonary resuscitation would serve no useful purpose (i.e., there is no possibility for meaningful prolongation of life). (See Chapter 18.)

76. **False.**

In addition to the lay public, trained health care providers may also benefit from using the AED because it greatly facilitates the process of defibrillation. With the use of this device, the time from arrival on the scene until delivery of the first countershock by an experienced paramedic team may be reduced by *more than 1 minute*. (See Section A of Chapter 11.)

77. **True.**

Acute epiglottitis is a bacterial infection that usually occurs in children between 2 and 7 years of age. In contrast, the viral form of croup (laryngotracheobronchitis) tends to be seen in younger individuals between 3 months and 3 years old. (See Section A of Chapter 17.)

78. **False.**

The pediatric heart typically responds to hypoxemia by *slowing* its rate. As a result, significant bradycardia and asystole are by far the most common arrhythmias associated with cardiopulmonary arrest in children. (See Chapter 17.)

79. **False.**

Pacemaker insertion is almost always required for patients who develop 3° AV block as the result of acute *anterior* infarction. The escape pacemaker in this case tends to be idioventricular (i.e., associated with a wide QRS complex), and is often accompanied by a slow heart rate and signs of hemodynamic compromise.

In contrast, 3° AV block that develops in association with acute *inferior* infarction will often occur with a stable junctional escape rhythm (i.e., narrow QRS complex) that is able to maintain the patient's hemodynamic status. The mechanism of AV block in this setting may simply reflect increased parasympathetic tone and/or ischemia of the AV node rather than irreversible myocardial damage. As a result, the conduction defect will often be transient. If heart rate and blood pressure remain adequate, no treatment (other than close observation) may be needed. With slower heart rates, atropine may be used in an attempt to accelerate the ventricular response and/or improve AV conduction. Many cases will not require pacemaker insertion. (See Section D of Chapter 3 and Section D of Chapter 12.)

80. **False.**

The EOA is not inserted with the patient's head in the sniffing position. Instead, the head is gently flexed *forward* to assist in directing the tube into the esophagus. (See Chapter 7.)

81. **False.**

In the past it was thought that *"warning arrhythmias"* (≥5 PVCs/min, ≥2 PVCs in a row, multiform PVCs, and the "R-on-T" phenomenon) regularly preceded the development of primary ventricular fibrillation in patients with acute myocardial infarction. As a result, it was thought that one could wait for the occurrence of such arrhythmias *before* initiating antiarrhythmic therapy for patients who were admitted with acute chest pain.

We now appreciate that ventricular fibrillation may often occur in acute myocardial infarction *without* being preceded by any warning arrhythmias at all. Even when warning arrhythmias do occur, they do not appear to reliably predict which patients will subsequently develop ventricular fibrillation. (See Sections B and E of Chapter 12.)

82. **False.**

The treatment of choice for *hemodynamically significant* ventricular tachycardia is immediate cardioversion. Thus, time should not be lost instituting medical treatment when hypotension, chest pain, and/or altered mentation result from the tachyarrhythmia. Lidocaine should be started *after* cardioversion—or for patients with hemodynamically *stable* ventricular tachycardia who can be treated medically. (See Chapter 1.)

83. **False.**

The diagnosis of acute myocardial infarction is not only based on the finding of ECG changes and cardiac enzyme abnormalities, but perhaps most important—*on the history!* The ECG is most helpful when suggestive changes are present; however, it is essential to emphasize that a normal tracing does *not* rule out acute infarction. Practically speaking, cardiac enzymes should play little (or no) role in determining whether a patient with new-onset chest pain is admitted to the hospital. Many factors other than acute infarction may affect (and falsely elevate) CK values, and an initially normal CK value in no way rules out the possibility of acute infarction. This leaves *history* as the KEY diagnostic parameter in many cases for determining whether to admit the patient who presents with new-onset chest pain to the hosptial. (See Section A of Chapter 12.)

84. **True.**

Although in the past it was thought that thrombus formation occurred *secondary* to acute myocardial infarction, we now know that acute thrombotic occlusion is actually the cause (and not the result) in the vast majority of cases. (See Sections A and C of Chapter 12.)

85. **False.**

In the past it was taboo to perform cardiac catheterization and/or angioplasty in the setting of acute myocardial infarction. In practice, these procedures have been shown to be remarkably safe when appropriate precautions are taken. As a result, cardiac catheterization is performed almost routinely with acute myocardial infarction in many centers, and angioplasty is frequently utilized as the method of choice for reperfusion therapy. (See Chapter 12.)

86. **True.**

Under normal circumstances, most adults breathe through their nose. However, with respiratory distress, adults tend to breathe through their mouth. The value of providing supplemental oxygen through a nasal cannula would therefore be significantly reduced if the patient was breathing through their nose. (See Chapter 7.)

87. **False.**

    Contrary to popular belief, tidal volumes generated with BVM units in the unprotected airway are far less than those generated by mouth-to-mouth or mouth-to-mask ventilation. (See Chapter 7.)

88. **True.**

    End-tidal CO_2 detection devices are a rapid, noninvasive, and reliable method for confirming ET tube placement. (See Chapter 7 and Section C of Chapter 10.)

89. **True.**

    Patients with acute myocardial infarction who present with a normal initial ECG tend to have fewer complications and a better long-term prognosis than those who demonstrate acute ECG changes on their initial tracing. (See Section A of Chapter 12.)

90. **False.**

    The suction catheter should be passed *adjacent to* the oral pharyngeal airway (rather than through the lumen of the airway) when suctioning is performed. The lumen of the airway is not large enough to allow passage of a suction catheter. (See Chapter 7.)

91. **False.**

    Previously it was thought that the infant heart was situated higher in the chest than the heart of older children and adults. We now know that the heart of the infant lies over the lower third of the sternum—just as it does in older children and adults. Therefore, finger placement for external compression in infants should be one fingerbreadth *below* the nipple line. (See Section C of Chapter 17.)

92. **True.**

    Once the patient has been intubated, the risk of gastric insufflation with ventilation is essentially eliminated. As a result, synchronization of ventilation and compression is no longer needed. If anything, simultaneous ventilation and compression may be advantageous and result in *increased* blood flow to the heart and brain (because it increases intrathoracic pressure). (See Chapter 7.)

93. **True.**

    Bradycardia is the most common rhythm in pediatric cardiopulmonary arrest, and asystole is the most common terminal event. Ventricular fibrillation is rare. (See Chapter 17.)

94. **False.**

    The AED should be activated to begin defibrillation as soon as the diagnosis of cardiac arrest has been confirmed. (See Chapter 1.)

95. **False.**

    The recommended dose of atropine for infants and children is 0.02 mg/kg. Therefore, the appropriate dose for a 15-kg infant is 0.3 mg. (See Table 17C-2 in Chapter 17.)

96. **False.**

    Although higher doses of epinephrine should help to optimize coronary perfusion in the arrested heart (and may result in salvage of some patients who would not have responded otherwise), it is unlikely that this intervention will have a major impact on ultimate survival from out-of-hospital ventricular fibrillation. By far, the most important determinant of long-term survival in this situation is the amount of time it takes for the patient to be defibrillated. Failure to respond to defibrillation is a poor prognostic indicator *regardless* of whatever medical therapy is given. (See Section A of Chapter 11.)

97. **False.**

    Mobitz I 2° AV block is *much* more common than Mobitz II in the setting of acute myocardial infarction. In general, the former conduction disturbance is most often associated with acute inferior infarction, while the latter is seen with acute anterior infarction. The importance of distinguishing between Mobitz I and Mobitz II AV block is that the former is usually a benign, transient conduction disturbance, whereas the latter requires pacemaker insertion. (See Chapter 3.)

98. **True.**

    The KEY to successful resuscitation of a patient in EMD is to identify and correct the underlying cause. Hypovolemia (from blood loss, dehydration, shock, inappropriate vasodilatation, etc.) is the most common potentially reversible cause. As a result, an *empiric* trial of fluid resuscitation is indicated if no precipitating cause is apparent. (See Chapter 1.)

99. **False.**

    Bretylium has a complex mechanism of action, including adrenergic stimulation (that results in an initial release of norepinephrine), followed several minutes later by adrenergic blockade (in which uptake of norepinephrine and epinephrine into post-ganglionic adrenergic nerve endings is prevented). This latter effect becomes the predominant one and accounts for the fact that, following an initial increase in blood pressure, *hypotension* commonly occurs and is the most common adverse reaction to bretylium infusion. (See Section E of Chapter 2.)

100. **True.**

    Not all patients in ventricular tachycardia immediately decompensate. Sustained ventricular tachycardia may occasionally persist for hours (and even days!) in some patients—especially if the heart rate of the arrhythmia is not excessively fast (i.e., less than 160 beats/min), and the patient is able to maintain vital organ perfusion by compensatory vasoconstriction. Hemodynamic stability cannot be used as a criterion for distinguishing between sustained ventricular tachycardia and SVT with either aberration or preexisting bundle branch block. (See Section B of Chapter 3 and Chapter 15.)

Essentials of the Airway and IV Access

CHAPTER 7

MANAGEMENT OF AIRWAY AND VENTILATION

The importance of controlling the airway in patients presenting with cardiac and/or respiratory emergencies cannot be overemphasized. For outcome to be favorable, spontaneously breathing patients should be provided with supplemental oxygen, those who are not adequately ventilating must be assisted, and patients in respiratory arrest must be intubated and oxygenated. This chapter discusses the modalities and techniques used to accomplish these tasks.

Opening the Airway

The first priority in managing the patient with respiratory difficulty is to assure patency of the airway. The two maneuvers recommended for doing this are the chin-lift and jaw-thrust.

In the unconscious supine patient, the musculature that normally supports the tongue and epiglottis relaxes. As a result, one or both of these structures may fall back and occlude the airway *(Figure 7-1)*. This accounts for the fact

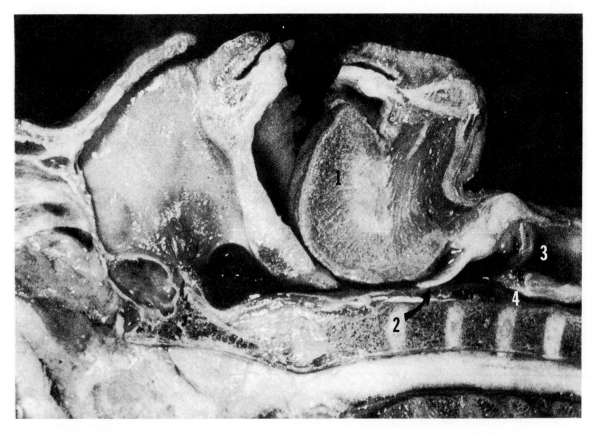

Figure 7-1.   Cross-section of the head demonstrating how the tongue and epiglottis may occlude the airway in the supine position when the musculature is relaxed. *(1)* tongue; *(2)* epiglottis; *(3)* trachea; *(4)* esophagus.
(Reproduced with permission from Yokochi C, Rohen JW: *Photographic anatomy of the human body*, Baltimore, 1978, University Park Press.)

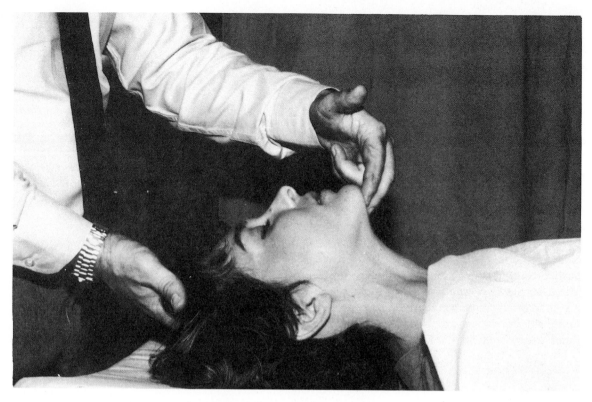

Figure 7-2.   Head tilt/chin-lift.

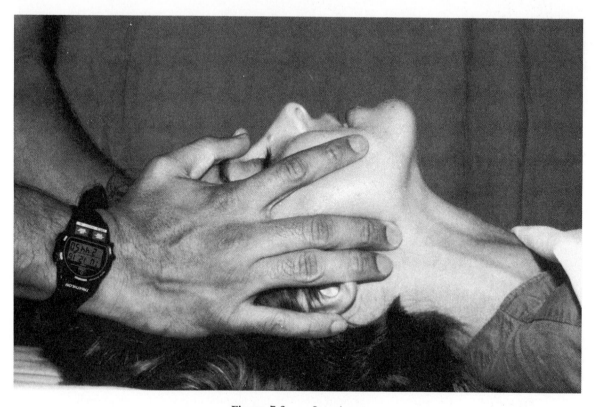

Figure 7-3.   Jaw-thrust.

that the most common cause of airway obstruction in the unconscious patient is soft tissue in origin.

The degree of airway obstruction may be aggravated in the patient who is making spontaneous attempts to breathe. Inspiratory efforts create a negative pressure that frequently draws the tongue and epiglottis back even more into the throat, further compromising the airway. Because the tongue and epiglottis are attached to the lower jaw, procedures aimed at displacing the mandible forward will lift these structures off the posterior pharynx and open the airway. This is the way in which the chin-lift and jaw-thrust maneuvers work.

THE HEAD-TILT/CHIN-LIFT

The *head-tilt/chin-lift* maneuver is the recommended method of choice for opening the airway because it is easier to learn and more effective than the jaw-thrust (Clinton and Ruiz, 1985). The technique is performed by placing the palm of one hand on the patient's forehead and the fingers of the other hand under the patient's chin. The fingers are positioned on the bony structure of the chin so as to avoid compression of soft tissues which might compromise the airway. With the hand on the forehead acting as a stabilizing force, the head is tilted backward by gently pushing the chin in a cephalad direction *(Figure 7-2)*.

> As the head is tilted back, the mouth will almost always open. When this occurs, resist the urge to force the mouth closed. Instead, concentrate on using the fingers under the chin to assist in supporting the head-tilt position.

THE JAW-THRUST

Although slightly more difficult to perform than is the head-tilt/chin-lift maneuver, the *jaw-thrust* is the procedure of choice when the possibility of cervical spine injury exists. This maneuver allows the rescuer to support the head and open the airway without flexing or extending the cervical spine. One hand is placed on each side of the patient's head and the index and/or middle fingers are used to displace the mandible anteriorly. This lifts the tongue off the hypopharynx *(Figure 7-3)*.

The Head-Tilt/Neck-Lift

> Although the *head-tilt/neck-lift* technique used to be the most commonly taught method for opening the airway, it is no longer recommended. Tilting the head back and lifting the neck is an indirect method of opening the airway and is much less effective than procedures that displace the mandible forward. It also poses the greatest risk when cerevical spine injury is a possibility.

Assessing the Adequacy of Ventilation

In order to determine optimal airway management, the emergency care provider must assess the adequacy of ventilation. The parameters to monitor include color, breath sounds, tidal volume, respiratory rate, and the work of breathing. Evaluating the patient's *color* is perhaps the easiest way to determine hypoxia. Cyanosis is an obvious indicator of inadequate oxygenation. Pallor and/or an ashen appearance suggests in addition diminished cardiac output.

All lung fields should be auscultated for *breath sounds*. The finding of good, symmetric breath sounds indicates that the airway is patent and that air movement is adequate. On the other hand, asymmetric or abnormal breath sounds suggest a problem in the airway. This may be due to obstruction (from foreign body, soft tissue, mucous plugging), cardiopulmonary disease (bronchospasm, pneumonia, congestive heart failure), or improper tube placement (right mainstem intubation, tracheal intubation with the esophageal obturator).

The next two parameters to monitor are *tidal volume* and *respiratory rate*. The product of these two make up the *minute ventilation*. Most adults breathe in about 500 ml of air an average of 12 times each minute. This results in a minute ventilation of 6 L (500 ml $\times$ 12 = 6000 ml). Because of the inverse relationship between tidal volume and respiratory rate, alterations in one of these parameters may be at least partially compensated by corrective alterations in the other. For example, minute ventilation may remain adequate despite a decrease in tidal volume provided the patient hyperventilates (and respiratory rate increases) proportionately.

Accurate assessment of tidal volume requires the use of a spirometer. In the absence of such equipment or in an emergency setting, one may surmise that the tidal volume is probably adequate if breath sounds are full and equal in the presence of good, symmetric chest excursion.

Respiratory rate should be counted. In our experience, failure to do so is the most frequently overlooked part of the physical exam of an acutely ill patient. We emphasize the importance of counting because of the ease with which one may overestimate or underestimate the frequency of respiration by casual inspection.

A conscious effort should also be made on the part of the observer to assess the *work of breathing*. This may be done at the bedside by looking for: (1) tachypnea, (2) suprasternal and substernal retractions, and (3) use of accessory chest and abdominal muscles. In addition to these respiratory changes associated with increased work of breathing, *cardiac changes* may also be evident.

> Cardiac changes associated with respiratory distress may be very different for adults compared to pediatric patients. In general, adults develop sinus tachycardia with respiratory distress. As a result of hypoxia, ventricular ectopy may develop,

sometimes progressing to ventricular tachycardia and/or cardiac arrest from ventricular fibrillation. In contrast, heart rate almost always *decreases* in pediatric patients who become hypoxemic. If uncorrected, heart rate continues to drop, leading to severe bradycardia and ultimately cardiac arrest from asystole. Fortunately, appropriate treatment with prompt correction of hypoxemia will usually reverse cardiac changes in both children and adults.

The above parameters must be frequently assessed while caring for patients in cardiac and/or respiratory distress. Unless frequent *serial examinations* are done, changes in hemodynamic or ventilatory status may easily pass unnoticed.

Monitoring the Adequacy of Oxygenation

In addition to assessing the adequacy of ventilation, the *efficacy* of ventilation (i.e., the adequacy of *oxygenation*) should also be assessed if at all possible. Serial **arterial blood gas (ABG)** analysis would seem to be the ideal evaluative method for accomplishing this. Unfortunately, a number of practical problems are associated with the use of ABG studies in an emergency setting.

Drawing ABGs is an invasive procedure that carries with it the risk of any of the complications that may arise from puncture of an arterial vessel. Finding the artery in a hypotensive or pulseless patient is often extremely difficult. Performing an Allen test in the upper extremity to verify collateral circulation (i.e., the presence of an ulnar artery pulse) may be impossible. Moreover, pulsations detected in the femoral area with external chest compression performed during cardiac arrest do not necessarily identify the femoral artery (because the lack of valves in the lower extremity venous system may result in retrograde transmission of pulsations to the femoral vein).

As discussed in Chapter 2, ABGs obtained during cardiopulmonary resuscitation do not reflect the true state of acid-base balance on a cellular level. This is because of the marked discrepancy that rapidly develops with cardiac arrest between arterial pH (as measured by ABGs) and the pH of mixed venous blood. A marked discrepancy is also seen between arterial $PaCO_2$ and the $PaCO_2$ of mixed venous blood. Readings from mixed venous blood rather than ABGs much more accurately reflect events at the cellular level during cardiac arrest.

PaO_2 readings obtained during cardiac arrest are often surprisingly high. It is well to remember that such readings result from slow passage of blood through the lungs (which allows more than adequate time for full saturation) and does *not* necessarily reflect satisfactory peripheral oxygenation.

A final limitation of ABGs as a reflection of the adequacy of oxygenation is that they cannot be analyzed in the field. Even if ABG samples could be drawn in the prehospital setting, the delay in delivery to the hospital laboratory for analysis would render the results meaningless.

An attractive alternative to ABG studies is the use of a noninvasive technique to monitor arterial oxygenation. Two types of devices are available: (1) *pulse oximetry,* and

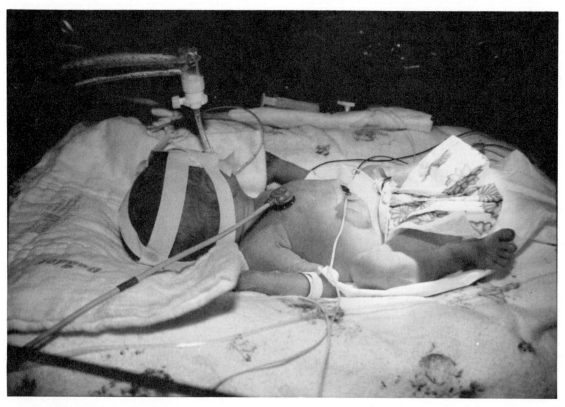

Figure 7-4.   Application of a transcutaneous sensor to the chest of this child for monitoring arterial oxygenation.

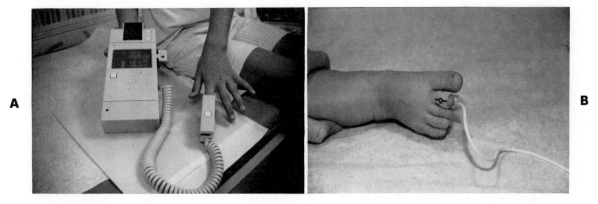

Figure 7-5. **A,** Application of a clip-on pulse oximeter to the finger; **B,** Application of a wraparound pulse oximetry sensor to the toe.

(2) *transcutaneous monitoring.* Both are effective, inexpensive methods for estimating the adequacy of oxygenation.

In emergency situations, *pulse oximetry* offers several advantages over transcutaneous oximetry. Transcutaneous oxygen sensors *(Figure 7-4)* must be pre-calibrated prior to collecting data, are heated (which may be uncomfortable to the patient), and require frequent site changes. Pulse oximeters are much easier to use. The device is simply attached to an ear lobe, toe, or finger, and sensing begins within seconds *(Figure 7-5).*

Pulse oximetry provides continuous measurement of oxygen saturation (SaO_2). Under normal conditions, the accuracy of this measurement is excellent (Taylor and Whitwarm, 1986; Hedges et al, 1987; Kulick, 1987). Oximetry may therefore be used as a noninvasive substitute for ABGs under certain circumstances.

> SaO_2 readings in the range of 95% to 100% generally correspond to high PaO_2 concentrations (i.e., >80 mm Hg). It is important to remember, however, that oxygen saturation is related to PaO_2 by the oxyhemoglobin dissociation curve, the slope of which changes sharply when SaO_2 drops into the range of 90% to 92%. A seemingly small decrease in SaO_2 from the 95% to 100% range, down to the 90% to 92% range may therefore correspond to a deceptively large drop in PaO_2 to as low a value as 60 mm Hg (Gordon, 1989). Clinically, this means that *oximetry should not be used to substitute for ABGs once SaO_2 readings drop below the 90% to 92% range.* Other drawbacks to oximetry are that this measurement becomes inaccurate with hypothermia (especially <35°C), hypotension (<50 mm Hg), severe vascular disease, vasopressor therapy, anemia, hyperbilirubinemia, and with abnormal hemoglobin as may be seen when there are increased concentrations of carboxyhemoglobin or methemoglobin (Gordon, 1989). Thus the use of oximetry has significant limitations in evaluating hemodynamically unstable patients and victims of cardiac arrest.

Rather than measuring oxygen saturation, *transcutaneous sensors* monitor the partial pressure of oxygen in the arterial blood. Because they are applied to the patient's chest or abdomen (instead of to an extremity area), transcutaneous sensors more accurately reflect arterial oxygenation when peripheral perfusion is poor.

Adjuncts for Improving Oxygenation

In the conscious, spontaneously breathing patient, one of the main priorities is to provide supplemental oxygen. Although many devices are available for accomplishing this, we will address only the four most commonly used modalities.

THE NASAL CANNULA

The *nasal cannula* is a piece of tubing with two ports designed to deliver supplemental oxygen through the nares. It is easily applied by slipping the tubing over the ears and sliding the prongs into the nares *(Figure 7-6).* Two to 6 L of oxygen may be administered per minute, providing the patient with inspired oxygen concentrations (F_IO_2) of 24% to 40%.

The advantage of this device is that it is well tolerated by most individuals. The nasal cannula is particularly valuable in patients with chronic obstructive pulmonary disease for whom low concentrations of oxygen (24% to 28%) are desirable. However, when higher concentrations of oxygen are needed, the non-rebreathing oxygen mask and Venturi mask are preferable.

> In normal persons, respiratory drive depends on arterial carbon dioxide concentration. In contrast, hypercarbia loses its value as a stimulus for respiration in many patients with chronic obstructive pulmonary disease (COPD). Such individuals come to depend on hypoxemia for their respiratory drive. Administration of high concentrations of oxygen to such patients is potentially dangerous because it may correct hypoxemia and suppress ventilation to the point of respiratory arrest. The F_IO_2 of supplemental oxygen should therefore be kept at low levels (2 L/min or less) for patients at risk of carbon dioxide retention.

The problem with the nasal cannula is that the actual amount of inspired oxygen varies greatly and depends on both tidal volume and whether the patient predominantly breathes through their nose or mouth.

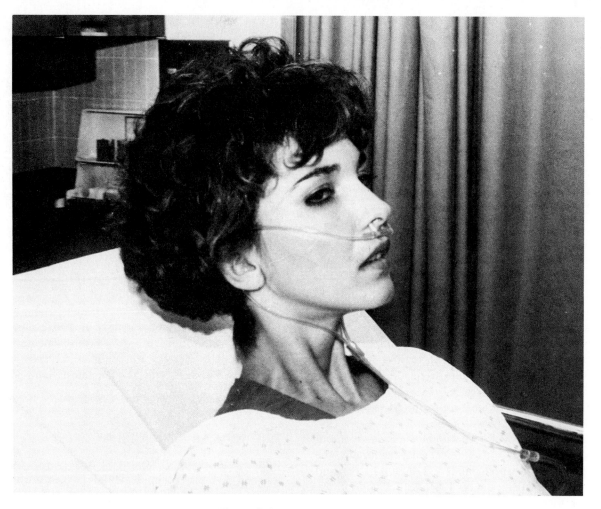

Figure 7-6.   Nasal cannula.

Under normal circumstances, most adults breathe primarily through their nose. In contrast, adults tend to change this pattern with respiratory distress, and breathe through their mouth. *The value of a nasal cannula is dramatically reduced if it is used in a patient who is breathing primarily through their mouth.*

Simply observing the patient will often suggest whether they are breathing primarily through their nose or mouth. In general, it is extremely difficult to breathe through the nose if one's mouth is open. (*Verify this statement by trying it out on yourself!*) As a result:

It is usually preferable to provide supplemental oxygen by *mask* rather than nasal cannula *for those individuals with respiratory distress whose mouths remain open.*

THE OXYGEN MASK

The *oxygen mask* is a plastic device with a number of small vents on each side which allow for inspiration and expiration of ambient air. There is also a port for delivery

of supplemental oxygen on the lower portion of the mask. Five to 10 L of oxygen may be administered, providing an F_IO_2 of up to 50%.

The principal drawback of this device is the tremendous variability in actual inspired oxygen concentration. This is because the amount of air entrained from the outside (that mixes with the supplemental oxygen) is dependent on the patient's inspiratory flow rate. Because of the variability in delivered F_IO_2 with the oxygen mask, a non-rebreather or Venturi mask is usually preferable when high concentrations of oxygen are required.

THE NON-REBREATHING OXYGEN MASK

The *non-rebreathing oxygen mask* is far superior to the basic plastic oxygen mask described above. It is the adjunct of choice when high concentrations of oxygen are needed, because it can consistently deliver an F_IO_2 of up to 90%.

Several modifications account for the superiority of this device (*Figure 7-7*). The first is that a *flutter* (one-way) valve has been added to each side of the non-rebreather mask.

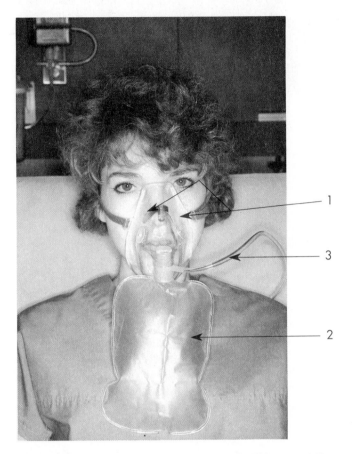

Figure 7-7. Nonrebreathing oxygen mask. This mask differs from the standard oxygen mask because it has flutter (one-way) valves (*1*) and an oxygen reservoir (*2*). Also shown is oxygen tubing (*3*) through which supplemental oxygen is directed into the reservoir.

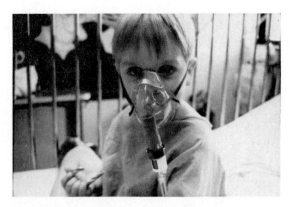

Figure 7-8. Venturi mask. The Venturi mask allows delivery of a *fixed* oxygen concentration of 24%, 28%, 35%, or 40%.

THE VENTURI MASK

The *Venturi mask* is similar in concept to the basic oxygen mask but features one important modification: it allows relatively fixed concentrations of supplemental oxygen to be inspired. Oxygen concentrations of 24%, 28%, 35%, and 40% can be delivered, using either 4 or 8 L/min flow rates. The advantage of this mask is *much greater control of the oxygen concentration administered to the patient.* Consistent oxygen delivery has made the Venturi mask the favored device for providing precise F_IO_2 rates to patients with COPD.

Airway Adjuncts

In the semiconscious or unconscious patient, invasive measures may be needed to maintain patency of the airway for ventilation. The two devices used are the oral and the nasopharyngeal airway.

THE ORAL PHARYNGEAL AIRWAY

The *oral pharyngeal airway* is a semicurved, tubular device that is placed on top of the tongue *(Figure 7-9)*. When properly positioned, the distal tip lies between the base of the tongue and the back of the throat. This prevents the tongue from occluding the airway and allows ventilation to occur through the lumen of the tube.

Appropriate sizing of the device may be estimated at the bedside or in the field by aligning the tube on the side of the patient's face and choosing an airway that extends from the tragus to the corner of the mouth *(Figure 7-10)*.

This allows exhaled air to escape but prevents ambient air from being inspired. In contrast, the open (air) holes on each side of the basic mask allow passage of both inspired and expired air. The other major difference between these two devices is that the basic mask directs the supplemental oxygen into the mask, while the *non-rebreathing* mask directs it into a *reservoir* bag. A one-way valve prevents exhaled air from entering this reservoir, so that the patient entrains 100% oxygen from the reservoir on inhalation. In contrast, the concentration of inspired oxygen from the basic mask is much less than 100% because supplemental oxygen has mixed with ambient air.

Special Considerations

The reservoir bag should remain completely filled when using the nonrebreathing oxygen mask so that ample supplemental oxygen is available for each breath. In order to assure that this occurs, high flow rates (10-15 L/min) must be used. In addition, the mask must fit snugly on the face to prevent ambient air from seeping in around the mask and mixing with oxygen inhaled from the reservoir bag.

Technique for Insertion

There are two ways to position the oral pharyngeal airway. The quickest method is to insert the device upside down into the mouth *(Figure 7-11A)*. As soon as the distal end reaches the hard palate, the airway is gently rotated 180° and slipped behind the tongue into the posterior pharynx *(Figures 7-11B and 7-11C)*.

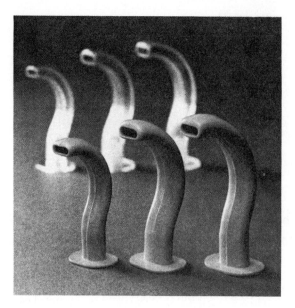

Figure 7-9.   Examples of oral pharyngeal airways.
(Reproduced with permission of Ambu, Inc from Lotz P, Ahnefeld FW, Hirlinger WD: *A systematic guide to intubation*, Atelier Flad, Eckental, West Germany.)

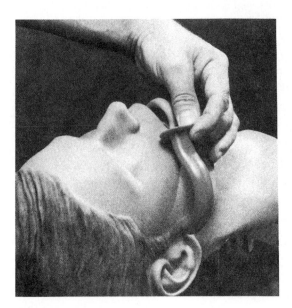

Figure 7-10.   Sizing the oral pharyngeal airway.
(Reproduced with permission of Ambu, Inc from Lotz P, Ahnefeld FW, Hirlinger WD: *A systematic guide to intubation*, Atelier Flad, Eckental, West Germany.)

The second technique for insertion of the oral pharyngeal airway requires a tongue blade. The tongue is depressed and the airway is inserted right side up into the oral pharynx. With either technique, the flange of the tube should sit comfortably on the lips if the device has been properly inserted (*Figure 7-12*).

Special Considerations

1. Although the second technique (i.e., direct visualization with the use of a tongue blade) may seem intuitively

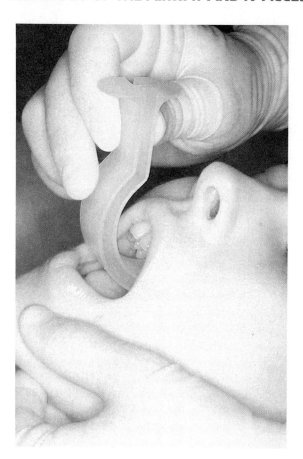

Figure 7-11A.   Insertion of the oral pharyngeal airway. The device is inserted upside down into the mouth.

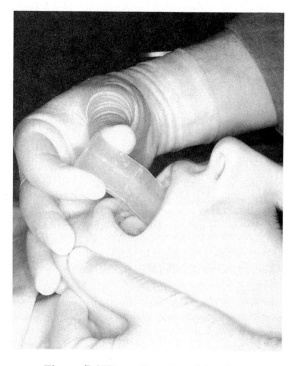

Figure 7-11B.   Rotation of the airway.

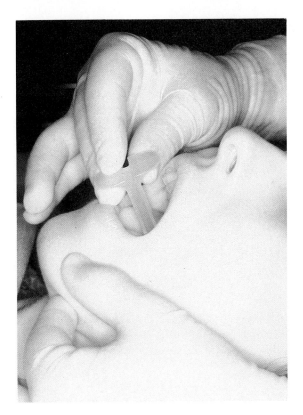

Figure 7-11C. Final position of the oral pharyngeal airway.

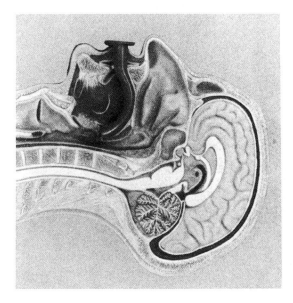

Figure 7-12. Correct final position of oral pharyngeal airway after insertion.
(Reproduced with permission of Ambu, Inc from Lotz P, Ahnefeld FW, Hirlinger WD: *A systematic guide to intubation*, Atelier Flad, Eckental, West Germany.)

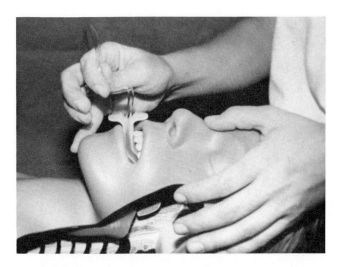

Figure 7-13. Although the lumen of the oral airway is adequate for *ventilation*, it is *not* large enough to allow passage of the suction catheter. In the above illustration, attempted passage results in kinking of the catheter.

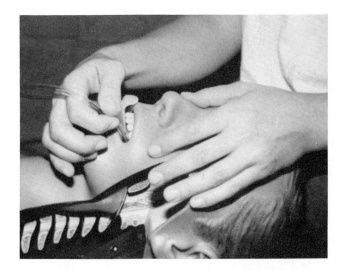

Figure 7-14. The correct way to suction a patient with an oral airway in place is to insert the suction catheter into the mouth adjacent to (but *not* through) the oral airway.

easier, one must be sure that the airway is inserted deep enough so as to come to rest *behind* the tongue. Unless careful attention is paid to doing this, it's all too easy to stop short—in which case the device may actually cause airway obstruction by pressing on the tongue and pushing it back to occlude the airway.

2. If the tube repeatedly comes out of the mouth, it is likely to be improperly seated (and compressing the tongue into the posterior pharynx). This may further obstruct the airway. Don't continue to force the airway in. Instead, *remove it entirely*; then try to insert it again.

3. Although the lumen of the tube is adequate for *ventilating* the patient, it should *not* be used for suctioning because the lumen is not large enough to allow passage of the suction catheter *(Figure 7-13)*. The suction catheter is instead inserted adjacent to the airway. Suction is then performed in the usual manner *(Figure 7-14)*.

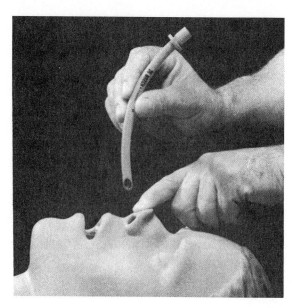

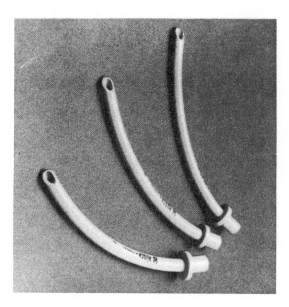

Figure 7-15.   Examples of nasopharyngeal airways. (Reproduced with permission of Ambu, Inc from Lotz P, Ahnefeld FW, Hirlinger WD: *A systematic guide to intubation*, Atelier Flad, Eckental, West Germany.)

Figure 7-16A.   Proper bevel position of the nasopharyngeal airway during insertion. In this illustration the bevel is placed against the septum as the airway is inserted into the right nares. (Reproduced with permission of Ambu, Inc from Lotz P, Ahnefeld FW, Hirlinger WD: *A systematic guide to intubation*, Atelier Flad, Eckental, West Germany.)

4. The oral pharyngeal airway should be used only in unconscious patients. Insertion of this device in a conscious or semiconscious patient is likely to activate the gag reflex (when the back of the tongue or posterior pharyngeal wall is touched) and precipitate vomiting. *Alert patients or semiconscious patients with an intact gag reflex are not suitable candidates for insertion of an oral pharyngeal airway.*

THE NASOPHARYNGEAL AIRWAY (NASAL TRUMPET)

The *nasopharyngeal airway* is an extremely compliant rubber tube approximately 15 cm in length *(Figure 7-15)*. The tube is designed so that its distal tip sits in the posterior pharynx while the proximal tip rests on the external nares. The lumen of this device permits the passage of air into the lower respiratory tract.

The principal advantage of the nasal pharyngeal airway is that it is usually well tolerated in the patient who retains a sensitive gag reflex. This makes it the airway adjunct of choice for the conscious or semiconscious patient with respiratory difficulty.

Technique for Insertion

The tube should be lubricated with 2% lidocaine gel prior to insertion. The purpose of the lidocaine is twofold: It anesthetizes the nasal mucosa in the posterior pharynx (so as to minimize sensitivity of the gag reflex), and lubricates the tube to facilitate insertion.

The nasopharyngeal airway is then advanced into the nares by placing the bevel against the septum of the nose *(Figure 7-16A)* and gently sliding the tube backward in line with the base of the ears *(Figure 7-16B)*. In this way the tube passes parallel to the floor of the nasal cavity *(Figure 7-17)*. When completely inserted, the distal end is seated in the posterior pharynx *(Figure 7-18)*.

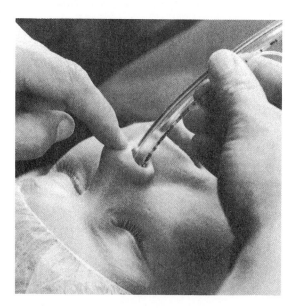

Figure 7-16B.   Careful sliding of the nasopharyngeal tube into the nasal cavity. (Reproduced with permission of Ambu, Inc from Lotz P, Ahnefeld FW, Hirlinger WD: *A systematic guide to intubation*, Atelier Flad, Eckental, West Germany.)

Special Considerations

1. Although in most cases proper insertion of the nasal trumpet will result in correct position of the distal end in the posterior pharynx, on occasion the tube may be too short or too long. Be alert to the fact that if this happens, adequate ventilation may not be achieved.

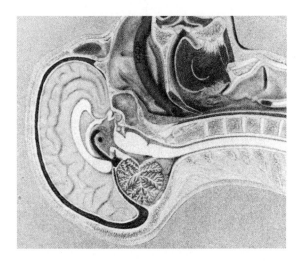

Figure 7-17.   Passage of the nasopharyngeal airway parallel to the floor of the nasal cavity.
(Reproduced with permission of Ambu, Inc from Lotz P, Ahnefeld FW, Hirlinger WD: *A systematic guide to intubation*, Atelier Flad, Eckental, West Germany.)

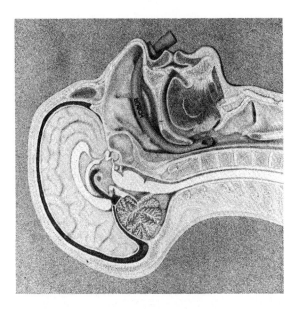

Figure 7-18.   Correct position of nasopharyngeal airway after insertion.
(Reproduced with permission of Ambu, Inc from Lotz P, Ahnefeld FW, Hirlinger WD: *A systematic guide to intubation*, Atelier Flad, Eckental, West Germany.)

2. While most conscious or semiconscious patients are able to tolerate this device, the gag reflex of certain particularly sensitive individuals may still be activated.
3. Forceful introduction of the airway into the nasal passage should be avoided, since this may cause abrasions or lacerate the nasal mucosa and produce significant bleeding.

SUCTION

Immediate accessibility to properly functioning *suction* equipment is equally important as availability of other airway adjuncts. Such equipment is needed to remove secretions and particulate matter that could otherwise be aspirated or compromise the airway. Suction units should be portable, durable, and capable of generating at least 300 mm Hg of negative pressure. When suctioning the oral pharynx, a large-bore catheter *and* tube should be used in order to assure that all large particulate matter will be evacuated. Smaller catheters are generally adequate for nasopharyngeal and/or endotracheal suction.

Suction Technique

Adequate ventilation does not occur during suctioning. As a result, patients should always be hyperventilated *before* beginning suctioning. The suction procedure itself should *never* be carried out for more than 15 seconds at a time to minimize the chance of hypoxemia.

Suction of the oral pharynx is performed by inserting the catheter in the patient's mouth and *intermittently* applying negative pressure. The key to endotracheal suctioning is not to apply negative pressure during insertion of the catheter down the endotracheal tube. Suction is applied intermittently, and *only* while slowly withdrawing the catheter.

Ventilatory Adjuncts

The devices described below are used to assist ventilation of patients in respiratory distress or to provide mandatory ventilation for those who are not breathing at all.

VENTILATION DURING CPR

Ventilating a patient during CPR is a special skill in itself that requires continuous monitoring and close attention to detail to assure proper performance. Incorrect ventilation (application of either excessive or inadequate inspiratory pressure) may result in hypoxemia, increased intracranial pressure, or gastric insufflation (especially in patients who are not intubated), as well as accompanying tachycardia or bradycardia.

For optimal oxygenation during CPR, it is extremely important for ventilations to be administered *slowly* and smoothly. Only by doing so can one avoid generation of turbulent air flow and assure even distribution to all lung fields. In addition, the parameters of respiration should ideally remain constant. Thus each ventilation should be administered at the same speed and pressure to result in as constant a minute ventilation* as possible.

CPR is not a benign procedure. In addition to fracturing ribs or the sternum, it may cause cardiac or pulmonary parenchymal changes (contusions), liver laceration, and/or pneumothorax or hemothorax. Some of these complications are not amenable to

---

*__Minute ventilation__ = tidal volume × respiratory rate.

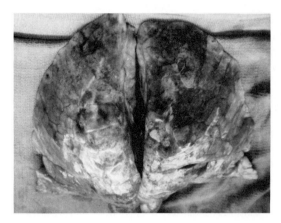

Figure 7-19.   Example of typical pulmonary changes that occur during CPR. There are numerous areas of contusions and hemorrhage (*dark areas in the figure*).

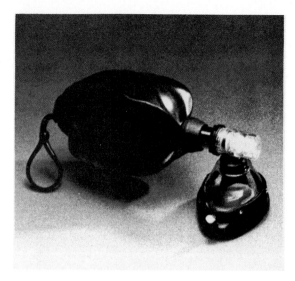

Figure 7-20.   Example of a self-inflating resuscitation (Ambu) bag.
(Reproduced with permission of Ambu, Inc from Lotz P, Ahnefeld FW, Hirlinger WD: *A systematic guide to intubation*, Atelier Flad, Eckental, West Germany.)

immediate treatment. Resuscitative efforts (including external chest compression) need to continue if a patient remains pulseless, regardless of whether there are cardiac contusions or fractured ribs. In contrast, other potential complications such as tension pneumothorax or cardiac tamponade mandate prompt recognition and immediate treatment if resuscitation is to have any chance for success.

Unfortunately, the goal of optimal ventilation during CPR is a task much easier wished for than accomplished. Pulmonary parenchymal changes are a common (expected) accompaniment of even perfectly performed CPR. This fact is made abundantly clear from inspection of *Figure 7-19*, which illustrates the typical appearance of the lungs after a short period (less than 15 minutes) of CPR. Numerous areas of pulmonary contusion, hemorrhage, and atelectasis are evident. As a result of these anatomic alterations, pathophysiologic changes are produced which lead to increased pulmonary vascular resistance with impaired pulmonary flow and suboptimal oxygenation. Parenchymal damage (and associated pathophysiologic changes) would likely be even more significant in patients with underlying pulmonary disease who undergo CPR. As might be expected, lung compliance is dramatically reduced by this process and continues to decrease (i.e., the lungs become stiffer) the longer resuscitation is in progress. Accordingly, ventilation during CPR becomes progressively more difficult and less effective.

Obviously, the best way to minimize the deleterious pathophysiologic alterations produced in the pulmonary parenchyma by CPR is to minimize the duration of the resuscitative process. Short of this, attention to several other factors may be helpful. Undue emphasis is often placed on strict interposition of ventilation after every fifth compression during basic life support. Practically speak-

ing, blood flow is *not* decreased when a portion of the ventilatory cycle overlaps with the next chest compression. In fact, blood flow to the arrested heart is actually *increased* by simultaneous ventilation and compression (Melker and Cavallaro, 1983; Cavallaro, 1990). While we are *not* suggesting to disregard AHA recommendations for basic life support (to administer ventilations during the pause after each fifth chest compression), we *are* emphasizing the tremendous importance of being sure that ventilation is not unduly hurried. Instead, it must be delivered *slowly* and smoothly to assure as even distribution of air to all lung fields as possible.

For patients who remain in cardiac arrest, intubation should be accomplished as expeditiously as possible. Subsequent ventilation (which is usually accomplished by compression of a bag-valve device) should continue to be smooth with a slow and even delivery, keeping respiratory parameters as constant as possible while maintaining the flexibility to adapt to alterations in lung compliance as the resuscitative process goes on.

SELF-INFLATING RESERVOIR BAGS

The *self-inflating resuscitation bag* (*bag-valve mask* or *BVM*) is a unit consisting of a bag and an adapter that can be attached to a mask or endotracheal tube (*Figure 7-20*).

The ideal BVM unit should have the following characteristics:

1. A *clear* mask
2. A self-inflating, easy-to-grip bag
3. A system for delivery of supplemental oxygen
4. An oxygen reservoir
5. No pop-off valve

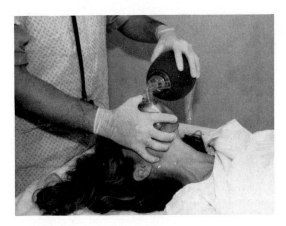

Figure 7-21A.   Use of a BVM unit by a single rescuer. This requires *simultaneous* accomplishment of three tasks (maintaining a patent airway *and* tight face seal with one hand, while ventilating the patient with the other hand).

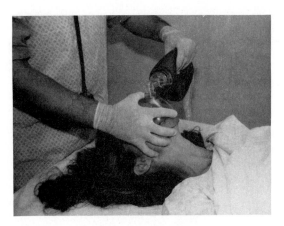

Figure 7-21B.   Follow-up picture to Fig. 7-21A, illustrating actual ventilation as the single rescuer squeezes the bag.

The reason for the *clear mask* is that it allows the emergency care provider to see if regurgitation has occurred. The bags of most BVM units are made of smooth rubber that becomes especially slippery when wet. An *easy-to-grip bag* would facilitate handling the unit when ventilating the patient.

A *system* for delivery of *supplemental oxygen* is important. An F_IO_2 of up to 40% may be provided by attaching a high-flow source of supplemental oxygen to the bag. With the additional attachment of an *oxygen reservoir* and a flow rate of 10 to 15 L/min, an F_IO_2 of up to 90% may be delivered.

Pop-off valves are not desirable for BVM units used to manage the airways of patients in cardiac arrest because of the dramatic decrease in lung compliance that occurs in this setting. As we have already mentioned, much higher than usual airway pressures are often needed to ventilate such patients. Pop-off valves could be self-defeating, as they might prevent generation of sufficient peak airway pressure to overcome this increase in airway resistance.

BVM units are the most commonly employed ventilatory adjunct in emergency situations. Nevertheless, significant drawbacks are associated with their use. These include fluctuations in peak airway pressure, tidal volume, and ventilatory rate; variability in delivered oxygen concentrations when a reservoir is not used; and face mask leaks.

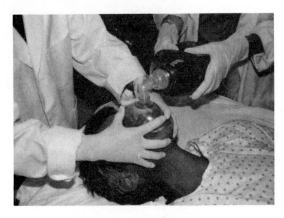

Figure 7-21C.   Addition of a second rescuer greatly facilitates proper ventilation with a BVM unit. One rescuer concentrates on maintaining a patent airway and tight face seal, while the second rescuer is able to use both hands to deliver ventilation.

> Contrary to popular belief, tidal volumes generated with BVM units in the unprotected airway are far less than those generated by mouth-to-mouth or mouth-to-mask ventilation. This is not true for intubated patients, since leakage of air through (around) the face mask is no longer a problem and both of the rescuer's hands are now free to squeeze the bag.

Technique for Use

The most difficult part about ventilating a patient who is not intubated using a BVM device is that one rescuer must simultaneously perform three tasks *(Figure 7-21A)*. A patent airway and tight face seal must be maintained with one hand,

while the other hand is used to ventilate the patient. Unless each of these tasks is performed correctly, inadequate ventilation is likely to result.

Insertion of an oral or nasopharyngeal tube may assist in maintaining patency of the airway. The mask of the BVM unit is then applied to the patient's face and secured by positioning the index finger on the portion that covers the chin, while the thumb holds the upper part of the mask firmly against the bridge of the nose (pushing down to ensure a good face seal). The remaining three fingers are placed on the base of the mandible and support the head in the tilt position (by careful upward pressure). Once the fingers are correctly in place, their action is similar to that when squeezing a rubber ball. The other hand is used to squeeze the bag *(Figure 7-21B)*.

To prevent high peak airway pressures and decrease the likelihood of gastric distention in the patient with an unprotected airway, the bag must be squeezed *slowly*. Use of a second rescuer is extremely helpful in this regard since it allows one rescuer to concentrate on securing a good face seal with the use of both hands, while the second rescuer may also use both hands to squeeze the bag *(Figure 7-21C)*. When proper ventilation is being administered, the chest will be observed to rise and fall with each insufflation of the bag. (An advantage of the BVM unit is that it provides the rescuer with a sense of the compliance of the patient's lungs.)

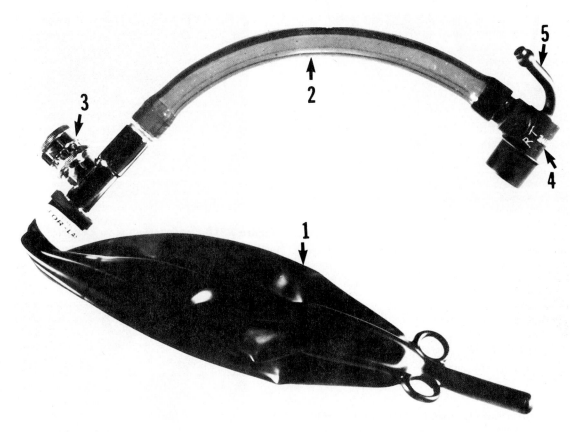

Figure 7-22.   Flow-inflation reservoir bag: (*1*) anesthesia bag; (*2*) plastic tubing; (*3*) exhaust valve; (*4*) standard ET tube connector; (*5*) connector for manometer (used to measure airway pressures).

FLOW-INFLATION RESERVOIR BAG

The *flow-inflation reservoir (anesthesia) bag (Mapelson-D bag)* requires even more skill to operate than does a BVM. It consists of an anesthesia bag, a piece of plastic tubing (that is approximately 1 foot long), an exhaust valve, and a standard endotracheal tube connector *(Figure 7-22)*. The latter is usually attached to the oxygen source and an endotracheal tube. Advantages of this bag over the standard BVM are that you can apply CPAP (continuous positive airway pressure) and PEEP (positive end-expiratory pressure). In addition, ventilation with 100% oxygen is guaranteed. In contrast, one is never entirely sure of the concentration of oxygen delivered with the BVM because of the variability in the amount of entrained room air.

> In general, Mapelson-D bags are used much less commonly than BVM units. This device should be operated *only* by individuals highly trained in its use. In the hands of an inexperienced provider, the risk of barotrauma (and tension pneumothorax) is great.

OXYGEN-POWERED BREATHING DEVICES (O₂PBD)

The *oxygen-powered breathing device* has been used to ventilate the victim in respiratory arrest and provide supple-

mental oxygen to spontaneously breathing patients. When used in the former setting, the O$_2$PBD functions as a manually cycled, pressure-limited ventilator *(Figure 7-23)*. Activation of the unit by the rescuer provides spontaneous flow rates of up to 120 L/min. Ventilation is terminated either by release of the activation button or when peak airway pressure attains 40 mm Hg (54 cm H$_2$O).

> Concerns about the use of this device relate to the high inspiratory flow rates it generates (and turbulent flow it produces) when manually operated, as well as the potential for producing gastric insufflation in the patient with an unprotected airway (AHA ACLS JAMA Suppl, 1986). Recent modifications in newer models (and manufacture of conversion kits for older models) have improved the safety of the O$_2$PBD by allowing reduction of flow rates to 40 L/min. Nevertheless, the device *must* still be used with extreme caution in adults (especially in patients who are not intubated), and it is not recommended for use in children.

The O$_2$PBD may be most useful when employed as a demand valve for spontaneously breathing patients. In this capacity, generation of as little as 1 cm H$_2$O negative airway pressure activates a flutter valve within the unit that allows the patient to inhale 100% oxygen. This aspect of the device is extremely advantageous in providing spontaneously breathing patients supplemental oxygen without requiring large volumes of stored oxygen.

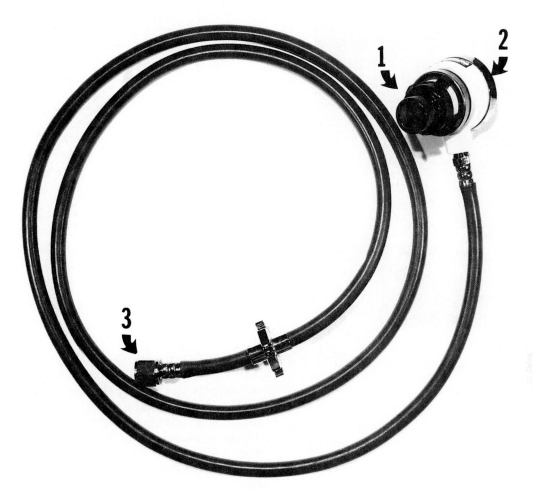

Figure 7-23. Oxygen-powered breathing device: (*1*) 15/22 mm connector for attaching endotracheal tube; (*2*) flow regulator; (*3*) oxygen source connector.

THE POCKET MASK (MOUTH-TO-MASK)

The *pocket mask* is very similar to the mask used in conjunction with the bag-valve devices (*Figure 7-24*). The major difference is that the mouth-to-mask unit has an additional port where supplemental oxygen can be administered, providing inspired oxygen concentrations of 50% when the flow rate is 10 L/min. The port used for attachment of the reservoir bag with the bag-valve device is the port through which the rescuer ventilates the patient with the pocket mask.

The most attractive feature of the pocket mask is that it allows the rescuer to perform mouth-to-mouth ventilation *without* the need for direct contact with the mouth of the victim. Addition of a disposable, inexpensive exhalation (one-way) valve further assures the safety of the rescuer (by diverting the victim's stream of exhaled air), and should alleviate concerns about contracting an infectious disease (such as AIDS or tuberculosis). As noted earlier, tidal volumes attainable by ventilation with the pocket mask are superior to those achieved from ventilation with a BVM unit.

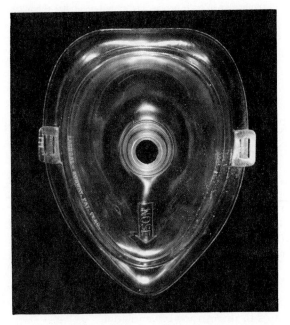

Figure 7-24. Pocket mask.

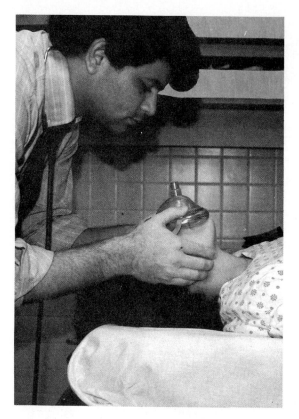

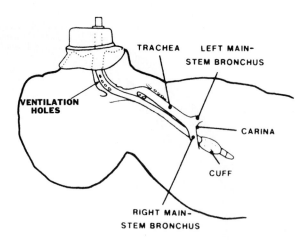

Figure 7-26. Correct positioning of esophageal obturator airway (EOA) after insertion. The cuff of the EOA lies just below the carina.
(Reproduced with permission from McIntyre KM, Lewis JA, editors: *Textbook of advanced cardiac life support*, Dallas, 1981, American Heart Association.)

Figure 7-25. Proper application of the pocket mask. The rescuer is at the head of the bed in good position to deliver breaths through the ventilation port.

Technique for Use

When using the pocket mask, the rescuer positions himself/herself above the head of the patient. The mask is placed on the patient's face and secured through a coordinated interplay of the fingers of both hands. The thumbs stabilize the mask over the bridge of the nose, while the index fingers hold the mask in place over the chin. The three remaining fingers of each hand are positioned under the chin and act in concert to maintain the head tilt which keeps the airway patent *(Figure 7-25)*.

Advanced Airway Management Techniques

ESOPHAGEAL OBTURATOR AIRWAYS

The principle of the *esophageal obturator* is to occlude the esophagus so that gastric insufflation is prevented and the ventilatory efforts of the rescuer can be directed into the trachea. Two types of obturators are currently available: the *esophageal obturator airway (EOA)* and the *esophageal gastric tube airway (EGTA)*. Although similar in appearance, important differences exist between the two types of obturators in the method of ventilation.

The EOA is the original esophageal obturator airway. This device was first described in 1968. It consists of a tube approximately 37 cm in length with a blind tip on its distal end. Inflation of a cuff just above this tip occludes the esophagus. When properly inserted, the cuff should lie slightly below the level of the carina of the trachea *(Figure 7-26)*.

The proximal end of the tube is open and fits snugly into a specially designed face mask. Small ventilation holes are present in the upper third of the tube. When the EOA is correctly positioned, the holes lie at the level of the posterior pharynx. It is through these small holes that ventilation occurs.

The EGTA was developed in 1977. It improved on the design of the EOA by adding a route for decompression of the stomach *(Figure 7-27)*. This lessens the chance of regurgitation and aspiration. Instead of having a blind tip on the distal end of the obturator tube, an opening was made through which a nasogastric tube could be passed into the stomach. The small holes which had previously been used for ventilation with the EOA are no longer present with the EGTA tube. Instead, a second port has been added to the mask through which ventilation occurs in a similar fashion as with the bag-valve mask *(Figure 7-28)*.

Technique for Insertion

The principle for insertion of the EOA and the EGTA is the same. The mandible is lifted forward by the rescuer's hand as the patient's head is gently flexed to assist passage of the tube into the esophagus *(Figures 7-29A and 7-29B)*. The EOA/EGTA is inserted into the oral pharynx and *blindly* advanced. It should follow the natural curvature of the pharynx and enter into the esophagus *(Figure 7-29C)*. At this point the mask should be seated on the face *(Figure 7-29D)*.

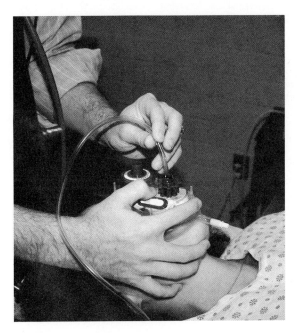

Figure 7-27. Inserting a nasogastric tube through the lumen of the EGTA tube to decompress the stomach.

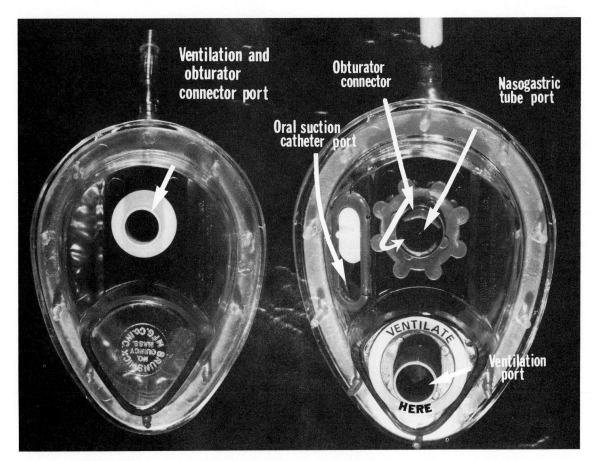

Figure 7-28. Comparison of EOA (*left*) and EGTA (*right*) face masks. Ventilation with the EOA is accomplished via the ventilation holes shown in Figure 7-26. In contrast, ventilation with the EGTA is accomplished through a special ventilation port. In both cases, air is directed into the trachea by virtue of the fact that the esophagus is occluded.

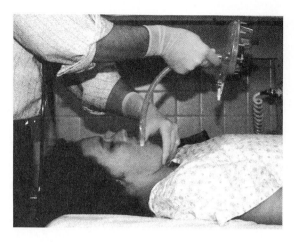

Figure 7-29A.   Position of the head (gently flexed forward) while inserting the obturator airway.

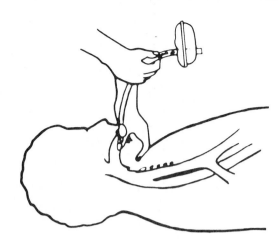

Figure 7-29B.   Schematic representation of Figure 7-29A. (Reproduced with permission from McIntyre KM, Lewis JA, editors: *Textbook of advanced cardiac life support*, Dallas, 1981, American Heart Association.)

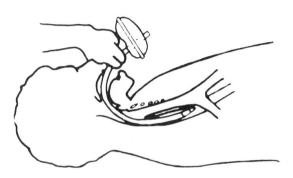

Figure 7-29C.   Advancing (blindly) the obturator airway, which follows the natural curvature of the pharynx to enter the esophagus.
(Reproduced with permission from McIntyre KM, Lewis JA, editors: *Textbook of advanced cardiac life support*, Dallas, 1981, American Heart Association.)

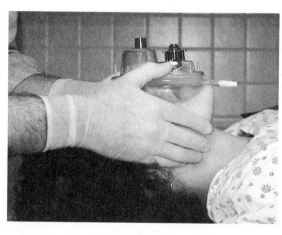

Figure 7-29D.   Final position of the obturator airway mask.

Never force advancement of the tube. If resistance is encountered along the way, simply withdraw the tube slightly, reposition the patient's head, and try again to advance the tube.

Confirming proper position of the tube is critical. If the trachea is inadvertently intubated and the cuff of the tube inflated with 20 to 30 ml of air, significant damage may occur to this structure. Several positive pressure ventilations should be delivered to test for tube position. Even though some of this air will enter the esophagus, enough should go into the trachea to produce a rise and fall of the chest wall if the tube is properly situated in the esophagus. The cuff may now be inflated with 30 ml of air. Further confirmation of proper tube placement can be obtained by auscultating over the apices and lateral lung fields for good bilateral breath sounds and observing for symmetric chest excursion.

Another way to confirm proper tube placement is by ET CO_2 monitoring. Extremely low CO_2 readings suggest that the obturator may have inadvertently intubated the trachea, whereas increasing CO_2 readings are consistent with proper tube placement.

Special Considerations

As was the case for ventilating a patient with a BVM, obtaining a good face seal is essential for ensuring adequate ventilation with the EOA/EGTA. Realize that head positioning in preparation for EOA/EGTA insertion is the *opposite* of that for preparing to intubate endotracheally. That is, the neck is slightly extended back, and the chin is flexed forward. Doing so minimizes the chance of inadvertently entering the trachea when the tube is inserted.

Although distinctly uncommon, esophageal rupture may complicate EOA placement. As a result, Clinton and Ruiz (1985) suggest that inflation of the EOA cuff be limited to 20 ml of air instead of the customary 30 ml. In their experience, doing so has not resulted in leakage around the cuff, and has virtually eliminated the risk of esophageal rupture.

The EOA/EGTA was initially advocated as an alternative method of endotracheal intubation. Its greatest application has been in the prehospital setting where operators skilled in endotracheal intubation are not always available. Advantages of the EOA are that insertion may be accomplished rapidly (in less than 10 seconds) by trained individuals (Clinton and Ruiz, 1985), and that neck extension is not needed for the procedure. However, significant problems have been associated with its use. These include:

1. Inadequate tidal volumes due to face mask leak
2. Inadvertent endotracheal intubation
3. Esophageal laceration and rupture
4. High incidence of gastric regurgitation on removal of the tube.

Because of these problems, *endotracheal intubation is universally acknowledged as the procedure of choice for managing the unprotected airway.*

Use of the EOA/EGTA is *contraindicated* if:
1. The victim is conscious.
2. There is suspicion of caustic ingestion.
3. The victim is less than 16 years of age.
4. There is known esophageal disease.

Additional Considerations

The EOA/EGTA has been used much less commonly in recent years, probably because of the increased ability of paramedical personnel to successfully perform endotracheal intubation. Nevertheless, they still comprise an alternative method for securing an airway.

Practically speaking, most emergency care providers will probably never have the opportunity to *insert* an EOA/EGTA. However, they are likely at some time to be involved with the removal of this device, especially if they work in an emergency facility. It is therefore essential to at least gain familiarity with the technique for *removal* of the tube.

If the patient is still not breathing spontaneously on arrival in the emergency department, endotracheal intubation must be performed *before* the esophageal obturator is withdrawn in order to protect the airway. Because of the extremely high incidence of gastric regurgitation with removal of the EOA/EGTA, the patient's head should be turned to the side, and suction must be readily available.

Hyperventilate the patient prior to any manipulation. The face mask of the obturator is then detached by squeezing the connector on the proximal end of the tube that protrudes through the mask *(Figure 7-30)*. To make room for the laryngoscope, the obturator tube is pushed to the left side of the mouth with the rescuer's index finger. Intubation can now be performed in the usual fashion. Due to the fact that the EOA/EGTA is still in place in the esophagus, the rescuer is far less likely to mistakenly intubate this structure.

Once correct placement of the endotracheal tube has been confirmed, the EOA/EGTA may be removed. This should be done by deflating the balloon, turning the patient on the side, and vigorously suctioning the oral pharynx at the same time that the tube is withdrawn.

Intubation

Intubation is the definitive method of managing the airway of patients who are not breathing, or who are unresponsive with an unprotected airway. The advantages of intubation are:

1. Prevention of aspiration
2. Lower risk for gastric insufflation
3. Allows for administration of high inspired oxygen concentrations and positive pressure ventilations

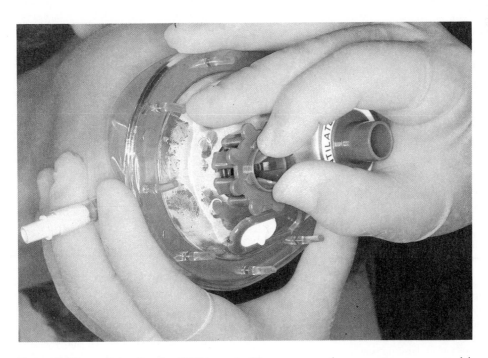

Figure 7-30.   Releasing the EGTA mask. The prongs on the connector are squeezed in the rescuer's thumb and index finger to release the mask.

CURVED BLADE

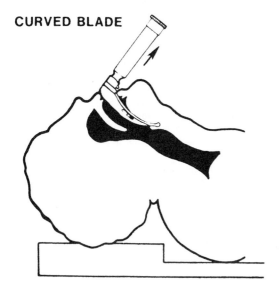

STRAIGHT BLADE

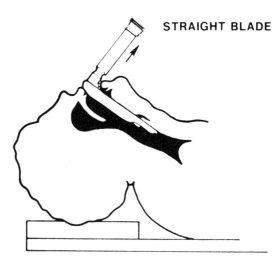

Figure 7-31. Proper placement of the curved blade in the vallecula.
(Reproduced with permission from McIntyre KM, Lewis JA, editors: *Textbook of advanced cardiac life support*, Dallas, 1981, American Heart Association.)

Figure 7-32. Proper placement of the straight blade. The epiglottis is lifted to provide visualization.
(Reproduced with permission from McIntyre KM, Lewis JA, editors: *Textbook of advanced cardiac life support*, Dallas, 1981, American Heart Association.)

4. Provides access for drug administration (with endotracheal intubation)
5. Provides access for suctioning of the tracheobronchial tree (with endotracheal or nasotracheal intubation)

ENDOTRACHEAL INTUBATION

The most definitive means of managing the airway for the nonbreathing, unresponsive patient is with *endotracheal intubation*. Two types of laryngoscope blades may be used to perform this procedure: the *Miller (straight) blade* and the *MacIntosh (curved) blade*.

The technique for visualization of the vocal cords is similar regardless of which blade is used. *The only difference in the procedure is in the placement of the tip.* When using the curved blade, the tip is inserted into the vallecula. The soft tissue is then lifted, and the laryngeal opening is visualized *(Figure 7-31)*. In contrast, when the straight blade is used, the epiglottis itself is lifted to provide visualization *(Figure 7-32)*. *It matters little which blade is chosen for intubation.* Far more important for the emergency care provider is to decide on his/her preference, and to become comfortable in the use of that *one* type of blade.

An advantage of the curved blade is its relatively large surface area compared to the straight blade. This facilitates manipulation of the tongue and provides a larger space in the oral cavity for passage of the endotracheal tube. It may also be somewhat easier technically to use the curved blade. On the other hand, visualization of the larynx may not be quite as good because the presence of the epiglottis below the curved blade may partially block the operator's view. With the straight blade the epiglottis is lifted up and out of the line of view. *Each blade has its advocates.* As indicated above, the choice of which one to use is simply a matter of personal preference.

The size of the endotracheal tube most commonly used to intubate adults is 7.5 to 8 mm in diameter for females, and 8 to 8.5 mm for males.

Prior to Intubation

All equipment must be routinely checked at frequent intervals. The time to find out that a laryngoscope bulb has burned out is not *after* the blade has been inserted into the pharynx. Similarly, the time to find out that the cuff is defective is not *after* the patient has been intubated.

Hyperventilation should always precede attempts at intubation. At no time should a patient remain unventilated for more than 15 to 20 seconds. If intubation is not successful within this time frame, withdraw the tube, reventilate the patient, and try again.

Positioning the Patient

It is commonly assumed that hyperextension of the head and neck will facilitate endotracheal intubation. In reality, hyperextension produces the opposite effect because it causes the axes of the oropharynx and trachea to become misaligned *(Figure 7-33)*. One technique that may make intubation easier is to place a small pillow or towel under the patient's occiput so as to lift the head slightly without extending it. This posture is known as the *sniffing* position *(Figure 7-34)*. As can be seen from *Figure 7-35*, a much more direct line for visualization of the vocal cords (due to alignment of the axes of the oropharynx and trachea) is now evident.

As an aid to conceptualizing the "**sniffing position**," pretend you are holding a wonderfully fragrant flower in front of you. *Now imagine how you would position yourself to take a sniff.* Do so. Now consider what you have done to achieve the position—*flexed your neck forward, and slightly extended it.*

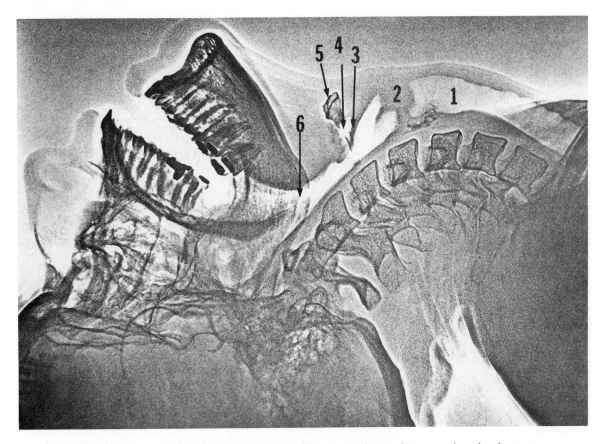

Figure 7-33.   Hyperextension of the neck. The axes at the oropharynx and trachea become misaligned with hyperextension, making endotracheal intubation more difficult: *(1)* trachea; *(2)* vocal cords; *(3)* epiglottis; *(4)* vallecula; *(5)* hyoid cartilage; *(6)* oropharynx.
(Reproduced with permission from Applebaum EL, Bruce DL: *Tracheal intubation,* Philadelphia, 1976, WB Saunders.)

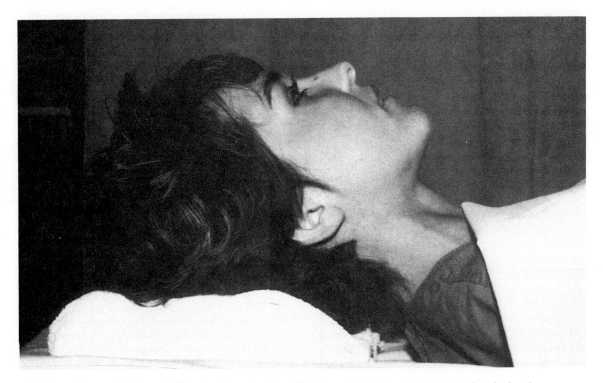

Figure 7-34.   Sniffing position. A pillow lifts the occiput without hyperextending the head.

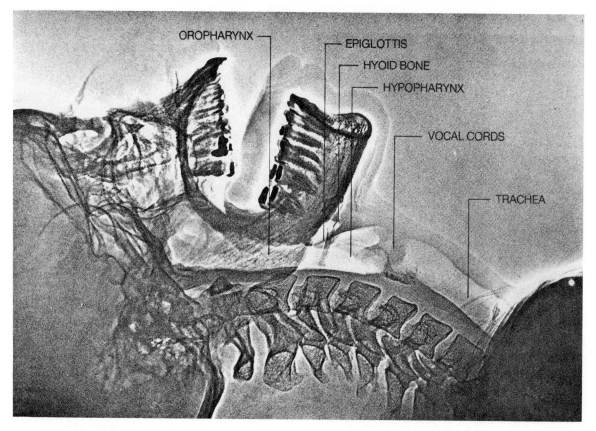

Figure 7-35.   X-ray demonstrating anatomic relationships in the sniffing position. Compared to Figure 7-33, a much more direct line for visualization of the vocal cords is now evident. (Reproduced with permission from Applebaum EL, Bruce DL: *Tracheal intubation*, Philadelphia, 1976, WB Saunders.)

Technique for Intubation

The key priorities for endotracheal intubation are speed of insertion (to minimize the time of hypoxia) and proper technique. *The two are equally important* (and closely interrelated). Thus, attention to proper technique naturally improves speed as operator familiarity and confidence increase and the need for repetitive intubation attempts becomes less.

A common mistake is to rapidly insert the full length of the laryngoscope blade without attention to placement. This frequently puts the tip of the blade *beyond* the epiglottis and vallecula, making it extremely difficult for the operator to identify the anatomy. The operator is then forced to search for key structures on withdrawal of the blade. *It is far simpler and more effective to insert the blade in a more controlled manner.* This allows visualization of structures in their natural sequence as the blade is advanced through the airway.

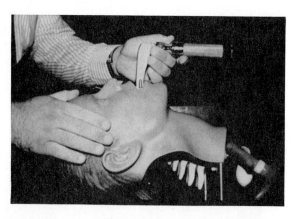

Figure 7-36.   Inserting the laryngoscope into the patient's mouth, following the natural curvature of the tongue.

Remember that the vallecula lies *at the base of the tongue* and is not nearly as deep in the throat as is commonly believed. It is therefore *not* necessary to insert the entire length of the laryngoscope blade into the patient's mouth for successful intubation.

After equipment has been checked and the patient properly positioned and hyperventilated, you are ready to begin the procedure. Insert the laryngoscope blade carefully into the patient's mouth, following the natural curvature of the tongue *(Figure 7-36)*. The hard palate and uvula are visualized as one tracks through the oral pharynx *(Figure 7-37)*. On arrival at the posterior pharynx, the tip of the blade is lifted. In most cases the epiglottis will now become readily visible *(Figure 7-38)*. If you are using the straight blade, the epiglottis itself is

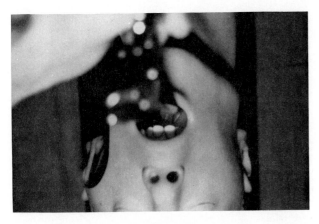

Figure 7-37.   Visualizing the hard palate and uvula as one tracks through the oral pharynx.

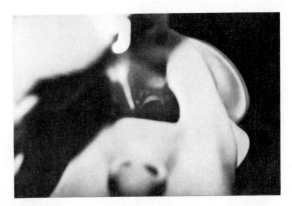

Figure 7-38.   Visualizing the epiglottis as the blade tip is lifted.

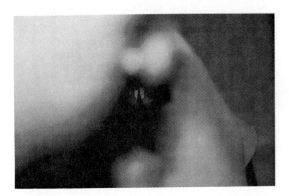

Figure 7-39.   Lifting the epiglottis with the straight blade to visualize the cords.

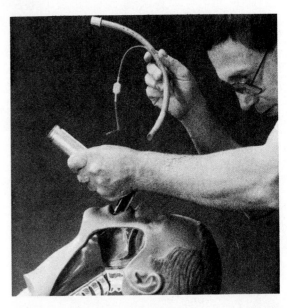

Figure 7-40.   Correct technique for insertion of the endotracheal tube, lifting the laryngoscope handle *forward* and *anteriorly*. *(Reproduced with permission of Ambu, Inc from Lotz P, Ahnefeld FW, Hirlinger WD: A systematic guide to intubation, Atelier Flad, Eckental, West Germany.)*

lifted to visualize the cords *(Figure 7-39)*. If the curved blade is used, the blade tip is inserted into the vallecula and then lifted a little higher to visualize the cords.

The teeth must not be used as a fulcrum to pry up the mandible when attempting to visualize the cords. Doing so makes it likely that a tooth will be fractured or dislodged. Instead, the operator should concentrate on lifting the laryngoscope handle *forward* and *anteriorly* as if reaching to touch the point where the ceiling and wall meet *(Figure 7-40)*. In doing so, the principal movement is from the arm and elbow. Excessive wrist flexion does *not* help visualization, *and it predisposes to trauma.*

Once the epiglottis has been lifted and the laryngeal opening is in view, the following structures should be seen:
1. The arytenoid cartilages
2. The vocal cords
3. The glottic opening

The *arytenoid cartilages* lie at the bottom of the rescuer's field of vision *(Figure 7-41)*. Behind them are found the white, glossy *vocal cords*, which are separated by the dark glottic opening. It is through this opening that the endotracheal tube is inserted. One should be extremely deliberate in *watching the tube pass through this opening.* Advance the endotracheal tube until the cuff *just* disappears from sight, which is approximately 2 cm beyond the cords *(Figure 7-42)*. Advancement beyond this point

should be avoided because it may result in intubation of the right mainstem bronchus.

Once the tube is properly seated in the trachea, is is held in position with the operator's right hand. Care must be taken not to dislodge the endotracheal tube or fracture any teeth while removing the laryngoscope.

The cuff is now inflated with 5 to 10 ml of air. Correct position of the tube should be verified by auscultating the lung fields and epigastric areas as several ventilations are administered. One listens for the presence of good bilateral breath sounds and looks for symmetric chest excursion. Absent or diminished breath sounds on the left side of the chest suggest intubation of the right mainstem bronchus. This can usually be rectified by withdrawing the tube a short distance until breath sounds equalize. Should gurgling sounds be heard over the epigastrium, the tube is in the stomach. Immediately deflate the balloon and remove the tube. Final confirmation of

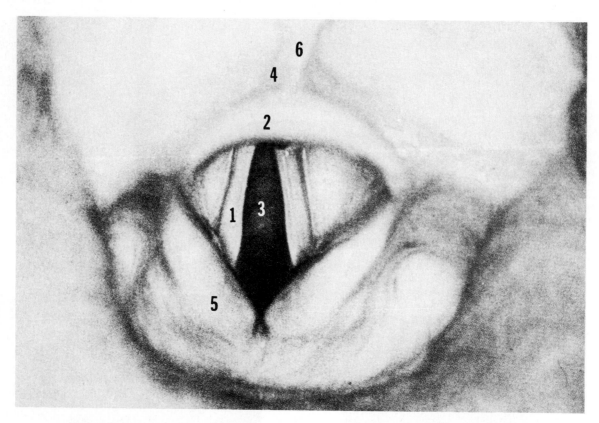

Figure 7-41.   Anatomy of the area around the entrance to the trachea: *(1)* vocal cords; *(2)* epiglottis; *(3)* aperture of the cords; *(4)* vallecula; *(5)* arytenoid cartilage; *(6)* tongue. (Reproduced with permission from Yokochi C, Rohen JW: *Photographic anatomy of the human body,* Baltimore, 1978, University Park Press.)

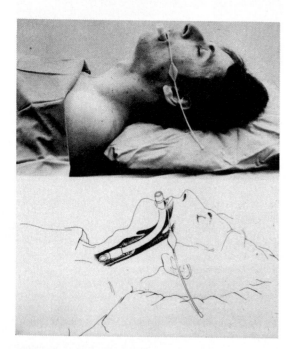

Figure 7-42.   Correct position of the endotracheal tube after insertion. The tube has been advanced through the cords until the cuff just disappears from sight.
(Reproduced with permission from Applebaum EL, Bruce DL: *Trahceal intubation,* Philadelphia, 1976, WB Saunders.)

proper tube placement is demonstrated radiographically.

Unfortunately, if at any time the cuff ruptures, the ET tube must be removed and the patient reintubated.

Use of a Stylet

Insertion of an endotracheal tube may sometimes be aided by the use of a *stylet*. This malleable, firm wire is inserted into the endotracheal tube, with the distal end of the stylet lying at least 1 cm proximal to the distal end of the endotracheal tube. The reason for recessing the distal end of the stylet is to avoid traumatizing the airway. Molding the stylet so that the distal end of the endotracheal tube takes on a "hockey stick" appearance, and then guiding this curvature in an anterior direction usually facilitates entry through the cords.

The Sellick Maneuver

Another technique that may greatly assist the operator during endotracheal intubation is application of cricoid pressure (the *Sellick maneuver*). This technique serves the dual function of facilitating visualization of the glottis and preventing regurgitation of gastric contents until intubation can be completed. Unlike other tracheal cartilages which have a soft membranous posterior portion, the cricoid is a full cartilaginous ring. As a result, pressure on this structure can occlude the esophagus by compressing it against the vertebral bodies that lie below (Sellick, 1961; Natanson et al, 1985).

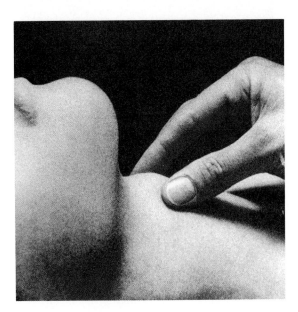

Figure 7-43. Application of the Sellick maneuver. Firm *downward* pressure is applied to the *anterolateral* aspect of the cricoid cartilage.
(Reproduced with permission of Ambu, Inc from Lotz P, Ahnefeld FW, Hirlinger WD: *A systematic guide to intubation*, Atelier Flad, Eckental, West Germany.)

To perform the Sellick maneuver, one must first identify the cricoid cartilage. This is done by walking one's hands down in the midline from the thyroid cartilage (Adam's apple) into the depression below (the cricothyroid membrane) and onto the next lying structure. This is the cricoid cartilage. Apply firm, *downward* pressure on the *anterolateral* aspects of this cartilage with the thumb and index finger of either hand *(Figure 7-43)*. Be sure to maintain this downward pressure until *after* the endotracheal tube has been inserted and the cuff is inflated (or else gastric regurgitation will occur)!

Proper hand placement is essential for the Sellick maneuver to work. Pressure must *never* be applied directly over the cricoid cartilage. Doing so will only compress the larynx and make intubation more difficult. Instead, the site for downward pressure application is along the outer edge (anterolateral aspect) of the cricoid cartilage.

Special Considerations

An interesting phenomenon to be aware of (and prepared for) is the development of *hypotension* immediately following the intubation of certain patients in acute respiratory distress. Considering the sequence of events leading up to emergency intubation, this phenomenon should not be unexpected. Endogenous catecholamines rise markedly in patients with acute air hunger as a natural result of the anxiety, fear, and severe stress they experience. Elevated catecholamines promote tachycardia and/or hypertension.

Sedation will often be needed to facilitate intubation of acutely anxious patients with severe air hunger. This may cause hypotension by two mechanisms: (1) the sedative drug shuts off the patient's endogenous catecholamine surge, and (2) many sedative drugs exert a direct vasodilatory effect on the arterial vasculature. Hypotension may be further aggravated by application of positive pressure ventilation after intubation which increases intrathoracic pressure and leads to a reduction in venous return.

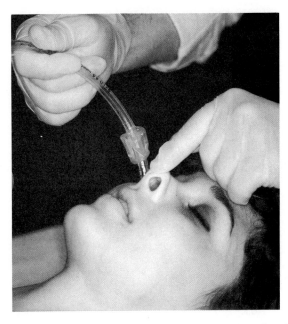

Figure 7-44. Insertion of nasotracheal tube into the right nares.

BLIND NASOTRACHEAL INTUBATION

The advantage of *nasotracheal intubation* is that it provides an alternative method for achieving definitive control of the airway in the spontaneously breathing patient who exhibits teeth clenching and/or who retains a sensitive gag reflex.

A slightly smaller (6.5 to 7.5 mm in diameter) endotracheal tube is recommended for this procedure than for endotracheal intubation.

Technique for Insertion

The technique for insertion is initially the same as that described for placement of a nasopharyngeal airway. The nasotracheal tube is lubricated with 2% lidocaine gel. It is inserted into the nares and advanced by placing the bevel against the septum of the nose and gently sliding the tube backward in line with the base of the ears *(Figure 7-44)*. In this way the tube passes parallel to the floor of the nasal cavity.

In passing from the nasopharynx to the posterior pharynx, the tube must take a downward turn. Occasionally it may get hung up trying to negotiate this turn and abut against the posterior pharyngeal wall. Clinically, this should be suspected if resistance to further advancement is encountered or there is loss of air movement through the tube. Should this happen, immediately withdraw the tube a short distance, reposition (slightly extend) the patient's head, and reattempt to advance the tube. Do *not* try to force the tube forward, as this may result in mucosal injury and bleeding (or even in retropharyngeal perforation)!

At this point, direct your attention to listening (or feeling) for air movement through the tube *(Figure 7-45)*. As the distal end of the tube gets closer and closer to the laryngeal opening, the sound of air movement should become increasingly louder *(Figure 7-46)*. Continue to gently guide the tube toward the

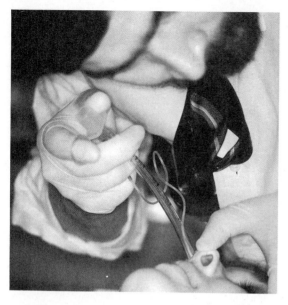

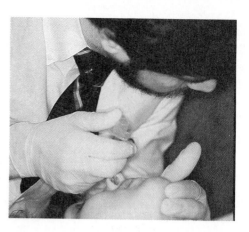

Figure 7-46.   As the final position of the nasotracheal tube is approached, the sound of air movement becomes increasingly louder. Manipulation of the trigger at this point may facilitate tracheal intubation.

Figure 7-45.   Listening for air movement as the tube is advanced.

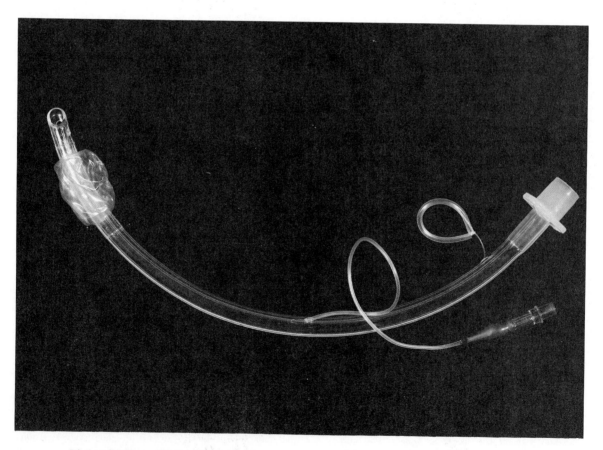

Figure 7-47.   Endotrol tube. A trigger mechanism at the proximal end of the tube allows controlled flexion of the distal end.

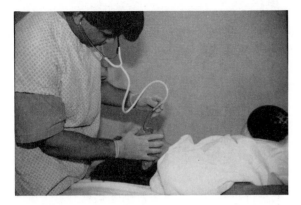

Figure 7-48. Use of the stethoscope for distancing oneself from the patient while listening for air movement during blind nasotracheal intubation.

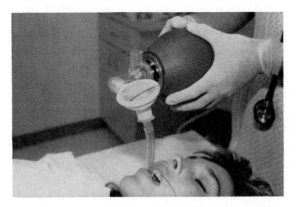

Figure 7-49. ET CO_2 monitor. The device is readily attached on-line between the endotracheal tube and the ventilatory support unit.

glottis. If at any time air movement ceases, withdraw the tube slightly, reposition the patient's head (if needed), and resume the process. When air movement sounds are at their loudest, hold the tube still and try to anticipate the next inspiratory effort of the patient. The moment this effort begins, attempt to advance the tube into the trachea. This often stimulates the patient's cough reflex. If the attempt is successful, inspiratory and expiratory air flow will be heard through the tube. If not, the esophagus may have been intubated. The tube should be immediately withdrawn, and another attempt made.

Once the patient has been intubated, final tube placement should be confirmed in the same manner as for endotracheal intubation.

Special Considerations

Recently a device has been made available that greatly facilitates blind nasotracheal intubation (*Endotrol*, National Catheter Corporation, Brunswick, New York). By means of a *trigger mechanism* at the proximal end of the tube, controlled flexion of the distal end is now possible *(Figure 7-47)*. This allows the operator to direct the distal tip anteriorly in the direction of the laryngeal opening at the moment the tube is inserted into the trachea (Fig. 7-46).

It is important to emphasize that since accurate placement with blind nasotracheal intubation is predicated on hearing (or feeling) air movement in the tube, the procedure cannot be performed in an apneic patient.

At times the intubator may not desire having to place his/ her face in the close proximity to the proximal end of the endotracheal tube (and to the patient's face) as shown in Figure 7-46 in order to listen for air movement. This can be easily accomplished by use of a stethoscope *(Figure 7-48)*.

Simply remove the stethoscope head and place the distal end of the stethoscope tubing down the endotracheal tube. Then listen for breath sounds in the usual manner. The length of the stethoscope tubing allows the operator a much more comfortable distance from the victim's face during the procedure *(Figure 7-48)*.

Another way to facilitate blind nasotracheal intubation incorporates use of an endotracheal tube whistle (Beck Airflow Monitor MARK IV Endotracheal Tube Whistle—Great Plains Ballistics, Inc., Donaldsville, Louisiana). This small plastic device conveniently attaches to the 15-mm endotracheal tube adapter. Air flow through the tube produces sound that varies in *intensity* (becoming louder as the larynx is ap-

proached) and *pitch* (producing a higher-pitched sound on inspiration than expiration). This not only alerts the operator to the anatomic position of the ET tube relative to the cords, but also facilitates anticipation of the next inspiratory phase. In a pilot study by Krishel et al (1992), all of the physicians who tried the device endorsed its potential utility—especially when attempting blind nasotracheal intubation in the noisy environment that is so common in emergency care settings.

END-TIDAL CO_2 (ET CO_2) MONITORING

Capnography (the measure of end-tidal volume carbon dioxide concentrations in expired air) has long been used as a noninvasive method for evaluating the efficacy of respiratory function. Capnography equipment used to be cumbersome and too impractical for use in the prehospital setting. Recent development of an inexpensive, portable, easy-to-use end-tidal CO_2 (ET CO_2) monitor (by Fenem, New York, New York) has rekindled interest in this area.

The ET CO_2 monitor is readily attached on-line between the endotracheal tube and the ventilatory support unit *(Figure 7-49)*. The patient is given six or more breaths to prime the chemical indicator on the monitor, which will now register an accurate reading of the percentage of CO_2 in expired air. Color coding of the chemical indicator on the monitor facilitates recognition of baseline CO_2 concentration and of changes in ET CO_2 as they occur.

Clinically, capnography may be useful in a number of emergency settings. As discussed in Section C of Chapter 10, ET CO_2 monitoring is achieving increasing recognition as a noninvasive method for assessing the efficacy of ongoing cardiopulmonary resuscitation. In general, the prognosis for victims of cardiac arrest with persistently low ET CO_2 readings is extremely poor. None of the patients in the study by Sanders et al (1989) who consistently had ET CO_2 readings of less than 10 mm Hg survived. All survivors in the study eventually increased ET CO_2 readings to at least this level. While other factors obviously play an important role in determining the likelihood of survival from cardiac arrest, the finding of a low ET CO_2 reading during resuscitation seems to suggest the need for some additional intervention if there is to be a reasonable chance for survival.

ET CO_2 monitoring may also be helpful in confirming proper endotracheal tube placement, especially when intubation has been performed by paramedics in the field. Auscultation of the chest for adequate air movement and symmetric breath sounds may be quite difficult from the back of a moving ambulance or in midflight on a noisy aircraft. ET CO_2 readings should significantly increase if the endotracheal tube has been correctly placed. Persistently low readings suggest esophageal intubation, inadequate CPR, and/or nonviability of the patient.

In the same manner, ET CO_2 monitoring can be used in the prehospital setting to confirm proper EOA (or EGTA) placement.

IS THE ET TUBE *TRULY* PLACED CORRECTLY?

Throughout this chapter we have emphasized the importance of verifying proper endotracheal tube placement after intubation. Verification begins at the bedside (or in the field in the prehospital setting) with auscultation of the lungs for equal bilateral breath sounds. Final confirmation requires a chest x-ray. A sobering study by Brunel et al (1989) points out the potential fallibility of the physical exam as a means of confirming proper tube placement.

The authors prospectively studied 219 critically ill patients who were intubated in the hospital. On the basis of the physical exam (palpation of the endotracheal tube cuff in the suprasternal notch, notation of equal chest excursion, and auscultation for symmetric breath sounds), endotracheal tube placement was felt to be correct in 97% of cases. Follow-up chest x-ray suggested suboptimal tube placement (right mainstem intubation or final tube placement too close to the carina) in 14% of cases. Thus, *physical examination was not as reliable a method as one would like for confirming proper endotracheal tube placement!* Obtaining a chest x-ray remains essential for confirmation, especially for emergency intubations. While ordering a chest x-ray is easy to do in a hospital setting, it is obviously impossible in the field. Use of ET CO_2 monitoring (as discussed in the preceding section) may prove helpful in assessing tube placement in the prehospital setting. Another finding to be aware of that favors proper tube placement is condensation of moisture on the inside of the endotracheal tube during ventilation.

Algorithm for Management of the Adult Airway

To help conceptualize the material covered in this chapter, we have developed an Algorithm for Management of the Adult Airway *(Figure 7-50)*. The management sequence begins with the rescuer simultaneously assessing ventilation and the level of consciousness **(1)**.

> Many definitions exist for the terms *conscious, semiconscious,* and *unconscious.* For the purpose of determining optimal management of the airway, we have defined these terms in the following manner:
>
> **Conscious**—a patient who is alert, awake, and responding appropriately.
> **Semiconscious**—a less alert patient who may not be awake and only responds to verbal or painful stimuli. The gag reflex may still be intact.
> **Unconscious**—a patient who cannot be aroused and does not respond to either verbal or painful stimuli. The gag reflex is absent.

If a patient is *conscious* or *semiconscious and* spontaneously breathing in a normal manner, all that may be needed is supplemental oxygen **(1-2-4)**. The rescuer should then evaluate the adequacy of oxygenation **(5)**. This may be done by physical examination (as described earlier in this chapter), oximetry, and/or by arterial blood gas sampling (if indicated). If this evaluation suggests that oxygenation is inadequate, more definitive management of the airway (either by insertion of a nasopharyngeal airway or endotracheal intubation) is needed.

Unconscious patients, even if they are breathing normally, require definitive airway management with endotracheal intubation **(1-3-7)**.

For patients who are breathing abnormally (and for those who are not breathing at all), appropriate management of the airway is the same regardless of the state of consciousness **(1-2-6)** or **(1-3-6)**. In either case, the airway should be manually opened by either the chin-lift or jaw-thrust maneuver **(8)**. If this results in resumption of normal breathing **(9)**, supplemental oxygen should be administered. For the *unconscious* patient, definitive airway management with endotracheal intubation is again the treatment of choice **(6-8-9-11)**. On the other hand, if the patient is *conscious* or *semiconscious* **(10)**, less definitive therapy may be needed. Manually maintain the airway. Further management will then hinge on assessment of the adequacy of oxygenation **(6-8-9-10-12)**.

If after initially opening the airway, the patient continues to breathe abnormally (or is still not breathing at all), the rescuer should reposition the airway **(6-8-13-14)**. If this results in resumption of normal breathing, management should follow the course described above **(8-9-10-12)** or **(8-9-11)**. On the other hand, if breathing is still abnormal after repositioning the airway **(15)**, the rescuer should assume *incomplete airway obstruction* is present and treat accordingly **(6-8-13-14-15-16)**.

If the patient remains in respiratory arrest even after repositioning the airway, an attempt should be made to ventilate the patient **(14-17-18)**. If successful, definitive airway management with endotracheal intubation should be performed **(19)**. If unsuccessful, the rescuer should assume *complete airway obstruction* and treat accordingly **(20)**.

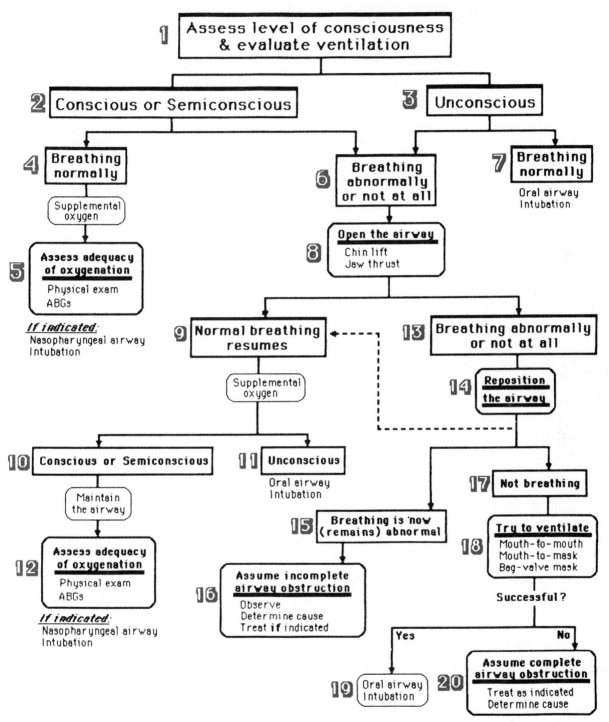

Figure 7-50.   Algorithm of **Adult Airway Management.**

References

American Heart Association (AHA) 1985 Conference (Montgomery WH, Donegan J, McIntyre KM, Albarran-Sotel R, Jaffe AS, Ornato JP, Paraskos JA, et al): Standards and guidelines for cardiopulmonary resuscitation (CPR) and emergency cardiac care (ECC), *JAMA* 255 (suppl):2990, 1986.

Auerbach PS, Geehr EC: Inadequate oxygenation and ventilation using the esophageal gastric tube airway in the prehospital setting, *JAMA* 250:3067, 1983.

Brunel W, Coleman DL, Schwartz DE, Peper E, Cohen NH: Assessment of routine chest roentgenograms and the physical examination to confirm endotracheal tube position, *Chest* 96:1043–1045, 1989.

Cavallaro DL: Personal communication (preliminary research data, 1990).

Clinton JE, Ruiz E: *Emergency airway management procedures*. In Roberts JR, Hedges JR, editors: *Clinical procedures in emergency medicine*, Philadelphia, 1985, WB Saunders.

Gordon K: Pulse oximetry in emergency medicine, *West J Med* 151:67, 1989.

Harrison RR, Maullo KI, Keenan RL, Boyan CP: Mouth-to-mask ventilation: a superior method of rescue breathing, *Ann Emerg Med* 11:74, 1982.

Hedges JR, Amsterdam JR, Cionni DJ, Embry S: Oxygen saturation as a marker for admission or relapse with acute bronchospasm, *Am J Emerg Med* 5:196, 1987.

Hochbaum SR: Emergency airway management, *Emerg med clin North Am* 4:441, 1986.

Krishel S, Jackimczyk K, Balazs K: Endotracheal tube whistle: an adjunct to blind nasotracheal intubation, *Ann Emerg Med* 21:33, 1992.

Kulick RM: Pulse oximetry, *Pediatr Emerg Care* 3:127, 1987.

Melker RJ, Cavallaro DL: Synchronous and asynchronous ventilation during cardiopulmonary resuscitation (CPR), *Ann Emerg Med* 12:142, 1983.

Montgomery WH: *Ventilation during cardiopulmonary resuscitation*. In Harwood AL, editor: *Cardiopulmonary resuscitation*, Baltimore, 1982, Williams & Wilkins.

Natanson C, Shelhamer JH, Parrillo JE: Intubation of the trachea in the critical care setting, *JAMA* 253:1160, 1985.

Sanders, Kern KB, Otto CW, Milander MM, Ewy GA: End-tidal carbon dioxide monitoring during cardiopulmonary resuscitation: a prognostic indicator for survival, *JAMA* 262:1347, 1989.

Sellick BA: Cricoid pressure to control regurgitation of stomach contents during induction of anesthesia, *Lancet* 2:404, 1961.

Taylor MB, Whitwarm JG: The current status of pulse oximetry, *Anaesthesia* 41:943, 1986.

White RD: Controversies in out-of-hospital emergency airway control: esophageal obstruction or endotracheal intubation? *Ann Emerg Med* 13:778, 1984.

CHAPTER 8

INTRAVENOUS ACCESS

Dan Cavallaro, REMT-P
Ken Grauer, MD

Contributing Authors*
Jorge Gourid, MD
Al Saltiel, MD
Larry Kravitz, MD

SECTION A

BASIC APPROACHES TO IV ACCESS

Along with management of the airway and defibrillation, establishing intravenous (IV) access is one of the major priorities of cardiopulmonary resuscitation. Many techniques exist for accomplishing this goal, each with its own relative merits and drawbacks. The skill of the operator and individual preferences (tempered by personal experience) all play a large role in determining which technique is chosen for any given situation and how the technique is performed. *The best technique is the one that works for you.* We limit our discussion here to a brief overview of the standard methods for obtaining intravenous access, with an expanded commentary on the more complicated intravenous techniques that have been helpful in our experience.

Initial Priorities

Circulation of drugs in the arrested heart is most effectively accomplished when administered into a *central* vein such as the internal jugular or subclavian (Kaye and Bircher, 1988). These veins offer the advantage of having a fairly constant location with respect to easily identifiable anatomic landmarks. This usually allows rapid cannulation, even in a state of cardiovascular collapse (when peripheral veins may be exceedingly difficult to visualize). However, achieving access at these sites is not without problems such as:

1. The need for an operator skilled in the technique
2. The need to stop CPR
3. Significant risk of pneumothorax and hemothorax

Selection of the femoral vein as the site for central venous access avoids the latter two problems but raises an additional concern. Several studies suggest that blood flow during CPR is significantly diminished below the diaphragm (Niemann et al, 1981; Dalsey et al, 1983; Hedges et al, 1984). Thus drugs administered through this route during cardiopulmonary resuscitation may not adequately reach the central circulation.

Practically speaking, the most commonly chosen site for intravenous access during cardiopulmonary resuscitation is a *peripheral* line. This is particularly true when operators skilled in the insertion of central lines are not on the scene. One should remember that the smaller the catheter and the more distal the site, the less likely there will be adequate drug delivery to the central circulation. Three practical suggestions may be helpful to optimize drug delivery by this route (Kaye and Bircher, 1988):

1. Select a proximal site (antecubital fossa) if possible, as this is superior to using a vein on the dorsum of the wrist
2. Use a *large*-bore needle (ideally 16 gauge or larger, although this may not always be possible)
3. Follow administration of the medication with a 50- to 100-ml bolus of fluid (to help "flush" the medication toward the central circulation)

Finally, one should not forget the *endotracheal* route. Three of the most commonly used drugs in cardiopulmonary resuscitation (epinephrine, lidocaine, and atropine) are effectively given in this manner. Although the pharmacokinetics of these drugs are clearly more favorable when they are administered through a central venous route, one should not hesitate to give drugs endotracheally if this is the only route available (Quinton et al, 1987; Paradis and Koscove, 1990).

*We appreciate and acknowledge the contributions of Drs. Harry Sernaker, Jerry Diehr, and Paul Augereau to the original version of this chapter that appeared in the second edition of our book.

Technique for Endotracheal Drug Administration

Three techniques have been proposed for endotracheal drug administration (Ward, 1985). In each, the drug should be diluted to a volume of at least 10 ml. The first method is the simplest and probably the most commonly used. Drug is drawn up in a 10- to 20-ml syringe with an 18-gauge needle firmly attached to the end of the syringe. The drug is then rapidly injected down the lumen of the ET tube, followed by *at least* five full insufflations of the lungs. This promotes more distal delivery of drug into the tracheobronchial tree. External chest compressions should be stopped momentarily while the drug is injected, since this may result in expulsion of the medication. Medication may also be expelled if the patient happens to cough during the procedure. In this case it may be necessary to readminister the dose of the drug.

In the second method of endotracheal drug administration, instead of injecting the drug down the opening of the ET tube, the 18-gauge needle is inserted *into* the ET tube itself. An advantage of this method is that the ventilatory device need not be disconnected from the ET tube opening in order to administer the drug. Medication is injected through the side of the ET tube during the inspiratory phase of ventilation, in this manner being forcefully delivered to the distal tracheobronchial tree. Unfortunately, the hole made by the needle in the ET tube will not always seal, so that there may be a small leak left in the airway system.

In the final method of endotracheal drug administration, a long (at least 8 cm) intravenous catheter is attached to the syringe instead of the 18-gauge needle. The catheter is inserted down the lumen of the ET tube. In this way, drug may be injected directly into the distal trachea and bronchi, without loss of solution onto the lumen walls of the ET tube.

Although data demonstrating the superiority of one method over another are lacking, intuitive advantages of the latter two techniques are that they probably deliver drug more directly to the distal tracheobronchial tree.

OUR SUGGESTION FOR OBTAINING IV ACCESS

If on your arrival at the scene of a cardiac arrest the patient is already intubated or has a large-bore proximal

IV in place, medications should initially be administered by one (or both) of these routes. If the patient does not respond (or if neither of these routes have been established), it is certainly reasonable to stop CPR momentarily to attempt insertion of an internal jugular, external jugular, or subclavian vein, provided you are adept with these techniques.

Intravenous Access Systems: General Considerations

In general, four types of cannulas are used to achieve intravenous access:

1. Catheters inserted over a guidewire (*Seldinger technique*)
2. Catheter-*over*-the-needle units
3. Catheter-*through*-the-needle units
4. The double-lumen peripherally placed intravenous catheter ("*Twin Cath*")

The first three types are illustrated in *Figure 8A-1*, and the last type in *Figure 8A-2*. Catheter-over-the-needle units and the double-lumen catheter are used for obtaining peripheral venous access, while the other two types of catheters are used for central venous cannulation.

With the catheter-*over*-the-needle system, the catheter is larger in diameter than the needle. After cannulation of the vein with the needle, the catheter is then advanced over the needle and in through the puncture site of the vessel wall. But because the diameter of the catheter is a little larger than the diameter of the puncture site, the catheter may sometimes fail to enter the vein. This is a marked disadvantage of the system.

The chances of threading the catheter into the vein are much greater with the third system, because the catheter is advanced *through* the needle. However, this system is also marked by a number of disadvantages. Catheter size

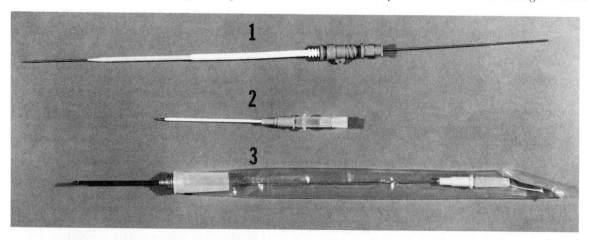

Figure 8A-1. Three types of catheter systems used to achieve intravenous access. (*1*) Guidewire and sheath dilator unit (Seldinger technique); (*2*) over-the-needle catheter; and (*3*) through-the-needle catheter.

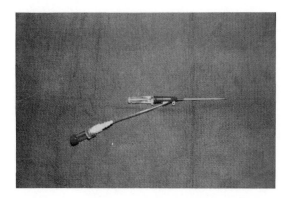

Figure 8A-2. Double-lumen peripherally placed intravenous catheter ("Twin Cath").

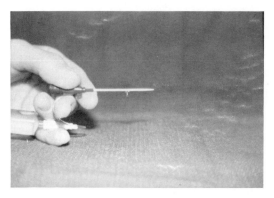

Figure 8A-3. Twin Cath showing a drop of fluid exiting from its proximal port of the catheter.

is limited by (and must be slightly smaller than) the diameter of the needle. If in the midst of an arrest situation the operator becomes momentarily distracted and *withdraws* the catheter back through the needle, a portion of the catheter may be sheared off and embolize distally in the vessel. Finally, because the catheter lumen is slightly smaller than the lumen of the needle, it will also be smaller than the diameter of the puncture site. Extravasation of fluid may therefore occur at the site where the catheter enters the vein.

> In the past, the catheter-through-the-needle system was a favored technique for achieving rapid access into the central circulation during an emergency situation. Because of the above disadvantages of the system, it is now being replaced by the Seldinger technique.

The *Seldinger technique* is the ideal system for obtaining intravenous access. It is not difficult to learn and provides rapid access (with a large-bore catheter) to the central circulation with a minimum of complications. Initially the vein is cannulated with a relatively small-bore introducing needle. The diameter of this needle may be small (i.e., 20 gauge)—*it only has to be large enough to accommodate the guidewire.* Because initial intravenous access is accomplished with a small-bore needle, the chances of successfully cannulating a vein in a state of cardiovascular collapse (when the lumen of the vein is small and hard to enter) are increased, while the potential for damaging surrounding structures by errant needle puncture is minimized. Once the guidewire is threaded through the introducing needle, the dilator and large-bore (8-8.5 French) catheter sheath may be inserted over the guidewire. The dilator and wire can then be removed, and access for rapid administration of medication, fluids, blood, or passage of a temporary transvenous pacemaker or Swan-Ganz catheter is secured. (We describe the Seldinger technique in more detail at the end of this chapter.)

> Another advantage of the Seldinger technique is that in a matter of moments an existing IV (such as an 18-gauge peripheral line placed by paramedics in the field) may be converted into a large-bore site of intravenous access. All one has

to do is slip the guidewire through the existing peripheral catheter, remove the catheter, and then proceed as above to insert the dilator/catheter sheath unit over the wire.

The last system (the "Twin Cath") is a double-lumen, peripherally placed intravenous catheter (Fig. 8A-2). This catheter is inserted in the same manner as standard peripherally placed IV catheters. Advantages of this catheter system are that it is relatively easy to insert, and that it allows two medications to be administered simultaneously through the two ports in the catheter. For example, lidocaine may be infused through the proximal port at the same time as dopamine is infused through the distal catheter port *(Figure 8A-3).* If only one medication is being given, the unused catheter port can then be "heplocked" until it is needed.

RATE OF FLUID ADMINISTRATION

The rate of fluid administration depends on the diameter and *length* of the particular catheter and IV tubing used. As an example of how dramatically these parameters affect the rate of fluid administration, consider the following (Sacchetti, 1985):

- Flow rate through an 18-gauge × 4.3-cm long catheter ≈ 55 ml/min
- Flow rate through a 16-gauge × 20-cm long catheter ≈ 25 ml/min
- Flow rate through a 16-gauge × 13.3-cm long catheter ≈ 57 ml/min
- Flow rate through a 16-gauge × 5.7-cm long catheter ≈ 83 ml/min
- Flow rate through a 14-gauge × 5.7-cm long catheter ≈ 94 ml/min
- Flow rate through an 8.5 French × 12-cm long catheter ≈ 108 ml/min

> *Thus the larger the bore and the shorter the catheter, the greater the flow rate.* Although this statement may seem intuitively obvious, it is surprising how commonly this principle is overlooked in

practice. For example, a 16-gauge, 20-cm long catheter-through-the-needle unit (as is commonly used for central venous cannulation) provides *less than one third the flow* of a 16-gauge, 5.7-cm long unit (as is commonly used for securing peripheral venous access). Clearly, cannulation of a central vein with a catheter-through-the-needle does not provide ideal access for rapid administration of large amounts of fluid.

COMPLICATIONS OF IV ACCESS SYSTEMS

Certain complications are common to all IV access systems. These include local complications (infiltration with resultant hematoma formation, infection, and thrombosis) and systemic complications (sepsis, pulmonary embolism, air embolism, and catheter fragment embolism). Technique-specific complications (such as pneumothorax, hemothorax) are addressed below.

Although strict aseptic technique is often not feasible during an emergency situation, one must remember to change contaminated IV lines as soon as possible in patients who have been successfully resuscitated.

Peripheral Lines

VEINS IN THE UPPER EXTREMITY

Most readers are thoroughly familiar with the techniques for insertion of a peripheral line in the upper extremity. Therefore we will limit our comments to a few selected points.

1. If unable to visualize a suitable vein for cannulation, apply a tourniquet, hang the arm off the bed, *and go to the other side*. If after 2 additional minutes you are unable to cannulate a vein on the other side, return to the original side (with the tourniquet). A vein may now be distended.
2. A trick for establishing a large-bore IV in a proximal upper extremity vein is first to establish distal access on the dorsum of the wrist with a 22-gauge butterfly. Then infuse 10 to 15 ml of fluid into this vein with a syringe. Frequently this will distend a larger, more proximal vein that can then be cannulated directly.
3. Perhaps the best method for facilitating insertion of a peripheral IV line is to apply a warm towel to the arm for several minutes. Alternatively, nitroglycerin ointment may be applied to the skin. The underlying veins will usually distend.

Unfortunately, the time involved with these techniques may preclude their use in an emergency situation.

EXTERNAL JUGULAR VEIN

The external jugular vein lies superficially along the lateral aspect of the neck. It extends from the angle of the mandible, and runs downward until it enters the thorax at a point corresponding to the middle of the clavicle. Shortly thereafter it terminates in the subclavian vein *(Figure 8A-4)*.

Under normal circumstances, the external jugular vein

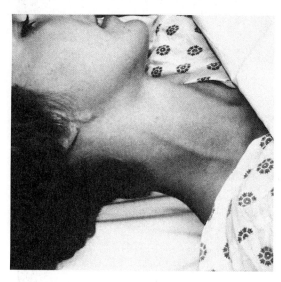

Figure 8A-4.   Anatomic location of the external jugular vein.

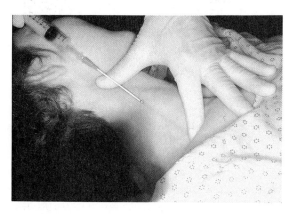

Figure 8A-5.   Cannulation of the external jugular vein.

is surprisingly easy to cannulate. Its advantage is that despite being a peripheral vein, it provides rapid access into the central circulation. The problem is that during a code situation, the external jugular is often not readily accessible, especially if rescuers are actively working on controlling the airway. Other drawbacks are that the vein tends to be very mobile and tortuous. Consequently, intravenous access may be tenuous (easy to dislodge) and positional (with flow sometimes varying greatly with even slight movement of the head).

Technique for Insertion

With the patient in the supine, head-down position, rotate the head to the opposite side. Applying digital pressure to the vein distally (just above the clavicle) will often assist in distending the vein. Insert the needle in the middle of the vein *(Figure 8A-5)*. Cannulation is then performed by essentially the same technique that is used with other peripheral veins.

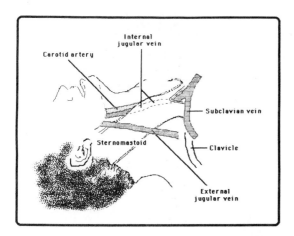

Figure 8A-6.   Anatomic location of the internal jugular vein.

VEINS IN THE LOWER EXTREMITY

As noted above, the lower extremity is not a preferred site for intravenous cannulation, since it appears that blood flow from below the diaphragm is significantly decreased during CPR.

Central Lines

INTERNAL JUGULAR VEIN

The internal jugular vein runs from the base of the skull downward along the carotid artery until it enters the chest to meet with the subclavian vein behind the clavicle *(Figure 8A-6)*. For those skilled in the technique, it is a favored site for obtaining intravenous access.

The right side of the neck is preferred for three reasons: (1) the dome of the lung and pleura are lower on the right side; (2) insertion of a cannula on this side follows a direct line to the right atrium; (3) the thoracic duct empties on the left side.

A major advantage of selecting the internal jugular instead of the subclavian vein is the significantly lower risk of pneumothorax. Unfortunately, during a code situation this site may not be readily accessible, especially if rescuers are actively working on controlling the airway.*

Special Considerations

One complication unique to internal jugular cannulation is *neck hematoma*. This may be due to extravasation from either

---

*Recently, Denys et al (1991) described an ultrasound-assisted technique using a portable transducer at the bedside for achieving central venous access in the internal jugular vein. Performance of Valsalva markedly enlarged the jugular vein in study subjects, and contributed to the 100% success rate in achieving access—in an average time of 11 seconds—with a 95% rate of entry into the vein on the first needle pass—and with minimal complications. With additional experience, strong consideration may be given in the near future to routine adoption of an ultrasound guidance system for achieving IV access.

the vein or inadvertent puncture of the artery. Fortunately, in either case local pressure will usually be sufficient to control the bleeding (although 10 to 20 minutes of firm pressure may be needed to control hemorrhage with arterial puncture). Should one suspect arterial puncture, *the operator must not attempt cannulation of the internal jugular vein on the other side*, since bilateral hemorrhage (with compression of the trachea) could occur. Instead, subsequent attempts at central venous cannulation should preferably be on the subclavian vein of the *same* side (to avoid the possibility of producing an iatrogenic bilateral complication).

Carotid artery disease is a relative contraindication to internal jugular cannulation for two reasons: (1) inadvertent arterial puncture may dislodge a plaque; and (2) should neck hematoma complicate the procedure, application of firm pressure to control the hemorrhage might further compromise carotid artery flow.

Body habitus may play a role in determining the likelihood of success with this technique. Cannulation is most difficult in patients with short, stubby necks. Finally, in conscious patients one should bear in mind that internal jugular cannulation is more uncomfortable than subclavian cannulation due to the restriction it places on neck movement.

Techniques for Insertion

There are three techniques for insertion of an internal jugular central line. *For each of them*, the patient is supine and in slight (15 to 30 degrees) Trendelenburg position with the head turned to the contralateral side. Additional maneuvers that may be helpful in distending the vein include asking the conscious patient to bear down (Valsalva), and having an assistant apply pressure to the abdomen of the unconscious patient.

POSTERIOR APPROACH

The needle is inserted at the junction of the middle and lower thirds of the lateral border of the sternomastoid muscle. It is then advanced *under* this muscle, aiming toward the suprasternal notch *(Figure 8A-7)*.

Most providers do not use this approach. It appears to be more difficult for the novice to master, is associated with potentially significant complications, and entails insertion of the needle a long way (5 to 7 cm) before the vein is entered.

ANTERIOR APPROACH

The index and middle fingers are placed on the carotid artery and retract it medially away from the anterior border of the sternocleidomastoid muscle. The needle is then inserted at the midpoint of the medial aspect of the sternocleidomastoid muscle at a 30- to 45-degree angle with the frontal plane, aiming for the ipsilateral nipple *(Figure 8A-8)*.

Most providers do not use this approach either. The major problem is the close proximity of the carotid artery. Because the carotid sheath is fairly well fixed to underlying structures, even the most diligent efforts to retract it medially are often less than successful. In the hands of the novice, the risk of arterial puncture appears to be significant.

CENTRAL (MIDDLE) APPROACH

The patient is supine and in slight Trendelenburg position, with the head rotated to the contralateral side. The needle is inserted at the apex of the triangle formed by the two heads

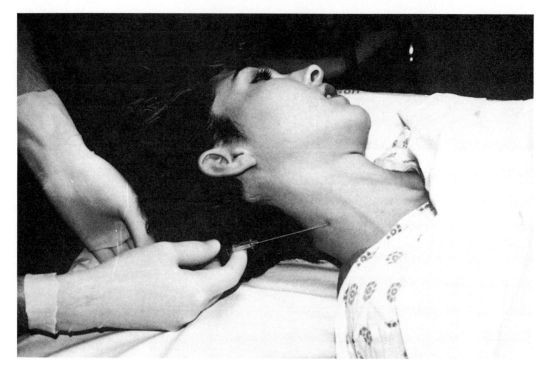

Figure 8A-7.   Posterior approach to the internal jugular vein.

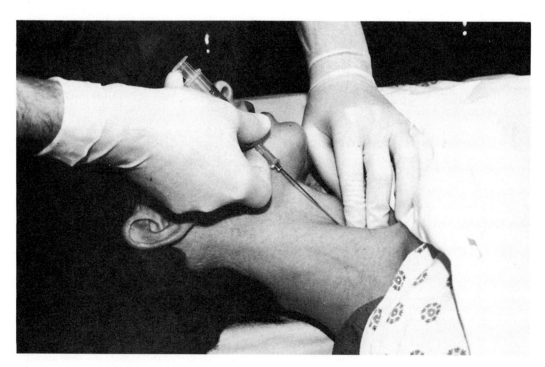

Figure 8A-8.   Anterior approach to the internal jugular vein.

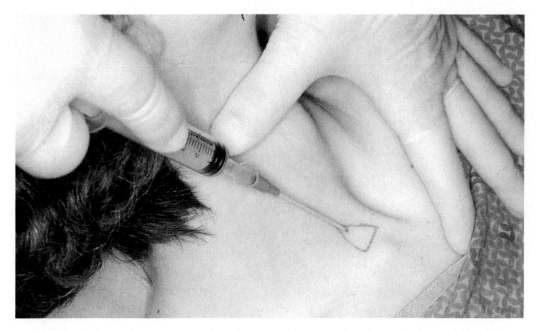

Figure 8A-9. Central approach to the internal jugular vein. The needle is inserted at the apex of the triangle formed by the two heads of the sternocleidomastoid muscle (here marked in ink).

of the sternocleidomastoid muscle and directed slightly lateral in the direction of the ipsilateral nipple. Although many texts suggest entering the skin at a 30-degree angle to the frontal plane, increasing the angle of entry to between 45 and 60 degrees may be more effective *(Figure 8A-9)*. The vein is usually entered within 1 to 3 cm. If unsuccessful, withdraw the needle and redirect it in a slightly more medial orientation on the next attempt.

This is the preferred approach of most emergency care providers who choose the internal jugular site, and the one we suggest. Anatomic landmarks (the two heads of the sternocleidomastoid muscle) are easy to identify on virtually all subjects, and the risk of carotid artery puncture is much less than with the anterior approach (since at this level of the neck the jugular vein lies lateral [and away from] the common carotid artery).

SUBCLAVIAN VEIN

The subclavian vein is the continuation of the axillary vein, beginning at the point where this vessel passes over the first rib and under the medial third of the clavicle. It then meets with the internal jugular vein to form the brachiocephalic (innominate) vein *(Figure 8A-10)*.

The subclavian vein is the central venous access site preferred by many providers because:

1. It may have been the only method taught during their training.
2. It may be more accessible than the internal jugular vein during cardiopulmonary resuscitation.
3. It may be easier for the novice to master than the internal jugular technique.

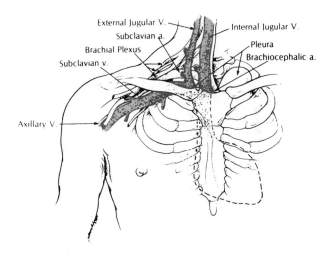

Figure 8A-10. Anatomic location of the subclavian vein. (Reproduced with permission from Roberts JR, Hedges JR, editors: *Clinical procedures in emergency medicine*, Philadelphia, 1985, WB Saunders.)

A significant drawback is the substantial risk of pneumothorax and other complications (hemothorax, subclavian artery puncture).

Additional contraindications to subclavian cannulation include anticoagulation and coagulopathy. Unlike the case for internal jugular cannulation, there is no way to locally tamponade bleeding should either venous extravasation or inadvertent arterial puncture occur.

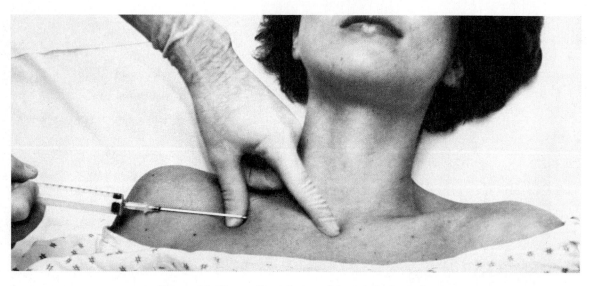

Figure 8A-11.   Cannulation of the subclavian vein.

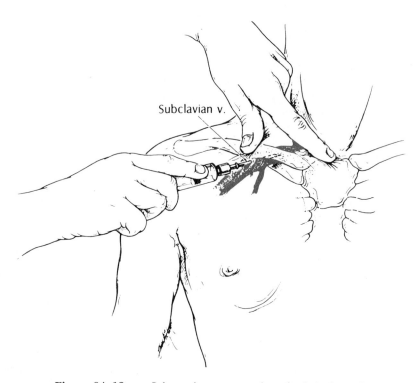

Figure 8A-12.   Schematic representation of subclavian vein cannulation. Aspirate until blood flash is obtained.
(Reproduced with permission from Roberts JR, Hedges JR, editors: *Clinical procedures in emergency medicine, Philadelphia, 1985, WB Saunders.*)

Special Considerations

As for the internal jugular vein, selecting the right side for the initial attempt at cannulation is favored, since this lowers the risk of pneumothorax (lower dome of the pleura on the right), and eliminates the possibility of thoracic duct puncture. Many clinicians feel these considerations outweigh the poten-

tial benefit offered by the smoother trajectory of the catheter when it is inserted from the left side.

Ideally, one should not make multiple attempts at cannulating the subclavian vein. Doing so only increases the risk of causing a pneumothorax. If unsuccessful on one side, instead of attempting subclavian cannulation on the opposite site (which invites the possibility of producing a bilateral iatrogenic complication), *it may be preferable to attempt internal jugular cannulation on the same side.*

Technique for Insertion

Again, the patient ideally is supine and in slight Trendelenburg position, with the head rotated to the contralateral side. Optimal positioning for subclavian cannulation may be further facilitated by placing a pillow or rolled towel between the scapulae; however, allowing the shoulders to fall too far back may be counterproductive by narrowing the space between the clavicle and the first rib. Make sure the arms are at the side of the patient and not hanging off the bed. (Having an assistant exert gentle downward traction on the ipsilateral arm [pulling toward the feet] sometimes helps maintain optimum positioning.)

Insert the needle at the junction of the middle and medial thirds of the clavicle. Then "walk" the needle down under the clavicle and advance it *parallel to the frontal plane.* Do not direct the needle downward, as this greatly increases the risk of pneumothorax. Position the index fingertip of the free hand in the suprasternal notch and use this as a reference point. The advancing needle should be aimed just above and posterior to this fingertip *(Figure 8A-11).* Aspirate on the syringe until a blood flash is obtained *(Figure 8A-12).* Then remove the syringe and feed in the catheter. *At no time expose the catheter hub to free air*, as this greatly increases the risk of air embolus.

In order to facilitate the catheter in making the downward turn into the brachiocephalic vein (instead of traveling up the neck), the bevel of the needle should be directed downward as soon as the lumen of the vein is entered. Aligning the bevel of the needle with the numerical markings on the syringe *before* beginning the procedure is a handy trick for knowing which way the needle will have to be rotated.

The catheter should thread easily. If it doesn't, it may have kinked, encountered an obstruction, or passed out of the vessel lumen. *Never force the catheter, and above all do not withdraw it through the needle if it does not thread.*

FEMORAL VEIN

As noted above, the femoral vein is no longer a favored site for central venous access during cardiac arrest.

SECTION B

THE SELDINGER TECHNIQUE

In recent years the Seldinger technique has become an increasingly popular method for central and peripheral venous cannulation. As discussed in our introduction, the advantages of this technique are that it provides rapid access with a large-bore catheter with minimal complications. Even under the extreme duress of trying to achieve intravenous access in trauma patients, peripherally placed catheters as large as 8.5 French can be readily inserted in a timely manner (Cavallaro—Personal communication from a study conducted with Arrow International).

A variety of prepackaged kits are commercially available. Some come complete with introducing needle, syringe, guidewire, dilator, and catheter sheath. Other kits do not contain the needle and syringe *(Fig. 8B-1)*. In either case, the technique for insertion is the same.

> Having the necessary equipment readily available in a prepackaged kit is most welcome in a code situation, as it avoids having to find and assemble material piecemeal during the haste of an emergency.

Guidewires may be straight or J-shaped. The purpose of the latter is to help negotiate vessel tortuosity if it is encountered. In general, straight guidewires are more than adequate for cannulation of the internal jugular or subclavian veins.

> As is the case for threading an intravenous catheter, guidewires should never be forced. Doing so only increases the chance that the wire may unwind, bend, or break (and possibly cause wire embolization). If gentle rotation of the wire does not facilitate easy advancement, remove the wire and try to confirm correct intravascular placement.

The *dilator* and *catheter sheath* function as a unit, with the 8 or 8.5 French catheter fitting over the dilator. The lumen through the dilator allows the unit to be threaded over the guidewire.

Technique for Insertion

Figure 8B-2 provides an overview of the entire procedure. The introducing needle with attached syringe is inserted into the vein in the standard fashion *(Figure 8B-3)*. Once the vein is cannulated as indicated by good blood return into the syringe *(Figure 8B-4)*, remove the syringe and insert the *soft* tip of the guidewire through the needle and into the vein *(Figure 8B-5)*. The guidewire should be inserted 5 to 10 cm, making sure that a substantial portion of it is still exposed. The needle is now removed *(Figure 8B-6)*.

A small nick should be made in the skin with a #11 scalpel blade *(Figure 8B-7)*. This nick must be deep enough to penetrate both the dermis and epidermis, since it must allow passage of the dilator through the skin. The dilator/catheter sheath unit is now slipped *over* the guidewire and into the incised area of skin *(Figure 8B-8)*. A twisting motion may facilitate skin penetration and subsequent entry into the vein. *The proximal tip of the guidewire should always protrude out of the distal end of the dilator/catheter sheath unit.* Advancing the unit without checking for the protruding wire tip may result in distal migration of the guidewire with embolization into the vessel.

After the dilator/catheter sheath unit is well into the vein, the wire and dilator are sequentially removed from the catheter. This leaves the large-bore catheter sheath in place in the vein, ready to be used as needed for administration of drugs, fluid, blood, or for passage of a transvenous pacemaker or Swan-Ganz catheter *(Figure 8B-9)*.

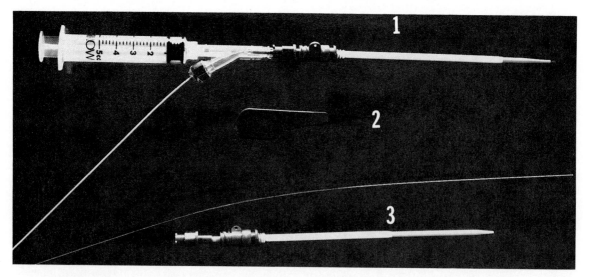

Figure 8B-1.   Pre-packaged kits for performing the Seldinger technique. (*1*) Combined kit containing syringe, needle, guidewire, dilator, and sheath; (*2*) small #11 blade for nicking the skin; (*3*) guidewire and dilator/sheath devices as separate units.

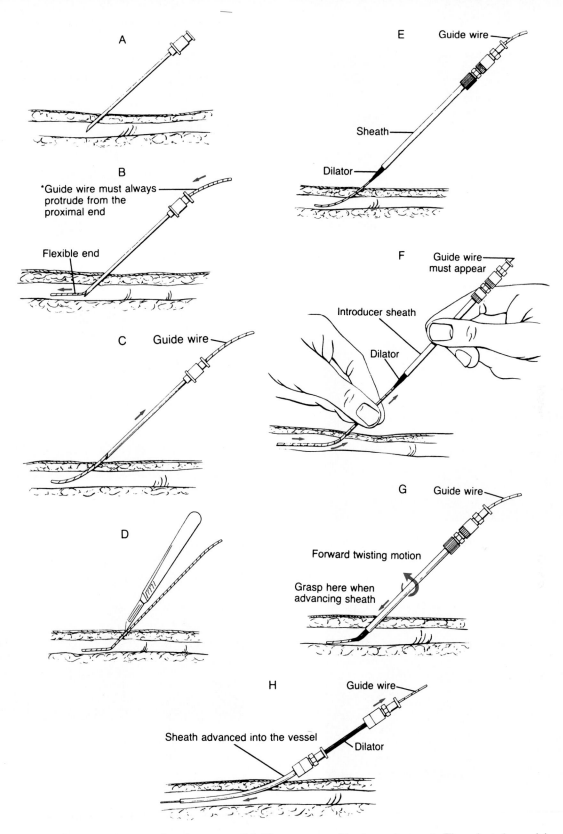

A

B

*Guide wire must always protrude from the proximal end

Flexible end

C Guide wire

D

E Guide wire

Sheath

Dilator

F Guide wire must appear

Introducer sheath

Dilator

G Guide wire

Forward twisting motion

Grasp here when advancing sheath

H Guide wire

Sheath advanced into the vessel

Dilator

Figure 8B-2. Procedure for placement of Seldinger-type guidewire catheter. *A,* The selected vessel is cannulated. *B,* The guidewire is threaded through the vessel with the flexible end first into the lumen of the vessel. *C,* The needle is removed so that only the wire now exits from the vessel. *D,* The skin entry site is enlarged with a #11 scalpel. *E,* The catheter sheath and the dilator are threaded over the wire and advanced to the skin. The wire must be visible through the back of the device. *F,* If the proximal wire is not visible, it is pulled from the skin through the catheter until it appears at the back of the catheter. *G,* The sheath and the dilator are advanced as a unit into the skin with a twisting motion. It is best to grasp the unit at the junction of the sheath and the dilator to prevent bunching up of the sheath. *H,* Once the sheath and the dilator are well within the vessel, the wire guide and the dilator are removed.

(Reproduced with permission from Roberts JR, Hedges JR, editors: *Clinical procedures in emergency medicine*, Philadelphia, 1985, WB Saunders.)

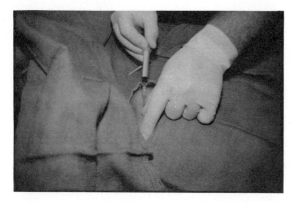

Figure 8B-3.   Insertion of the needle under the clavicle in the direction of the suprasternal notch (i.e., toward the subclavian vein). Negative pressure is applied to the syringe while inserting the needle.

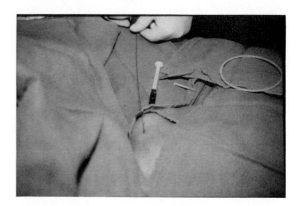

Figure 8B-6.   Guidewire after needle removal.

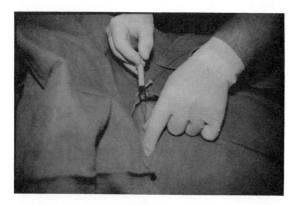

Figure 8B-4.   Upon entering the vein, blood will flow back easily into the syringe.

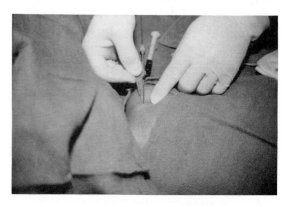

Figure 8B-7.   Nicking the skin with a #11 scalpel blade.

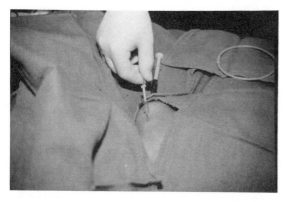

Figure 8B-5.   Insertion of guidewire into the needle.

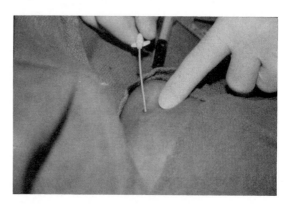

Figure 8B-8.   Slipping the dilator/sheath catheter unit over the guidewire into the vein.

Catheter Confirmation

One should always confirm correct placement of any central venous catheter. At the bedside this is done by immediately aspirating for blood after cannulation, or by lowering the IV bag below bed level to look for blood return.

One should be aware that in addition to suggesting arterial placement of the catheter, a *pulsating* flashback of blood may be due to ventricular tachycardia (if there is retrograde conduction to the atria), atrial fibrillation (when the right atrium contracts against the closed tricuspid valve), or tricuspid regurgitation (Wyte and Barker, 1985).

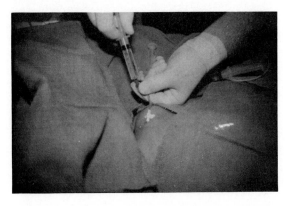

Figure 8B-9. Verifying the final position of the sheath in the vein by drawing back on the syringe. Correct positioning is confirmed by free blood flow into the syringe, followed by effortless flushing of the catheter.

Ultimate confirmation of correct central line placement in the superior vena cava (and reassurance that neither pneumothorax nor hemothorax was produced) should be by chest x-ray at the first convenient moment.

References

Becker A: *Central venous catheter placement and care.* In Rippe JM, Scete ME, editors: *Manual of intensive medicine*, Boston, 1983, Little, Brown.

Cavallaro DL: Personal communication (from study with Arrow International).

Dalsey WC, Barsan WG, Joyce SM, Hedges JR, Lukes SJ, Doan LA: Comparison of superior vena cava vs inferior vena cava access for delivery of drugs using a radioisotope technique during normal perfusion and CPR, *Ann Emerg Med* 12:247, 1983 (abstract).

Denys BG, Uretsky BF, Reddy PS, Ruffner RJ, Sandhu JS, Breisheatt WM: An ultrasound method for safe and rapid central venous access, *N Engl J Med* 324:566, 1991 (letter).

Dronen SC: *Subclavian venipuncture.* In Roberts JR, Hedges JR, editors: *Clinical procedures in emergency medicine*, Philadelphia, 1985, WB Saunders.

Hähnel JH, Lundner KH, Schürmann C, Prengel A, Ahnefeld FW: Plasma lidocaine levels and PaO$_2$ with endobronchial administration: dilution with normal saline or distilled water, *Ann Emerg Med* 19:1314, 1990.

Hedges JR, Baisan WB, Doan LA, Joyce SM, Lukes SJ, Dalsey WC, Nishiyama H: Central versus peripheral intravenous routes in cardiopulmonary resuscitation, *Am J Emerg Med* 2:385, 1984.

Hollinshead WH: *Textbook of anatomy*, New York, 1969, Harper & Row.

Kaye W: *Intravenous techniques.* In McIntyre KM, Lewis AJ, editors: *Textbook of advanced cardiac life support*, Texas, 1983, American Heart Association.

Kaye W, Bircher NG: Access for drug administration during cardiopulmonary resuscitation, *Crit Care Med* 16:179, 1988.

Niemann JT, Rosborough J, Hausknecht M, Ung S, Criley JM: Blood flow without cardiac compression during closed chest CPR, *Crit Care Med* 9:380, 1981.

Paradis NA, Kascove EM: Epinephrine in cardiac arrest: a critical review, *Ann Emerg Med* 19:1288, 1990.

Quinton DN, O'Byrne G, Aitkenhead AR: Comparison of endotracheal and peripheral intravenous adrenaline in cardiac arrest: is the endotracheal route reliable? *Lancet* 1:828, 1987.

Rosen P, Sternbach G: *Atlas of emergency medicine*, Baltimore, 1979, Williams & Wilkins.

Sacchetti A: *Large-bore infusion catheters (Seldinger technique) of vascular access.* In Roberts JR, Hedges JR, editors: *Clinical procedures in emergency medicine*, Philadelphia, 1985, WB Saunders.

Ward JT: *Endotracheal drug administration.* In Roberts JR, Hedges JR, editors: *Clinical procedures in emergency medicine*, Philadelphia, 1985, WB Saunders.

Wyte SR, Barker WJ: *Central venous catheterization: internal jugular approach and alternatives.* In Roberts JR, Hedges JR, editors: *Clinical procedures in emergency medicine*, Philadelphia, 1985, WB Saunders.

Pearls and Pitfalls in Management of Cardiac Arrest

CHAPTER 9

Pearls & Pitfalls in the Management of Cardiac Arrest

The techniques of basic and advanced cardiac life support have been taught to thousands of medical and paramedical personnel across the country. Yet despite widespread dispersion of knowledge, certain fundamental errors in the application of these techniques continue to be made.

It has been said that,

> *"Experience is errors."*

More appropriately, it might be said that:

Experience is having *learned* from the errors one has already made (and/or from errors already made by a trusted colleague).

As Wrenn and Slovis eloquently stated (1991), *"We all make mistakes of varying severity, REGARDLESS of our level of experience. The KEY to dealing appropriately with mistakes is not to deny them, but rather to embrace them and learn from them. It is NOT healthy to dwell on mistakes. It IS healthy to use a mistake to become an expert in a particular area."*

With these concepts in mind, we have developed this chapter. Our purpose is *purely* constructive. We hope that drawing attention to some of the more common pitfalls in management of cardiac arrest and cardiopulmonary emergencies will increase awareness of these problems and help to improve the delivery of emergency cardiac care.

Aspects in the management of cardiac arrest that are covered in this chapter include:

A. Overview of the General Management of Cardiac Arrest
B. Provision of Basic Life Support
C. Administration of Drugs
D. Defibrillation
E. Miscellaneous Pearls and Pitfalls in Management of Cardiac Arrest
F. Pearls and Pitfalls in Arrhythmia Interpretation

For each subject area, we'll attempt to list the most common *pitfalls* that are likely to be encountered. Helpful "pearls" in management are added along the way.

A. Overview of the General Management of Cardiac Arrest

Who hasn't (at one time or another) walked into the scene of a cardiac arrest in which there was general confusion and disorganization? In most such cases, one or more of the following pitfalls are likely to have contributed to the generation of this feeling.

1. **Failure of Anyone to Assume Command of the Resuscitation Effort.** The need for *someone* to take charge of the resuscitation effort is perhaps the most important determinant of the success of the code. The person who assumes command does *not* necessarily have to be a physician, but may be any qualified emergency care provider on the scene. Often it will be the first emergency care provider to arrive. Whether this role is subsequently passed on to others with more experience (as they arrive) is not nearly as important as having a *single* person clearly identified as the one responsible for making decisions.

As **code director** (or **team leader**), your roles are many. They include:

   a. To oversee and coordinate the overall resuscitative effort.
   b. *To clear the room of unnecessary personnel.*
   c. To verify that CPR is being performed correctly, and that a pulse is produced by external chest compressions.
   d. To make sure that the patient is adequately ventilated at all times (by bag-valve mask, pocket mask, mouth-to-mouth ventilation, or an endotracheal tube).
   e. Following endotracheal intubation, to be sure that equal bilateral breath sounds are heard.
   f. To see to it that the patient is promptly hooked up to a monitor, and to make sure that someone continuously monitors the rhythm.
   g. To be sure that a pulse is checked for whenever the cardiac rhythm changes. If a pulse is present, to check for a blood pressure.
   h. To order the administration of drugs in the appropriate dosage, and by the appropriate route.
   i. To delegate an experienced individual to inquire about the patient's history, his/her overall health status, and the events leading up to the arrest. Resuscitation of a patient with diabetes in ketoacidosis is vastly different from resuscitation of a patient who has overdosed or who is uremic. Moreover, how aggressively one proceeds with the resuscitative effort may be strongly influenced by

factors in the patient's history, such as whether or not he/she has a terminal disease (*and whether there is a Living Will or other advance directive!*).

j. To order appropriate radiographic and laboratory tests as they are needed. Blood for determining arterial blood gases (ABGs) should be drawn to help guide respiratory therapy (and assist in the decision of whether to administer sodium bicarbonate). Once a stable rhythm has been established, a chest x-ray film should be done to verify correct positioning of the endotracheal tube, central lines, and/or pacemaker wires, and to rule out pneumothorax. A 12-lead ECG should be obtained to look for evidence of infarction. Finally, serum electrolyte values and other blood work may be needed to help determine the etiology of the arrest and the need for corrective therapy.

k. **To talk to your colleagues.** It is important (and will be immensely appreciated) to let others know why various actions are being taken (e.g., *"The patient is in ventricular tachycardia with a pulse—so let's cardiovert with 200 joules"*). Orders should be clearly (and loudly) stated to avoid any possible misunderstanding of your intentions. Insist that other team members do the same, and announce completed tasks as they are accomplished (e.g., *"One ampule of epinephrine given by the ET route"*).

Announcing your actions enables everyone present to follow the course of the resuscitation in a more meaningful way. It also allows team members to anticipate future actions that will need to be taken. This not only facilitates coordination of the team effort, but also prevents needless duplication of tasks and improves accuracy of the code sheet recording.

l. To consult with the patient's primary physician at the earliest opportunity.

m. **To talk to the patient's family.**

n. To decide when the resuscitation effort should be terminated.

o. *After the code is over,* to concisely document (in a progress note) the events that have transpired.

p. To acknowledge the efforts of those who helped in the resuscitation process.

2. **Failure to Record the Sequence of Events As They Unfold During the Arrest.** The **code sheet** should reflect the following information:

   a. The various cardiac rhythms that occurred during the code, and whether or not they were associated with a pulse and blood pressure.

   b. The time of administration, dose, route, site, and indication for all medications given during the code.

   c. The number of countershock attempts and the energies used.

   d. The performance of any procedures (such as endotracheal intubation, pericardiocentesis, insertion of a pacemaker or of a central IV line)—including the name of the person performing the procedure, the time, and any complications.

   e. The names of those emergency care providers in attendance.

   f. The time the arrest began, as well as the time and reason the resuscitation effort was terminated.

Keeping track of the information listed above *as the code is taking place* is especially important with regard

to the use of drugs that are commonly administered on a *timed* basis (e.g., atropine, epinephrine, and boluses of lidocaine or bretylium). If sodium bicarbonate is given, correlation of the time of administration with respect to the timing of endotracheal intubation and drawing of ABGs is critical.

Medicolegally, the code sheet serves as a key source of documentation. For this documentation to be accurate, events must be recorded *as they happen*. Practically speaking, it is often difficult enough just trying to keep track of all that is happening *during* a code—*even when someone is specifically assigned to accomplish nothing but this task.* Trying to reconstruct the *exact* sequence of events that occurred *after the code* becomes almost impossible *unless events are recorded as they happen.*

Clearly, the KEY to accurate recording (and accurate documentation) of the events of a cardiac arrest is continuous notation of the precise *timing* of these events *as they occur.*

---

3. **Failure to Review the Resuscitation Effort.** The importance of this undertaking cannot be overemphasized. Ideally, review should be accomplished on at least two occasions: *immediately* after the resuscitation effort, and at a later date.

The last thing most emergency care providers want to do immediately following a code is to reflect on the process. This seems to be especially true for cases in which the patient died. Nevertheless, forcing oneself to go back over the code sequence, review events (and/or the actual ECG recordings), and *think about how things might have gone better* may be a source of invaluable feedback. Discussing the case with a trusted colleague—especially if they were also present during the code—may likewise be immensely insightful.

Periodic review of code sheets by ICU personnel or a code committee is another extremely helpful mechanism for assuring regular feedback with the intent of improving future resuscitation efforts. It is also a way of verifying that adequate documentation of code events is being obtained.

4. **Not Regularly Checking to See That All Crash Cart Drugs Are Restocked and All Emergency Equipment Is in Working Order.** Laryngoscope bulbs, Ambu bags, defibrillator gel or pads, and suction equipment all have a disturbing tendency to "disappear" at the very moment that they seem to be needed most (i.e., at the moment that an arrest is called). Similarly, the supply of essential drugs (such as epinephrine, dopamine, and bretylium) is likely to be "exhausted," and defibrillator function (and/or batteries) impaired *unless* provisions have been made in advance for regularly scheduled crash cart maintenance checks.

5. **Failure to Consider *"Do Not Resuscitate" (DNR)* Orders *BEFORE* the Arrest Occurs.** Ideally, the question of whether or not to initiate resuscitation in the event of a cardiopulmonary arrest will be *routinely* addressed for *all* patients who are admitted to the hospital. If this was regularly done *at the time of admission*, it would virtually eliminate the problem of not knowing what to do after the arrest is called.

> The decision of whether or not to initiate resuscitation may be arrived at in a number of ways. (For full discussion of this issue, *see Chapter 18 on Medicolegal Aspects of ACLS.*) If the patient is sufficiently competent to participate in the decision-making process, *their desires are given highest priority.* Input from the family and the medical health care team provide additional assistance. If it is felt to be in the patient's best interests not to initiate CPR (e.g., because of a terminal illness or because there is no chance of restoring the patient to a meaningful level of function by performing CPR), *this decision must be adequately documented on the chart and made clear to ALL hospital personnel involved in the care of the patient.*

Unless there is adequate documentation of DNR status, CPR will have to be initiated. Finally, it should be emphasized that the decision of whether to initiate resuscitation may need to be actively reconsidered if *(whenever)* the patient's clinical condition changes during the course of hospitalization.

6. **Failure to Inquire about a Living Will When Appropriate.** *Advance directives* in the form of a ***Living Will*** have become legal in many states. All that is required for completion of this document is that the patient be competent at the time he/she fills out the form. Specific aspects of resuscitation may be defined by the patient. For example, he/she may indicate a desire to be made "as comfortable as possible" (e.g., with analgesics) and a willingness to allow chemical and electrical resuscitation, but firm refusal to be intubated.

> While it may not always be appropriate/feasible to ask each patient at the time of admission to the hospital whether he/she has filled out a Living Will, awareness of the existence of such documents (if they are legal in the state where you practice) and sensitivity to the issues encompassed by them will go a long way toward helping the emergency care provider elicit such information at the earliest opportune moment. Available family that are close to the patient may occasionally assist if they know of the patient's desires (or if they know of advance directives that have already been filled out).

B. Provision of Basic Life Support

1. **Delay in Making the Diagnosis of Cardiopulmonary Arrest *(and in Beginning Treatment).*** In view of the critical importance of *time* as the KEY deter- minant of survival from cardiopulmonary arrest, as soon as a victim is found to be unresponsive, it is essential to:
   a. Call for help/activate EMS
   b. Check for the adequacy of spontaneous ventilation and circulation
   c. Initiate basic life support (BLS) measures as needed for pulselessness and/or apnea.

If the patient is not breathing and no airway adjunct is immediately accessible, *mouth-to-mouth ventilation will have to be started within very short order if the patient is to survive.*

> In this day and age of heightened concern over the possibility of AIDS transmission, the decision of whether YOU would (will) perform mouth-to-mouth resuscitation on a stranger in need is one that must be made by each of us. Reasonable options include:
>
> a. *Categorical refusal* to perform mouth-to-mouth resuscitation on *any* stranger.
> b. *Categorical acceptance* of any potential risk of disease transmission by a decision to perform mouth-to-mouth resuscitation on anyone in need of this procedure.
> c. *Selective refusal* to perform mouth-to-mouth resuscitation on an unknown victim in need depending on:
>   • clinical circumstances (i.e., site of occurrence, presumed duration, and/or probable precipitating cause of the arrest)
>   • physical characteristics and age of the victim (i.e., whether the victim is a child, an elderly person, or someone who may be perceived as having an increased likelihood of HIV-positivity)
>   • the amount of time likely to pass before help (in the form of a bag-valve mask) arrives.

We wish to emphasize that we are *not* advocating one of these options over another. However, what we are advocating is to set aside a moment for *anticipatory reflection* on how YOU feel it will be most appropriate to act in the event that you are one day confronted with this problematic clinical dilemma. *A moment of anticipatory reflection at this time may be invaluable for facilitating the decision-making process (as well as EXPEDITING your actions) in the event that you encounter this situation at some time in the future.*

> The reluctance of trained health care professionals to ventilate the nonbreathing victim of cardiopulmonary arrest would probably be minimized by more ready availability of a pocket mask in health care settings where rapid application of other respiratory adjuncts and/or intubation is not feasible.

(See discussion on "Mouth-to-Mouth Resuscitation: An Extinct Art?" in Section 10D for additional thoughts on our approach to management of the apneic patient in the absence of respiratory adjuncts.)

2. **Overlooking the Possibility of Foreign Body Airway Obstruction as the Cause of Apnea.** If despite repositioning the nonbreathing victim, you are still

unable to ventilate (resistance is met and the chest will not rise), *assume airway obstruction until proved otherwise*. Treatment for foreign body obstruction (i.e., with subdiaphragmatic or chest thrusts as appropriate according to the Heimlich maneuver) should be immediately administered.

3. **Unnecessarily Interrupting CPR.** CPR should not be stopped for more than 5 seconds except for intubating or moving the patient. *No more than a 15- to 20-second interruption should be permitted for these maneuvers.*

4. **Delay in Securing a Definitive Airway.** Practically speaking, the resuscitation effort is doomed to failure unless an airway can be established and maintained. Application of either the chin-lift or jaw-thrust maneuver should open the airway. Ventilation with a properly positioned pocket mask or BVM device will usually be sufficient to maintain adequate oxygenation until personnel experienced in intubation arrive. *CPR should not be repeatedly interrupted by inexpert attempts at intubation until such personnel arrive.*

5. **Failure to Place a Backboard under the Patient.** Cardiac massage is not effective when performed on a mattress.

6. **Improper Application of External Chest Compression.** The technique recommended for performing chest compression is as follows:

   The rescuer should be correctly positioned over the patient's sternum with arms extended. Pressure is then applied to the lower sternum with the heels of both hands, displacing it downward by 1.5 to 2 inches toward the spine. Standing on a stool may help to optimize body mechanics. The rescuer should not remove his/her hands from the sternum between compressions, but must be sure to release pressure completely. Fingers should not rest on the patient's chest, and jerking or bouncing movements must be avoided. Instead, external chest compression should be delivered in as smooth and regular a manner as possible. *The actual period of chest compression should ideally occupy at least 50% of the cycle* (to assure maximum blood flow during CPR).

   In the past, great emphasis had been placed on delivering compressions at a precisely defined rate (i.e., 60 times a minute). Undue attention was commonly focused on complying with this rate criterion— all too often at the cost of improper technique. Practical considerations suggest:

   a. that proper technique is extremely important
   b. that the optimal rate for chest compression is not yet known
   c. that a *range* (of between 80-100 compressions/min) is currently recommended—and that aiming for the *higher side* of this range will probably result in optimal flow
   d. that left to themselves, *many* (if not most) *emergency care providers tend to compress the chest at too slow a rate.*

Even if multiple emergency care providers are already on the scene, you can still provide valuable feedback to the resuscitation team by monitoring the compression rate (and seeing to it that *at least* 80 compressions are delivered each minute).

(See Section 10A for additional discussion on the performance of CPR.)

7. **Inadequate Ventilation during CPR.** Two KEY points should be kept in mind when administering ventilation during CPR:

   a. *Always make sure that the ventilatory device being used is connected to a supply of 100% oxygen.* With a self-inflating resuscitation (i.e., Ambu) bag, this means that a reservoir must be attached to the BVM device in order to ensure delivery of 100% oxygen to the patient.
   b. Be sure that ventilations are always delivered *S L O W L Y.* Prior to intubation, ventilations are delivered during the pause after each five compressions. Following intubation, it will no longer be necessary to sequence ventilations with compressions, but it will still be important to administer ventilations *slowly* to ensure optimal oxygen delivery.

8. **Ignoring Gastric Distention.** Even when performed correctly, administration of one- and two-person CPR will frequently result in *gastric distention*. This can compromise left ventricular filling and predispose the patient to regurgitation of stomach contents. *Increasing gastric distention should be actively looked for while CPR is being performed.* If found, it can usually be relieved by insertion of a nasogastric tube (*after* protecting the airway by endotracheal intubation). Intubation prevents further gastric distention from taking place.

   The amount of gastric distention that develops during one- or two-person CPR can be minimized by performing rescue breathing *S L O W L Y enough* (i.e., over a period of 1.5 to 2 seconds) to allow delivery of a *full* ventilation. Doing so significantly reduces airway inflation pressures, and minimizes the amount of air that will enter the esophagus.

9. **Forgetting about the Sellick Maneuver.** Application of downward pressure on the anterolateral aspects of the cricoid cartilage (with the thumb and index finger of one hand) serves the dual function of *facilitating intubation* (by making it easier to visualize the glottis) and *minimizing the chance of gastric regurgitation* (by occluding the esophagus).

   It is important to *maintain downward pressure* on the cricoid cartilage until *AFTER* the endotracheal tube has been

Table 9B-1

Parameters for *Pediatric* Basic Life Support			
BLS PARAMETER	**INFANTS** (<1 year old)	**CHILDREN** (1-8 years old)	**ADULTS**
Assessment			
• Pulse Check	Check the *brachial* pulse	Check the carotid pulse	Check the carotid pulse
Ventilation			
• Tidal Volume requirement	*Much less* than for adults (i.e., deliver *just enough* air to produce adequate chest rise)	*Less* than for adults (i.e., deliver *just enough* air to produce adequate chest rise)	
• Rate of Rescue Breathing (if a pulse is present)	20/min (i.e., 1 breath every 3 seconds)	15/min (i.e., 1 breath every 4 seconds	12/min (i.e., 1 breath every 5 seconds)
Chest Compression			
• Finger Placement Location	1 fingerbreadth *below* the nipple line	Lower half of the sternum	Lower half of the sternum
• Compression Delivery	*Two-finger technique* (using the index and middle fingers) *or* use of bimanual circumferential compression	Use the heel of *one* hand	Bimanual compression with the heels of both hands
• Depth of Compression	0.5-1 inch	1-1.5 inches	1.5-2 inches
• Rate of Compression	*At least* 100/min	80-100/min	80-100/min
• Compression-Ventilation Ratio	5:1	5:1	15:2 (1-person CPR) 5:1 (2-person CPR)

inserted and the cuff is inflated (or else gastric regurgitation is likely to occur!).

10. **Forgetting the Parameters for *Pediatric* Basic Life Support** *(Table 9B-1).* It is all too easy for the emergency care provider with limited exposure to pediatric patients to forget the different BLS parameters that are recommended for resuscitation of infants and children.

C. Administration of Drugs

1. **Unnecessary Concern with Sterile Technique during Resuscitation.** Although ideally all procedures would be performed with as sterile a technique as possible, clearly the more important concern of cardiopulmonary resuscitation must be to save the patient's life. Utilization of sterile technique may have to take a back seat role to this primary goal.

2. **Forgetting about the Endotracheal Route.** The onset of action of *intratracheally* administered (i.e., en-

dotracheal) epinephrine in patients with cardiovascular collapse is almost comparable to that when the drug is given intravenously. Consequently, in the event that a patient is intubated but an IV line cannot be started, *one should not hesitate to administer epinephrine by the endotracheal tube. Higher doses may be needed.*

Atropine and lidocaine may also be given endotracheally, although the pharmacokinetics of these two agents is clearly more favorable when they are administered intravenously. (The mnemonic *A L E*—**a**tropine, **l**idocaine, and **e**pinephrine—may help recall that these three drugs can be given by the ET route.)

Other medications that can be given by the endotracheal route include Narcan and Valium. (Expansion of the mnemonic to *NAVEL*—**N**arcan, **a**tropine, **V**alium, **e**pinephrine, and **l**idocaine—may help you remember these five drugs.)

3. **Preoccupation with Inserting a Central Line.** During closed-chest compression, circulation of drugs by a central IV line is preferable to using a peripheral IV. This is because administration of drugs through a central IV line allows more immediate access to the central circulation. Insertion of a central IV line dur-

ing cardiopulmonary resuscitation is not without drawbacks, however, and *other routes CAN be used for drug administration* (albeit with slightly slower entry into the central circulation).

> Insertion of an internal jugular or subclavian line requires temporary cessation of CPR, and exposes the patient to a significant risk of pneumothorax. These concerns do not apply to the insertion of a femoral line, but diminished blood flow below the diaphragm during CPR makes the femoral route an undesirable one for administration of medications during a code.

As noted above (in #2), three of the medications most commonly used during cardiopulmonary resuscitation can be given by the endotracheal route. In contrast, circulation of drugs that are administered through an IV line inserted in a *distal* peripheral site (such as the dorsum of the wrist, hand, or lower leg) may not be reliable in the arrested heart. Establishment of a peripheral IV in a *more proximal* site (such as the antecubital fossa) is much more likely to provide adequate access for blood flow to the central circulation. Thus, if an operator skilled in the insertion of central lines is not immediately available, *administration of medications through either an antecubital vein or the endotracheal route will usually result in adequate (albeit less than optimal) drug delivery*. Practically speaking, use of either of these alternative routes is far preferable to repeated inexpert attempts at cannulation of a central vein. *Higher doses may be needed with the ET route.*

> A third (commonly overlooked) alternative route for drug delivery is the *external* jugular vein. Although cannulation of this vein may necessitate temporary cessation of CPR, drug delivery is almost comparable to that with the use of a central IV line *without* the associated risk of producing a pneumothorax.

4. **Failure to Optimize Drug Delivery through a Peripheral IV.** As implied above (in #3), *the more distal the site of a peripheral IV, the less likely it is that there will be adequate drug delivery to the central circulation.* Thus, insertion of a tiny "butterfly" IV in the dorsum of the wrist may not really provide much better access for drug delivery to a patient in cardiac arrest than having no access at all!

Drug delivery through a peripheral IV may be optimized by attention to the following three factors:

---

a. *Selection of the most appropriate site.* In general, the more proximal the site, the better drug delivery will be. Perhaps the most ideal site for insertion of a peripheral IV is the antecubital fossa.
b. *Use of a short-length/large-bore catheter for the IV.* According to the Laws of Poiseuille and Hagen, fluid flow is proportional to the *fourth power* of the diameter of the catheter, and *inversely* proportional

---

to its length. Thus, *a small increase in IV lumen diameter may make a substantial difference in the rate of fluid administration.* Optimal flow will be obtained when large-bore catheters of *short* length are used.
c. *Elevation of the extremity and injection of a bolus of fluid following administration of the medication.* These actions may help to "flush" medication toward the central circulation.

---

5. **Failure to Flush the IV Line After Administration of Sodium Bicarbonate.** Catecholamines (epinephrine, dopamine, isoproterenol) and calcium salts are inactivated when mixed with sodium bicarbonate. It is therefore essential to thoroughly flush the IV line after giving sodium bicarbonate *before* infusing any additional drugs.

6. **Inappropriate Administration of Medication by Intracardiac Injection.** Administration of drugs by the intracardiac route is associated with an extremely high incidence of serious complications (including induction of intractable ventricular fibrillation, laceration of a coronary artery, pneumothorax, and hemopericardium with tamponade). As a result, use of this route is probably best reserved *as a last resort* after all other measures have failed *(if it is used at all)*.

7. **Dosing Atropine Inappropriately.** Administration of atropine in a dose of 0.5 mg every 5 minutes (up to a total dose of 2 mg) has been recommended for treatment of hemodynamically significant bradyarrhythmias. However, atropine is *not* a benign medication, and errors occur in both underdosing and overdosing the drug.

> Many patients with acute myocardial infarction and cardiac arrest manifest increased activity of *both* sympathetic *and* parasympathetic divisions of the autonomic nervous system. Clinically, if parasympathetic activity predominates (as is commonly the case with acute *inferior* infarction), bradycardia is likely to be seen. The rationale for administering atropine to such patients is in the hope that the parasympatholytic action of this drug will counteract any excess in parasympathetic tone and restore the heart rate to normal. Unfortunately, the effect of the drug may backfire in some patients by unmasking underlying sympathetic hyperactivity (that is no longer held in check by opposing parasympathetic tone). This may result in sinus tachycardia (with an associated increase in oxygen consumption and/or ischemia), or even precipitate ventricular tachycardia or fibrillation.

Because of these potential adverse effects, use of atropine should be reserved for treatment of bradyarrhythmias that are truly *hemodynamically significant*. In addition, special caution in dosing is urged when treating patients with only *minimal* signs of hemodynamic compromise. Thus, it would not be prudent to administer more than 0.5 mg of atropine to a patient with a heart rate of 50 beats / min and a blood pressure of 80 mm Hg until adequate time had passed to observe the full effect of the drug. In contrast, administration of a 0.5-mg dose at 5-minute intervals (as recommended) to a patient with more severe bradycardia and hypotension (i.e., with a heart rate of less than 40 beats / min and a blood pressure of 60 mm Hg or less) would require *no less* than 15 minutes to deliver the usual 2-mg atropinization dose. In this latter situation, administration of a larger dose (i.e., 1 mg at a time) at more frequent intervals (i.e., repeating the dose in 2 to 3 min if there is no response) may be preferable. *Occasionally, more than 2 mg is needed.*

8. **Forgetting that Drug Administration During (or Preceding) Cardiac Arrest May Alter Pupil Size and Responsiveness.** Although in most cases therapeutic doses of atropine will not completely abolish pupillary responsiveness, administration of this drug may produce a degree of pupillary dilatation and alter the pupillary reaction to light for a period of at least several hours. As a result, interpretation of pupillary responsiveness must be made with caution in patients who receive atropine during cardiopulmonary resuscitation.

> Other drugs may also alter pupillary responsiveness (including narcotics, amphetamines, cocaine, and tricyclic antidepressants). Overdose from any of these agents can precipitate cardiac arrest.

9. **Reflexive Use of Sodium Bicarbonate— *And Depending on the Results of ABG Studies to Guide Acid-Base Therapy.*** In the past, sodium bicarbonate was liberally administered during cardiac arrest— and arterial blood gas (ABG) studies were frequently obtained to monitor the efficacy of this therapy. In recent years, use of sodium bicarbonate has been strongly deemphasized. It is now appreciated that standard ABG studies *cannot* be relied upon in the setting of cardiac arrest because they do not accurately reflect the true state of *intracellular* homeostasis.

> There are many reasons why sodium bicarbonate is no longer routinely recommended for treatment of the patient in cardiac arrest. First, despite the intuitive logic that acute buffering of acidosis should be beneficial, objective data demonstrating improved survival from such treatment are lacking. Clinically, we now appreciate that the acidosis seen during the early minutes of cardiopulmonary arrest is primarily *respiratory* in nature. Development of metabolic acidosis appears to require a lag time of *at least* 5 to 15 minutes in this setting. Consequently, it would seem far more appropriate to correct acidosis by improving ventilation (i.e., *hyperventilating* the patient) rather than by administering sodium bicarbonate—at least during the initial phase of the resuscitation process. Moreover, *sodium bicarbonate therapy is far from being benign.* Adverse effects of excessive administration of this agent include development

of alkalosis, hyperosmolality, hypokalemia, sodium overload, shifting of the oxyhemoglobin dissociation curve to the left (with consequent impaired oxygen release to the tissues), and precipitation of convulsions, ischemia, and/ or arrhythmias. In addition, sodium bicarbonate administration may lead to development of a *paradoxical intracellular acidosis*. This last effect is particularly problematic because the clinician may be led into thinking that the patient is improving (since the pH of ABG studies may return toward normal), whereas the degree of *intracellular* acidosis is actually becoming worse. Thus, it is well to remember:

In the setting of cardiac arrest, ABG studies do NOT accurately reflect the true state of intracellular homeostasis.

Practically speaking, then, it would seem that the use of sodium bicarbonate for treatment of the patient in cardiac arrest should be limited to cases of *severe* metabolic acidosis (i.e., pH ≤7.15) that persist *beyond* the initial phase (i.e., beyond the first 5-15 minutes) of the resuscitation process—and/or for selected patients known to have a *severe preexisting* metabolic acidosis—*IF* any bicarb is indicated at all. . . .

10. **Continued Use of Calcium Chloride for Asystole or EMD.** Calcium chloride is no longer recommended for treatment of asystole or EMD. Clinical data supporting the efficacy of this agent are lacking, and the use of calcium in this setting has been associated with an adverse outcome in certain cases. As a result, the *only* remaining indications for the use of calcium chloride in the setting of cardiac arrest or emergency cardiac care are:

   a. treatment of hypocalcemia
   b. treatment of hyperkalemia
   c. treatment of asystole (or severe bradycardia) that follows the use of a calcium channel blocking agent
   d. as an adjunct to verapamil administration (to minimize the hypotensive effect of this antiarrhythmic agent)

11. **Continued Use of Isoproterenol in the Arrested Heart.** The use of isoproterenol in the setting of cardiac arrest / emergency cardiac care has been greatly deemphasized.

> Potential problems associated with isoproterenol administration are many. They include excessive acceleration of heart rate, arrhythmogenicity, increased myocardial oxygen consumption, hypotension, and decreased myocardial and vital organ perfusion. The drug is contraindicated in the arrested heart because its pure β-adrenergic stimulating action produces vasodilatation, which is likely to result in a lowering of aortic diastolic pressure and impaired coronary perfusion.

At the present time, the *only* indication for the use of isoproterenol is as a *stopgap measure* (i.e., until pacemaker therapy can be initiated) in the treatment of hemodynamically significant bradyarrhythmias that have not responded to atropine. Other pressor agents (i.e., epinephrine and dopamine) appear to be preferable to isoproterenol because of their more favorable effect on coronary flow in this setting.

12. **Indiscriminate Use of Verapamil as a Diagnostic/ Therapeutic Trial for Treatment of Wide Complex Tachyarrhythmias of Unknown Etiology.** If the etiology of a regular, wide QRS complex tachyarrhythmia is uncertain, *ventricular tachycardia MUST always be assumed until proved otherwise.* This dictum holds true *regardless* of the patient's blood pressure or level of consciousness at the time of the tachycardia. In such situations, the all too common practice of administering verapamil (as a diagnostic/therapeutic trial to help distinguish between a supraventricular and ventricular etiology) is clearly *NOT* advised. Granted, if the tachyarrhythmia turns out to be supraventricular, administration of verapamil is likely to result in conversion to sinus rhythm. On the other hand, if the etiology of the wide complex tachycardia is ventricular, the vasodilatory and negative inotropic effect of verapamil is extremely likely to precipitate ventricular fibrillation.

> It should be emphasized that *ventricular tachycardia is a much more common cause of a regular wide complex tachycardia than PSVT with either aberration or bundle branch block.* This is especially true in adults with a history of underlying heart disease (e.g., prior infarction, angina pectoris, or heart failure).

Two alternatives to the indiscriminate use of verapamil should be strongly considered in this situation:

a. *Closer electrocardiographic scrutiny* in the hope of picking up additional clues (such as telltale atrial activity or diagnostic QRS morphology) that may point toward the true etiology of the arrhythmia. Obtaining a 12-lead ECG and/or use of special lead systems may be invaluable in this regard.
b. Use of *IV procainamide* as a therapeutic trial. This type IA antiarrhythmic agent may work regardless of the etiology of the arrhythmia since it is often effective for *both* supraventricular and ventricular tachyarrhythmias. Even in cases of ventricular tachycardia that are not converted by the drug, procainamide will often slow the rate of the ventricular response (and thus improve the patient's ability to tolerate the arrhythmia).

13. **Withholding Oxygen for Fear of Causing Carbon Dioxide Retention.** Carbon dioxide retention is extremely unlikely to occur in an acutely ill patient who is being closely monitored. *Such patients are simply not left alone long enough for this to happen.* Administration of high-flow oxygen in the acute care setting is therefore safe (and often essential), and may be empirically given until ABG studies and/or clinical evaluation indicates otherwise.

14. **Not Optimally Monitoring Patients on Potent Cardioactive Agents.** Blood pressure cuff readings obtained on patients who are in shock are not always accurate (and may not truly reflect intraarterial pressure). As a result, an *arterial line* may need to be inserted to ensure accurate recordings. Similarly, clinical assessment of hemodynamic status on patients with acute myocardial infarction, shock, or just after resuscitation from cardiopulmonary arrest, is frequently subject to error. In such situations, use of invasive hemodynamic monitoring (with a *Swan-Ganz catheter*) may be needed to obtain more reliable information.

15. **Inappropriate Use of Bretylium as an Antiarrhythmic Agent.** Although bretylium is potentially a very effective antiarrhythmic agent, there are a number of caveats to its use.

a. *Dosing of bretylium for treatment of refractory ventricular fibrillation is largely empiric.* If standard treatment measures (i.e., repeated defibrillation, epinephrine, and lidocaine) have failed—and the decision is made to administer a trial of bretylium—it is important to realize that *more than one dose* of the drug may be needed for therapeutic effect. Thus, if an initial 5-mg/kg bolus is ineffective, a second dose (of 10 mg/kg) may be given. Additional boluses (up to a total dose of 30 mg/kg) may be considered if ventricular fibrillation persists.

   Chemical conversion (i.e., spontaneous conversion of ventricular fibrillation by the drug itself) is rare. It is therefore essential to circulate the drug with CPR for *at least* 1 to 2 minutes following administration of each dose *before* defibrillating. Finally, it should be remembered that *the onset of action of bretylium may sometimes be delayed (for as long as 10-15 minutes)!* Thus, once the decision is made to try the drug, adequate time should be allowed for bretylium to have an *opportunity* to work before concluding that it has been ineffective. Resuscitation efforts should therefore continue for *at least* this amount of time after the first dose is given.
b. *Use of bretylium for treatment of PVCs and/or ventricular tachycardia has been de-emphasized.* Because of bretylium's mechanism of action (i.e., initial adrenergic stimulation—followed by adrenergic blockade)—ventricular ectopy may paradoxically worsen when the drug is first given, and orthostatic hypotension may limit continued use. As a result, other antiarrhythmic agents (i.e., lidocaine, procainamide) are preferable to bretylium for treatment of PVCs and/or ventricular tachycardia.

(Additional information on the use of bretylium is found in Section 2E.)

16. **Forgetting to Administer Lidocaine *Prophylactically* Following Successful Conversion of Ventricular Fibrillation.** Because of the altered pharmacokinetics of lidocaine in the setting of cardiac arrest, only bolus therapy is needed for as long as the patient remains in ventricular fibrillation. As soon as the patient is converted out of ventricular fibrillation, however, it is essential to rebolus with lidocaine, and to initiate a maintenance infusion. Failure to do so significantly increases the risk that ventricular fibrillation will recur.

> Practically speaking, it may be easier to develop the habit of *always* initiating a lidocaine infusion *whenever* bolus therapy of this drug is begun (*regardless* of the clinical situation). The advantage of this practice is that it eliminates having to remember to start the infusion at the moment the patient is converted out of ventricular fibrillation.

17. **Failure to Use the Lowest Possible Dose of a Pressor Agent.** For many patients, use of a pressor agent (such as dopamine, isoproterenol or epinephrine) will be essential for supporting the circulation either during and/or immediately after the process of cardiopulmonary resuscitation. Nevertheless, a strong effort should still be made to use the *lowest possible dose* of these agents. Once spontaneous circulation is restored, attention should be *redirected* at reducing the rate of infusion of the pressor agent as soon as this is possible. Failure to taper the rate of infusion of these catecholamines (especially *after* restoration of spontaneous circulation) may predispose to development of tachyarrhythmias that could precipitate a recurrence of the arrest.

18. **Failure to Appreciate the Role of Epinephrine in the Treatment of Cardiac Arrest.** Epinephrine is an endogenous catecholamine with both α- and β-*adrenergic* stimulating properties. Although the drug's β-adrenergic effect acts to increase the force and rate of myocardial contraction, *its α-adrenergic effect appears to be far more important in the treatment of patients in cardiac arrest.*

> α-Adrenergic stimulation produces vasoconstriction. This results in an increase in aortic diastolic pressure, which translates into improved coronary perfusion during CPR. The α-adrenergic effect of the drug also appears to promote a favorable redistribution of blood flow to the cerebral circulation.

> The optimal dose of epinephrine for treatment of cardiac arrest remains unknown. Factors such as individual patient characteristics (e.g., age, body weight, presence of underlying heart disease), the precipitating mechanism of the arrest (e.g., ventricular fibrillation, asystole, or EMD), and arrest du-

ration may all influence the dose of epinephrine required to achieve optimal effect. The point to emphasize is that *epinephrine appears to be the one drug capable of producing a favorable effect on blood flow to BOTH* the coronary and cerebral circulations.

Full discussion of our rationale for epinephrine dosing in the setting of cardiac arrest is found in *Section 2B.* In general, we favor beginning with a *standard dose* of 1 mg (i.e., **SDE,**—or **S**tandard-**D**ose **E**pinephrine)—and then *rapidly increasing this dose as needed* (to **HDE**—or **H**igh-**D**ose **E**pinephrine) until the desired clinical effect is achieved.

19. **Failure to *At Least* Consider the Use of Magnesium Sulfate.** The use of magnesium sulfate in emergency cardiac care remains controversial. Nevertheless, we feel one should *at least consider* use of this drug in the presence of the following conditions:

a. Selected cardiac arrhythmias in the acute care setting (i.e., PVCs, MAT, PSVT) that occur in patients who are (or who are likely to be) hypomagnesemic—*especially if conventional measures have failed.*

b. Ventricular arrhythmias associated with *digitalis toxicity* (especially if serum magnesium or potassium levels are low or in the low-normal range).

c. Ventricular arrhythmias in association with cardiac arrest (including refractory ventricular fibrillation and/or sustained ventricular tachycardia)—*especially if other measures have failed* (and *regardless* of whether prearrest serum magnesium levels were known or suspected to be low).

> The one indication for which the use of magnesium sulfate is no longer controversial is in the treatment of torsade de pointes. At the present time, magnesium sulfate is the medical treatment of choice for this condition.

(*Full discussion on our recommendations for the use of magnesium sulfate may be found in Section 2B.*)

20. **Failure to *At Least* Consider Use of an IV β-Blocker as Treatment in *Refractory* Cardiac Arrest.** Most cases of cardiac arrest are effectively managed without the use of an IV β-blocker (propranolol, esmolol, or metoprolol). However, in certain situations, other treatment simply will not work, and the use of this agent may prove to be *truly* lifesaving. *IV β-blockers should NOT be forgotten.*

> Clinical situations for which use of an IV β-blocker is most likely to be successful are treatment of ventricular arrhythmias associated with (or caused by) *excessive sympathetic tone* or *ischemia.* Clues suggestive of the presence of these factors include sinus tachycardia and/or hypertension occurring in the minutes prior to the onset of the

arrhythmia (or arrest)—especially in the setting of acute *anterior* infarction (which is commonly associated with sympathetic hyperactivity early in its course). Two other clinical settings that may predispose to development of catecholamine-induced tachyarrhythmias (refractory to other treatment) are *cocaine overdose* and *severe psychologic stress states*. Finally, use of an IV β-blocker might also be considered purely on an *empiric* basis for treatment of patients with malignant ventricular arrhythmias / cardiac arrest of unknown etiology that has not responded to other measures.

(Additional information on the use / dosing of IV β-Blockers may be found in Chapter 14 [for propranolol and esmolol] and Section B of Chapter 12 [for metoprolol].)

D. Defibrillation

1. **Forgetting to Clear the Area Before Defibrillation.** Although seemingly obvious, careless application of countershock without first verifying that no one is in direct (or indirect) contact with the patient still results in accidental defibrillation of hospital personnel. Standing in spilled IV fluids and "the hanging stethoscope" are two nemeses that may catch the unaware rescuer who is holding the paddles.

2. **Failure to Apply 25 lb of Firm Pressure to Each Paddle When Defibrillating.** Application of firm downward pressure on each defibrillator paddle reduces transthoracic resistance (TTR) of the chest wall, and therefore increases the efficacy of defibrillation.

3. **Unfamiliarity with the Defibrillation Equipment.** The time to learn about the specifics of your defibrillator / cardioverter is *not* during a cardiac arrest.

4. **Failure to Use the Quick-Look Paddles.** Most defibrillators are equipped to provide a *quick look* at the cardiac rhythm on contact of the paddles to the patient's chest. Use of this time-saving feature allows more rapid diagnosis of ventricular fibrillation, and therefore results in more rapid initial defibrillation.

5. **Failure to Hook the Patient Up to a 12-Lead ECG.** Although application of quick-look paddles (followed by use of the defibrillator monitoring lead) is extremely helpful for expediting delivery of initial countershocks, subsequent monitoring is probably best performed by *continuous* recording from a 12-lead ECG machine. Thus, the patient should ideally be hooked up to a 12-lead ECG machine *at the earliest opportunity* during the resuscitation process.

Monitoring from the single lead displayed on the defibrillator may be problematic in a number of ways. Introduction of artifact on the recording is common, and sometimes difficult to differentiate from the irregular baseline of ventricular fibrillation. Undetected reduction of the amplitude gain may "convert" coarse ventricular fibrillation to very fine ventricular fibrillation, or even asystole. Conversely, undetected augmentation of the gain may produce the opposite effect, and convert a flat-line recording into one that simulates ventricular fibrillation. Finally, rhythm analysis may be quite difficult from the limited (narrow) view afforded by the oscilloscope of the defibrillator. Use of a continuous ECG recording (from a 12-lead ECG machine) facilitates the process and enhances the accuracy of rhythm interpretation by the additional information it provides and the ready availability of supplemental leads (for assessment of QRS morphology, P wave detection, etc.).

6. **Delay in Defibrillation.** The chance for successful conversion of ventricular fibrillation is inversely proportional to the time from the onset of this rhythm until the time that countershock is applied. As a result, *as soon as the diagnosis of ventricular fibrillation is made, the patient should be defibrillated.*

Precious time should not be wasted trying to intubate the patient or secure an IV line prior to defibrillation. Neither of these interventions will exert a favorable effect on fibrillation threshold. On the contrary, delaying defibrillation until completion of these procedures is likely to *adversely* affect fibrillation threshold (and make it that much more difficult to resuscitate the patient). Moreover, if defibrillation is promptly delivered and if it is successful in restoring spontaneous circulation, intubation may no longer be needed. Establishment of IV access is also likely to be achieved much more easily if there is resumption of spontaneous circulation.

7. **Use of Excessive Energy with the Initial Defibrillation Attempt.** *Defibrillation is not benign.* Use of excessive energy for defibrillation not only risks causing additional injury to the conduction system (that may only be evident in the postconversion rhythm), but may also paradoxically make it even more difficult to convert the patient out of ventricular fibrillation (Weaver et al, 1982; Kerber et al, 1988). As a result, *the amount of delivered energy selected for the initial countershock attempt should ideally be limited to the lowest amount likely to be successful.* An initial energy level of 200 joules is currently recommended for this purpose. Higher energies may be used if this is unsuccessful.

Defibrillation using even lower energy levels (i.e., 100 joules) may be successful in a surprising number of cases. This is especially true for patients who have low TTR values, since a significantly greater amount of current will penetrate the chest wall of such individuals with defibrillation at any given energy level. Although increased use of current-based defibrillators (able to instantaneously measure TTR and adjust current delivery accordingly) is likely in the near future, present guidelines still favor 200 joules as the energy level selection for the initial countershock attempt when standard defibrillators are used.

8. Failure to Minimize Time Between Successive Countershock Attempts. Minimizing the time between successive countershock attempts lowers TTR. As a result, an *increased* amount of current will pass through the chest wall with each defibrillation attempt. This increases the *efficacy* of defibrillation at any given energy level.

> Practically speaking, the *ONLY* interventions that should be performed between successive countershock attempts in the *initial* defibrillation series are:
> a. Verification of continued unresponsiveness and pulselessness (in association with persistance of ventricular fibrillation)
> b. Recharging of the defibrillator
> c. Clearing the area
> d. Defibrillating

9. Failure to Use *Synchronized Cardioversion* Appropriately. Synchronized cardioversion is indicated for the treatment of patients with supraventricular tachycardias and/or ventricular tachycardia if (when) they manifest evidence of hemodynamic compromise and/or they fail to respond to other measures.

> By delivering the electrical impulse during that portion of the cardiac cycle when the ventricles are most refractory, synchronized cardioversion is less likely to inadvertently precipitate ventricular fibrillation than would be the case with delivery of an unsynchronized countershock. The procedure is extremely effective in converting patients in atrial flutter or ventricular tachycardia, and use of relatively low energy levels (of 50 joules or less) will often be successful for treatment of these conditions. Synchronized cardioversion is less effective in converting atrial fibrillation, even when higher energy levels (of 200 joules or more) are appropriately used. However the real KEY to the procedure lies with becoming *thoroughly familiar with the operation of the defibrillator/synchronizer unit* in your particular clinical setting *BEFORE* the time that you need to use it.

If for whatever reason the synchronized electrical impulse does not discharge when activated (and a rapid attempt at troubleshooting does not resolve the problem), *synchronization should be abandoned in favor of delivery of an unsynchronized countershock.*

(See Section 2D for additional discussion on the use of synchronized cardioversion.)

10. Failure to Adequately Address the Problem of Defibrillator Failure. A recent report by the Defibrillator Working Group of the Food and Drug Administration suggests that the incidence of ***defibrillator failure*** during clinical use is significantly greater than is generally appreciated—and may be unacceptably high (Cummins et al, 1990).

Surprisingly, *operator errors* in defibrillation appear to be much more common than equipment malfunction. Even in cases in which equipment malfunction is initially suspected as the primary problem, operator oversight and/or errors of omission are often found on later review. Examples of personnel-related errors include attempting to deliver a shock before the defibrillator is fully charged, allowing the charge to "bleed" down before discharging the capacitors, failure to have a replacement battery readily available, and inability to obtain an ECG tracing suitable for rhythm diagnosis and shock decisions.

Clearly, the frequency of operator error decreases as experience with defibrillation and frequency of use increase. Thus, the problem is greatest with personnel who only infrequently have occasion to apply their skills in defibrillation. It is exacerbated even more in institutions that possess a variety of defibrillator makes and models—many of which are older, infrequently used devices. As might be expected, the emphasis of the recommendations put forth by the Defibrillator Working Group was that many (if not most) episodes of defibrillator failure could be prevented if a regular schedule of equipment checks and periodic maintenance was adhered to, and a more concerted effort was made to train personnel and maintain their skills with regular "hands-on" practice sessions (Cummins et al, 1990).

11. Failure to Take Appropriate Precautions When Defibrillating a Patient with a *PERMANENT PACEMAKER.* It is important to realize that the electrical discharge produced by defibrillation may have serious consequences when delivered to a patient who has a permanent (implanted) pacemaker. Pacemaker function may be adversely affected by countershock in such individuals either *directly* (i.e., from damage to the pacemaker circuitry itself), or *indirectly* (i.e., with loss of normal pacing function *despite* the fact that internal pacemaker circuitry remains intact).

> Pacemaker malfunction that develops as a *direct* result of damage to internal pacemaker circuitry may manifest in a number of ways, including alteration in the pacing threshold, failure in the ability of the pacemaker to capture or sense appropriately, and/or sudden changes in the rate, mode, or output of the pacemaking device (Zullo, 1990).
> Surprisingly, *indirect causes* of pacemaker malfunction appear to be *at least as common* clinically as direct causes. In this situation, an *external event* is the cause of impaired pacing function. For example, localized myocardial injury (at the pacemaker lead site) produced from the countershock itself may alter the ability of the myocardium to respond to otherwise normal pacemaker stimuli. Other potential "indirect" causes of impaired pacemaker function (that are likely to be seen in patients who undergo cardiopulmonary resuscitation) include pacemaker lead fracture or displacement of the lead wire from its site on the myocardium. Trauma, seizure activity, and/or performance of external chest compression may all be contributing factors to this type of pacemaker malfunction.

Fortunately, pacemaker malfunction following defibrillation appears to occur less commonly with modern pacemaking devices than it did in the past. Development of effective suppressor circuits within the pacemaker itself is now able to limit the amount of current that enters the pulse generator. This greatly reduces the chance of damaging internal pacemaker circuitry, although it does not completely eliminate the risk. Thus, pacemaker malfunction may still occur—*either directly or indirectly*—in any of the forms noted above. As a result, one may want to consider the following precautions when caring for the acutely ill patient who has a permanent pacemaker (Owen, 1983):

---

a. Documenting the type of pacemaker, the manufacturer, and the model number of the pulse generator *at the time that the patient is admitted to the hospital.*
b. Determining the *baseline* function of the pacemaker *(ideally at the time of admission to the hospital)*—including notation of currently set parameters for pacing rate and output. *Establishing that baseline function of the pacemaker was normal is essential for ruling out the possibility that subsequent cardiac arrest was caused by antecedent pacemaker malfunction.*
c. If defibrillation is required, consider adjusting placement of the defibrillator paddles so as to minimize the amount of energy that will pass through the pacing system. Use of an anterior-posterior paddle pacement orientation is ideal for this purpose because it results in a defibrillation vector that is *perpendicular* to the plane of the pacemaker's sensing apparatus. If this is not possible, both paddles may still be placed on the anterior chest (over the apex and right side of the sternum)—but care should be taken to assure that each paddle is placed *at least 10 cm away* from the pulse generator.
   Finally, the amount of energy selected for defibrillation should be limited to as low a level as possible since the likelihood of developing pacemaker malfunction is directly related to the amount of energy that passes through the pacing system.
d. Having a temporary pacemaker readily available (as a backup) in the event that the patient's permanent pacemaker malfunctions after defibrillation.
e. Being sure to carefully reevaluate the function of the permanent pacemaker at the earliest opportunity after defibrillation.

E. Miscellaneous Pearls and Pitfalls in Management of Cardiac Arrest

1. **Misuse of the Precordial Thump.** The precordial thump has been recommended for treatment of ventricular tachycardia/fibrillation because it may occasionally be effective in restoring normal sinus rhythm. The problem is that the thump is *not* a benign procedure, and that it appears to be much more likely to precipitate deterioration of these arrhythmias than to convert them to sinus rhythm. Thus, use of the precordial thump to treat ventricular tachycardia may result in ventricular fibrillation, and use of the thump to treat ventricular fibrillation may result in asystole.

Physiologically, the reason that a precordial thump may precipitate deterioration of the rhythm is that the emergency care provider has absolutely no control over when in the cardiac cycle the energy will be delivered. As a result, there is no way to guard against inadvertent delivery of energy during the vulnerable period. This is in distinct contrast to what happens with synchronized cardioversion, where delivery of the electrical impulse is programmed to arrive at a specific point in the cardiac cycle (i.e., on the upstroke of the R wave), at which time aggravation of the arrhythmia is exceedingly unlikely to occur.

We find it easiest to think of the thump as a "***No-Lose Procedure.***" That is, *we do not favor its use for treatment of any arrhythmia that is associated with a pulse* (as may be the case for sustained ventricular tachycardia). There is simply "too much to lose" in this situation (i.e., *you may lose the pulse!*). On the other hand, we see nothing against trying a precordial thump for treatment of pulseless rhythms (such as ventricular fibrillation, asystole, or pulseless ventricular tachycardia)—since there is "nothing to lose" in these situations.

---

2. **Forgetting about Cough Version.** Although the mechanism of action for cough version remains uncertain (conversion of the mechanical energy of a cough into electrical energy? activation of sympathetic tone? enhanced coronary perfusion from the increase in intrathoracic pressure produced by a cough?)—*the procedure may definitely be effective in converting some cases of sustained ventricular tachycardia to sinus rhythm.* Unlike the thump, aggravation of the arrhythmia from coughing is uncommon.

Don't forget about cough version. Consider its use in conscious, hemodynamically stable patients who are in sustained ventricular tachycardia.

---

3. **Failure to *At Least Consider* the Possibility that Positional Changes May Precipitate Cardiac Arrhythmias in Certain Patients.** In general, physicians tend to downplay the possibility that patient positioning may play a role in inducing certain cardiac arrhythmias in susceptible patients. A survey conducted by us suggests that a *majority* of critical care nurses have witnessed this phenomenon at least once in their career, and that more than one third of them have seen it occur on at least five occasions (Grauer, Green, and Cavallaro, 1990). *Can the observations of so many caregivers at the bedside be ignored?*

> Unfortunately, the literature is lacking on this subject, and we are unaware of other studies that have examined the effect that patient positioning might have on induction of cardiac arrhythmias. In our experience, the rhythm most commonly induced by patient positioning is ventricular tachycardia. The phenomenon seems to occur most often in critically ill patients with severe heart failure who are turned to their left side—although it may also occur with assumption of the Trendelenburg position.
>
> We do not know the mechanism responsible for induction of arrhythmias with patient positioning. We suspect it may be related to the anatomic change in position of an already irritable (and arrhythmia-susceptible) heart when the patient moves.

It should be emphasized that we are *NOT* implying that every time a critically ill patient is turned on his or her left side, that ventricular tachycardia will result. Nevertheless, we feel it is important to appreciate that *in selected, critically ill patients, positioning on the left side (or in Trendelenburg) may sometimes precipitate potentially life-threatening arrhythmias.* Awareness of this phenomenon is especially important if a medical care provider *suspects* that an arrhythmia may have already been induced by patient positioning. In this case, *prudence would dictate avoidance of turning the patient in that particular position again!* When turning the patient, preference might be given to the right side.

---

4. **Failure to Take Routine Vital Signs During Cardiac Arrest.** Temperature is the most frequently forgotten vital sign in the setting of cardiac arrest (Harris and Smith, 1988). In our survey of critical care nurses, a majority indicated that they had *never* seen a temperature recorded at the scene of a cardiac arrest (Grauer, Green, and Cavallaro, 1990). In view of the special treatment considerations necessary for successful resuscitation of hypothermic victims, this oversight may have potentially important prognostic implications.

> Hypothermia *CAN* be the cause of cardiopulmonary arrest—and its presentation may sometimes be subtle. Thus,

it will *not* always be detectable from physical appearance, or even from touching the patient to "see if they are cold." The condition can occur—*even in warm weather areas*—and even during the *warmer months* of the year. It is especially likely to occur in the elderly, young children, victims of cold water immersion or drug overdose, and patients with a history of hypothyroidism, stroke, sepsis, and/or alcohol abuse.

Don't forget about the possibility of hypothermia. Because diagnosis of this disorder can't be made unless the temperature is taken, strongly consider routinely recording this vital sign on all victims of cardiac arrest (at the earliest opportunity during the resuscitation process).

---

5. **Failure to Consider the Possibility of a "Special Situation" as the Cause of Cardiac Arrest—*and Failure to Adjust Treatment Accordingly.*** Consideration should always be given to the *possibility* that a "special situation" may be the precipitating cause of (or at least a contributing factor to) the cardiopulmonary arrest. Although in many cases, the presence of such precipitating factors will be quite obvious from the history or physical examination of the patient, this is not always the case.

> In addition to hypothermia, other "special situations" to consider include drug overdose (especially from tricyclic antidepressants, cocaine, or narcotics), electrical injuries, lightning, near-drowning, heat exhaustion or heat stroke, and trauma (which may be unsuspected). Because of potential subtleties in presentation and significantly different considerations in management, maintaining a high index of suspicion for the possibility of a "special situation" is essential.

(Detailed discussion of each of the above "Special Situations" is included in Chapter 13.)

6. **Failure to Actively Seek out an Underlying Cause of Electromechanical Dissociation (EMD).** Practically speaking, resuscitation of a patient in EMD is unlikely to be successful *unless* the underlying cause of the disorder can be determined and corrected. Potentially correctable causes of EMD to consider include:

  a. *Inadequate ventilation* (from intubation of the right mainstem bronchus, tension pneumothorax, bilateral pneumothorax)
  b. *Inadequate circulation* (from pericardial effusion with tamponade, or hypovolemia from acute blood loss, dehydration, septic, neurogenic, or cardiogenic shock, etc.)
  c. A *metabolic disorder* (persistent acidosis, hyperkalemia, drug overdose, etc.)

(See Case Study D in Chapter 4 for additional discussion on evaluation and management of EMD.)

7. Delay in Arranging for Emergency Pacing. A patient with a hemodynamically significant bradyarrhythmia who has not responded to atropine is in need of cardiac pacing. The use of a pressor agent should be only employed as a *stopgap measure* for hemodynamic support until cardiac pacing (with either an external or transvenous pacemaker) can be achieved.

> If an external pacemaker is readily available, it may be preferable to use it instead of atropine—especially in settings where increased parasympathetic tone is unlikely to be the cause of the bradyarrhythmia (i.e., for treatment of Mobitz II 2° AV block, or 3° AV block that occurs in association with acute *anterior* infarction).

F. Pearls and Pitfalls in Arrhythmia Interpretation

A host of pearls and pitfalls on the various aspects of arrhythmia interpretation are contained within the text of Chapters 3, 15, and 16—as well as in Section 17D (which discusses pediatric arrhythmias from the viewpoint of *"How Children Are Different"*). We limit the section here to brief mention of some of the most salient points about arrhythmia interpretation.

1. Forgetting that the most common "cause of a pause" is a *blocked PAC* (premature atrial contraction) **and *NOT* some type of AV block.**

> Blocked PACs are extremely easy to overlook *unless they are specifically looked for*. The two *KEYS* to increasing your ability to detect their presence are:
> a. To always maintain a high index of suspicion (i.e., to remember that *"the commonest cause of a pause is a blocked PAC"*).
> b. To regularly look for this phenomenon *whenever* you are confronted with an arrhythmia that contains one or more "pauses" (i.e., to always focus on the T wave at the beginning of the pause to see if any subtle deformity that may be indicative of a blocked PAC is present).

> Remember:—*Blocked PACs are FAR more common in clinical practice than any of the AV blocks!*

2. Not distinguishing between AV dissociation and complete (3°) AV block.

> The diagnosis of AV dissociation is commonly misunderstood. All that the term means is that atrial activity is *unrelated* to ventricular (or junctional) activity—*at least* for a moment in time.
> AV dissociation is *never* a primary disorder. Instead it is always *secondary* to (i.e., the result of) some other rhythm disorder. Thus, AV dissociation may be the result of *"usurpation"* (from an *accelerated* junctional rhythm that has taken over the pacemaking function), *"default"* (if the rate of the sinus pacemaker drops *below* that of the AV nodal or ventricular escape rate), or *AV block*. AV dissociation that occurs as a result of

AV block may be *transient* and/or intermittent (as is likely to be seen with various forms of 2° AV block), or *complete* (when 3° AV block is present).

Clinically, AV dissociation by usurpation is often the result of digitalis toxicity. In contrast, AV dissociation by default may be a purely physiologic phenomenon (as commonly occurs in association with the normal sinoatrial slowing during sleep). Neither of these forms of AV dissociation necessarily implies the presence of any degree of AV block. As a result, treatment considerations for AV dissociation (*if any treatment is needed at all!*) may be very different than they are when true AV block is present.

> A pearl to remember in the diagnosis of 3° AV block is that *most of the time, the ventricular response will be REGULAR with this conduction disorder.* Because—*by definition*—AV dissociation is *complete* with 3° AV block, no supraventricular impulses are able to penetrate the AV node—and the resultant ventricular response will therefore reflect the rate and regularity of the previously subservient escape pacemaker (that had been "waiting in the wings"). *If the ventricular response is not regular, complete (3°) AV block is probably NOT present!* Strongly consider the possibility of 2° AV block (with transient/intermittent AV dissociation) and/or blocked PACs in this situation.

3. Misdiagnosing 2° AV block with 2:1 AV conduction as Mobitz II.

> Second-degree AV block with 2:1 AV conduction may be the result of *either* Mobitz I or Mobitz II type block. Statistically, Mobitz I is *far more common* than is Mobitz II. Differentiation is important because observation alone (or low-dose atropine) is often all that is needed for treatment of Mobitz I, whereas Mobitz II 2° AV block usually requires pacemaker therapy.

> Mobitz I 2° AV block is almost certainly present if the setting is that of acute *inferior* infarction, the QRS complex is narrow, and/or there is clear evidence of Wenckebach elsewhere on the tracing.

4. Failure to recognize and appreciate the diagnostic utility of *group beating*.

> The presence of "group beating" should suggest the *possibility* of some type of Wenckebach conduction. In addition to greatly facilitating the diagnosis of 2° AV block of the Mobitz I (Wenckebach) type, awareness of the phenomenon of group beating may also allow recognition of more subtle forms of Wenckebach conduction (such as SA Wenckebach and atrial fibrillation or flutter with Wenckebach conduction out of the AV node).

5. **Misdiagnosis of accelerated idioventricular rhythm (AIVR) as "ventricular tachycardia."**

AIVR is the term used to describe a regular (or fairly regular) ventricular rhythm with a heart rate of between 50 and 110 beats/min. It is often an "escape rhythm" that arises in response to slowing of the supraventricular pacemaker, and is especially common in the setting of acute inferior infarction. Much of the time, the patient remains hemodynamically stable. As a result, *treatment is usually NOT needed.* On the contrary, treatment of AIVR with either lidocaine or countershock may be counterproductive by abolishing the only escape rhythm that the patient has! If treatment is needed (because of symptoms resulting from the loss of the atrial kick), the drug of choice would be atropine (with the aim of attempting to speed up the supraventricular pacemaker).

6. **Falsely assuming that a wide complex tachyarrhythmia is supraventricular** because the patient is alert and hemodynamically stable.

Patients may remain alert and hemodynamically stable despite the presence of sustained ventricular tachycardia for hours—*or even days!* Statistically, it is well to remember that ventricular tachycardia is a *far more common cause* of a regular, wide complex tachycardia in adults than supraventricular tachycardia (with either *aberration* or preexisting bundle branch block). As a result, *one should ALWAYS assume that a wide complex tachycardia is ventricular in etiology until proved otherwise.* The patient should be treated accordingly (i.e., verapamil should *never* be used as a "diagnostic/therapeutic trial"!).

7. **Not suspecting atrial flutter** in the presence of a supraventricular tachycardia at a rate of about **150 beats/min.**

It is extremely easy to overlook atrial flutter unless one constantly maintains a high index of suspicion for the diagnosis. This is because flutter waves may often be occult—and may only be evident in certain leads.

The KEY to diagnosis of atrial flutter lies with remembering that the atrial rate of untreated flutter is almost always close to 300 beats/min in adults. Normally the AV node is *unable* to conduct impulses at this fast a rate. As a result, only *half* of these impulses are usually conducted. This leads to a 2:1 ratio for AV conduction, and a ventricular response of approximately 150 beats/min (i.e., 300 ÷ 2 = 150/min).

The possibility of atrial flutter should ALWAYS be strongly considered in the presence of a regular, supraventricular tachycardia at a rate of approximately 150 beats/min when *normal* atrial activity (i.e., an upright P wave in lead II) is not clearly present.

---

8. **Failure to appreciate the *subtleties* of arrhythmia diagnosis associated with atrial fibrillation:**

a. Not recognizing atrial fibrillation when the rhythm is rapid (i.e., between 150-200 beats/min) and only a *minor* degree of irregularity exists.
b. Not considering the possibility of an accessory pathway

(i.e., WPW) when the QRS complex is wide and the rate of atrial fibrillation is *unusually fast* in certain places (i.e., up to 250-300 beats/min).
c. Not ruling out the possibility of subtle atrial activity (and another diagnosis such as MAT) by failing to examine the arrhythmia in more than one lead. This is an especially important consideration in the evaluation of patients with COPD (in whom MAT is probably equally common as a cause of an irregularly irregular rhythm as atrial fibrillation).
d. Not suspecting sick sinus syndrome or acute myocardial infarction when the rate of *untreated* atrial fibrillation is unusually slow (i.e., *less* than 50-60 beats/min).
e. Not suspecting *digitalis toxicity* when the rhythm of a patient who was in atrial fibrillation becomes "regularized."

9. **Falsely assuming that anomalous** (i.e., widened) **beats are aberrantly conducted *without convincingly* demonstrating "a reason" for aberration** (such as the presence of typical RBBB morphology in a right-sided monitoring lead, a *premature* P wave, a relatively narrow QRS complex, etc.).

An anomalous beat should always be presumed "guilty" (i.e., a PVC) until *proved* to be innocent (i.e, supraventricular with aberration)—*rather than the other way around.* In general, doing so will significantly improve accuracy in arrhythmia diagnosis.

Early beats that are "only a little bit wider" than normal should *not* be presumptively labeled as PJCs (premature junctional contractions) simply because they "don't look wide enough to be ventricular." *PJCs are much less common in practice than is generally appreciated.* QRS morphology of true PJCs is usually identical (or *almost* identical) to that of normally conducted beats. And although PJCs may occasionally be conducted with aberration, *most of the time* early beats that "look a little different" (and are not preceded by premature P waves) will be *ventricular* in origin.

10. **Failure to use more than one monitoring lead** (or to obtain a 12-lead ECG) **for arrhythmia interpretation**—*especially when the patient is hemodynamically stable and the diagnosis is somewhat in doubt.*

Additional monitoring leads are particularly valuable for detecting flutter waves (*see #7 above*), ruling out the possibility of MAT when the rhythm is irregular (*see #8 above*), distinguishing fine ventricular fibrillation from asystole, confirming that beats that look "just a little bit different" in one lead are PVCs rather than PJCs (*see #9 above*), and differentiating between PVCs and aberrantly conducted beats (*see #9 above*).

11. **Failure to appreciate the difference in pediatric arrhythmias.**

All of the norms are different in children! Thus, heart rates are normally much faster, intervals (PR and QRS) are normally much narrower, and the usual rate limits for the various rhythm disorders are different (i.e., the atrial rate in flutter may easily *exceed* 400 beats/min). In addition, the prevalence of certain cardiac arrhythmias is quite different. For example, ventricular arrhythmias are generally far less common in children than in adults (with the possible exception of the postoperative setting, and/or in children who have congenital heart disease). Thus, *the mind-set of the emergency care provider must change significantly* when he/she is presented with an arrhythmia from an infant or child.

(See Section 17D for a detailed discussion on "Pediatric Arrhythmias: How Children Are Different.")

References

Cummins RO, Chesemore K, White RD, and the Defibrillator Working Group: Defibrillator failures: causes of problems and recommendations for improvement, *JAMA* 264:1019, 1990.

Grauer K, Green E, Cavallaro D: Less publicized aspects of cardiac arrest: a survey of caregivers at the bedside, *Fam Prac Recert* 12:32, 1990.

Harris ML, Smith J: Temperature determination during CPR, *Ann Emerg Med* 17:296, 1988 (letter).

Kerber RE, Martins JB, Kienzle MG, Constantin L, Olshansky B, Hopson R, Charbonnier F: Energy, current, and success in defibrillation and cardioversion: clinical studies using an automated impedance-based method of energy adjustment, *Circulation* 77:1038, 1988.

Owen PM: The effects of external defibrillation of permanent pacemakers, *Heart Lung* 12:274, 1983.

Weaver DW, Cobb LA, Compass MK, Hallstrom AP: Ventricular defibrillation: a comparative trial using 175-J and 320-J shocks, *N Engl J Med* 307:1101, 1982.

Wrenn K, Slovis CM: The ten commandments of emergency medicine *Ann Emerg Med* 20:1146, 1991 (editorial).

Zullo MA: Function of ventricular pacemakers during resuscitation, *PACE* 13:736, 1990.

ACLS POETRY ADDENDUM: "THE NIGHT BEFORE MORNING"

Fred Langer, RN
Ken Grauer, MD
Ellie Green, RN

On a lighter note, we conclude this book with a verse on ACLS.

T'was the night before morning in MICU,
Not a patient was stirring and the call lights were few.
The housestaff were finally supinely positioned,
Attempting to remedy their critical condition.

The mood in the unit was divinely serene,
With a glow from the monitors of peaceful, pale green.
When all of a sudden, without any warning,
An alarm pierced the air—some thought it was morning.

With Pavlov response bodies lurched to and fro
While trying to focus to see where to go.
"Code blue" was the battle cry sounded with vigor
And the troop of the faithful grew ever bigger.

The doorway was jammed, the mood was of gloom
But a surge from the rear pushed them into the room.
"What's the rhythm?" a self-proclaimed leader demanded
As he turned to the troops that he now commanded.

"It looks like a heart block."—"No, atrial flutter!"
"It will soon be asystole," a pessimist muttered.
"Does he have a pulse?" someone nervously queried.
And five searching hands in the groin were soon buried.

"Yes!" "No!" came a flurry, and a quick vote was taken.
A recheck was done to see who was mistaken.
"There *IS* a faint pulse!" "Then what is the pressure?"
The sphygmomanometer soon gave the measure.

"Sixty systolic and the rate thirty-five!"
Above all they shouted, *"Let's keep her alive!"*
"Atropine!" "Epi!" "Get the external pacer!"
Syringes and needles flashed forth like a laser.

"The rate is increasing!"—brought a sigh of relief.
But what happened next caused a moan of "Good grief!"
That ominous, ubiquitous, wavering tracing
Signaled V Fib and sent their hearts racing.

"No pulse, start compressions . . . and YOU—intubate!
Give me those paddles before it's too late."
With the poise of a golfer beginning his swing,
He sent two hundred joules through the heart with a "zing."

Three hundred—three sixty—the leader was possessed,
He gave five more shocks before pulled from the chest.
"I'm sorry, forgive me, I got carried away."
Then they looked at the monitor—this just wasn't their day.

The V Fib continued—they bagged and they pumped.
They bolused, they dripped, they prayed, and they thumped.
When the last drop of bretylium entered the vein
Another defib and the rhythm had changed.

"Aha, there's a rhythm!"—but it still caused a fright.
It was wide, it was fast with no P waves in sight.
"It's V Tach!" "No, it's not!" "SVT led aberrantly?"
A battle ensued with no winner apparently.

"There's a pulse and a pressure of eighty or so!"
"Verapamil!" "Lidocaine!"—bantered back to and fro.
But just as the victor prepared his prescription,
The paper spewed forth with an ominous inscription.

Asystole—straight line—were all that were printed.
"Oh, *WHERE* is that pacer?" the leader lamented.
Someone assured it was being delivered,
So everyone paused, and bicarb was considered.

"How 'bout some calcium?" an old-timer shouted.
The laughter confirmed that his knowledge was doubted.
And then in a flash a new face in the room.
The cardiologist entered and lifted the gloom.

"What happened?" he asked just as cool as you please.
A nurse ventured forward and dropped to her knees.
"Oh, kind sir, please spare me!" was all she could squeak.
His stern stare entrapped her . . . . no one dared speak.

"So what have you given here, milk of magnesia?"
And everyone suddenly suffered amnesia.
"There is nothing so hard about saving a life.
You ALL can do it—just as well as my wife!"

He slipped in a pacer and then threw the switch,
It fired and captured without the first hitch—**_for the
   moment......_**
The patient awoke and gazed up at her savior
And asked how she ever could return him the favor.

The proud resurrector said, "Nothing to pay,
It's all in the work that I do every day."
His exit was swift, the TEAM in a hush,
Thinking what they had witnessed _was JUST a bit much._

And sure enough, just as soon as he parted,
The pacer malfunctioned and asystole restarted.
The TEAM thought a moment: "There's an EASY so-
   lution,
With an _external_ pacer will come resolution."

So they slapped on the pacer,
And they ALL threw the switch.
And _this_ time it worked
Without further glitch.

So the code was now over, and the case could be closed.
And all of the housestaff would soon be reposed.
While the nurses continued by the peaceful green light,
Till the end of their shift in the dawn's early light.

The whole TEAM had been tested and run through the
   mill,
Just as strenuous as any MEGA CODE will.
ACLS algorithms are all so forgiving
When the end result is that the patient is living.

INDEX

The letter *f* after a page number indicates a figure; *ff* indicates multiple tables; *t* indicates a table.

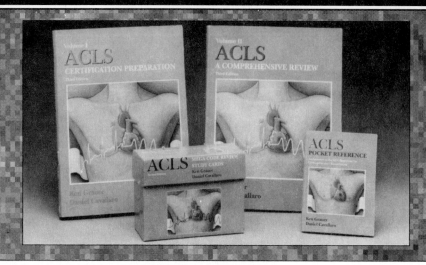

ACLS: MEGA Code Review/Study Cards, 2nd Edition
By Ken Grauer, MD, FAAFP, and Dan Cavallaro, REMT-P
February, 1993. 376 cards. (Book Code: 01980)

These unique cards facilitate preparation for the ACLS course in a time effective manner. Included is an extensive series of cards that simulate the testing conditions of the challenging Mega Code station. Other sections contain cards with a clinical question, drug, and/or arrhythmia on the front, with the appropriate answer and detailed explanation on the back. Material is complementary but does not duplicate information contained in the ACLS books.

All ACLS components contain the Author's commentary on the JAMA '92 CPR ECC Guidelines.

Practical Guide to ECG Interpretation, 1st Edition
By Ken Grauer, MD, FAAFP
1991. 416 pages, 278 illustrations. (Book Code: 02159)

From the earliest stages of ECG interpretation to accurate evaluation of the vast majority of ECGs you'll encounter, this book covers it all. The informal and clearly written text is accompanied by extensive and detailed illustrations.

Free with purchase of Practical Guide to ECG Interpretation
ECG Interpretation Pocket Reference
By Ken Grauer, MD, FAAFP
1992. 64 pages, 26 illustrations. (Book Code: 02002)

▲ contains the most essential information from the larger text in a convenient, quick reference format
▲ also available separately

For more information or to order, call Mosby Lifeline 1-800-325-4177.

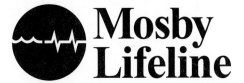

Mosby
Lifeline

Mosby Lifeline
11830 Westline Industrial Drive
St. Louis, MO 63146
Toll Free 1-800-325-4177
FAX# (314)432-1380